Helical/Spiral CT

A Practical Approach

Robert K. Zeman, M.D.
Professor and Clinical Director of Diagnostic Radiology
Co-Director, Abdominal Imaging and Computed Tomography
Director of CT, Georgetown University Medical Center
Washington, DC

James A. Brink, M.D.
Assistant Professor of Radiology
Washington University School of Medicine
Mallinckrodt Institute of Radiology
St. Louis, Missouri

Philip Costello, M.D.
Director of Computed Tomography and Chest Radiology
Department of Radiological Sciences
Deaconess Hospital
Associate Professor of Radiology
Harvard Medical School
Boston, Massachusetts

William J. Davros, Ph.D.
Diagnostic Medical Imaging Physicist
Division of Diagnostic Radiology
The Cleveland Clinic Foundation
Cleveland, Ohio

Bradford J. Richmond, M.D.
Head, Section of Musculoskeletal Radiology
Departments of Diagnostic Radiology and Orthopaedic Surgery
The Cleveland Clinic Foundation
Cleveland, Ohio

Paul M. Silverman, M.D.
Professor of Radiology
Co-Director, Abdominal Imaging and Computed Tomography
Co-Director of CT, Georgetown University Medical Center
Washington, DC

Pedro T. Vieco, M.D., FRCP (C)
Section Chief, Neuroradiology
Assistant Professor
Department of Radiology
Medical Center Hospital of Vermont
Burlington, Vermont

Helical/Spiral CT
A Practical Approach

Robert K. Zeman, M.D.
James A. Brink, M.D.
Philip Costello, M.D.
William J. Davros, Ph.D.
Bradford J. Richmond, M.D.
Paul M. Silverman, M.D.
Pedro T. Vieco, M.D., FRCP (C)

McGraw-Hill, Inc.
Health Professions Division

New York St. Louis San Francisco Auckland Bogotá Caracas Lisbon
London Madrid Mexico City Milan Montreal New Delhi
San Juan Singapore Sydney Tokyo Toronto

Helical/Spiral CT: A Practical Approach

Copyright 1995 by Robert K. Zeman, James A. Brink, Philip Costello, William J. Davros, Bradford J. Richmond, Paul M. Silverman, and Pedro T. Vieco. All rights reserved. Printed in the United States of America. Except as permitted under the United States Copyright Act of 1976, no part of this publication may be reproduced or distributed in any form or by any means, or stored in a data base or retrieval system, without the prior written permission of the publisher.

1234567890 KGPKGP 987654

ISBN 0-07-072653-1

This book was set in Times Roman by Monotype Composition Company, Inc.
The editors were Jane Pennington and Mariapaz Ramos Englis; the production supervisor was Clare Stanley; the project was managed by Tripp Narup, JIMA.
Quebecor Printing/Kingsport was printer and binder.
The book is printed on acid-free paper.

Library of Congress Cataloging-in-Publication Data

Helical/spiral CT: a practical approach / Robert K. Zeman . . . [et al.].
    p. cm.
   Includes bibliographical references.
   ISBN 0-07-072653-1
   1. Spiral computed tomography.   I. Zeman, Robert K.
   [DNLM: 1. Tomography, X-Ray Computed.   WN 200 H475 1995]
RC78.7.TBH45   1995
618.07'872—dc20
DNLM/DLC
for Library of Congress   94-31371

To our families
—*The Authors*

Contents

HELICAL/SPIRAL CT: TECHNICAL PRINCIPLES 1
    James A. Brink
    William J. Davros

HEAD, NECK, AND SPINE 27
    Pedro T. Vieco

THORAX 105
    Philip Costello

ABDOMEN AND PELVIS 153
    Robert K. Zeman
    Paul M. Silverman

MUSCULOSKELETAL SYSTEM 221
    Bradford J. Richmond

VASCULAR SYSTEM AND THREE-DIMENSIONAL CT ANGIOGRAPHY 265
    Robert K. Zeman

APPENDIX: COMPARISON OF HELICAL/SPIRAL CT SCANNERS 299
    William J. Davros
    Robert K. Zeman

INDEX 329

Notice

Medicine is an ever-changing science. As new research and clinical experience broaden our knowledge, changes in treatment and drug therapy are required. The authors and the publisher of this work have checked with sources believed to be reliable in their efforts to provide information that is complete and generally in accord with the standards accepted at the time of publication. However, in view of the possibility of human error or changes in medical sciences, neither the authors nor the publisher nor any other party who has been involved in the preparation or publication of this work warrants that the information contained herein is in every respect accurate or complete, and they are not responsible for any errors or omissions or for the results obtained from use of such information. Readers are encouraged to confirm the information contained herein with other sources. For example and in particular, readers are advised to check the product information sheet included in the package of each drug they plan to administer to be certain that the information contained in this book is accurate and that changes have not been made in the recommended dose or in the contraindications for administration. This recommendation is of particular importance in connection with new or infrequently used drugs. User manuals and technical information brochures should also be consulted to confirm product specifications and scanning protocols.

Preface

Helical/spiral CT has rapidly arrived on the imaging scene. This breakthrough technology significantly differs from conventional CT and has caused many of us in clinical practice to rethink our entire approach to how we perform CT examinations. Although the scientific literature in this field is rapidly growing, it has not yet addressed many of the issues that are important to the practicing radiologist.

Helical scanning is far more flexible than conventional scanning but entails more complex scanning protocols. Understanding contrast dynamics and scan parameters such as scan timing, length of exposure, collimation, and pitch are critical to performing high-quality helical CT. This book is primarily directed at the clinical radiologist, who has a good grasp of cross-sectional anatomy and pathology but is looking for scanning guidelines, real-life scanning protocols, and a finer appreciation of the unique attributes and pitfalls of helical CT. We have tried to prepare an up-to-date compendium of helical CT that is easy to read, contains numerous practical tips, and is lavishly illustrated with the types of cases that are frequently seen in day-to-day practice.

While the book is primarily directed at radiologists who already have helical CT in their practice, there are two other groups of radiologists that will find the book useful. If you are contemplating adding helical CT to your practice, this book will help you appreciate the indications and specific utility of helical scanning. Extensive tables comparing the devices that are currently commercially available will be most helpful in sorting out the important features to look for before you purchase a helical scanner. The book will also provide valuable information for a second group of radiologists, namely radiology trainees who are receiving their initial exposure to this field. By discussing the technical basis for helical scanning and providing an overview of the diseases commonly studied using helical methodology, the book will provide a solid foundation for learning about this very important imaging technique.

The book consists of six chapters and an appendix, which may all be read as "freestanding" sections. Because of this, some duplication is necessary but this has been kept to a minimum. Chapter 1 addresses the technical aspects of helical CT and focuses on the physical principles of scanning, reconstruction algorithms, and some of the common elements found in all helical scanners. Chapter 2 highlights the use of helical CT in neuroradiology. Emphasis has been placed on evaluation of the carotids and the circle of Willis since these are two areas where helical techniques will revolutionize our approach to cerebrovascular disease. Chapter 3 addresses the evaluation of the thorax. Significant savings in the use of contrast material, improved pulmonary nodule recognition, and evaluation of the major vessels is stressed and is of importance to all radiologists. Chapter 4 discusses the use of helical scanning in the abdomen and pelvis. Helical CT has had a profound impact on the assessment of the liver, pancreas, and kidneys. Chapters 4 and 6 review three-dimensional vascular applications and their relevance for surgical planning in the abdomen and elsewhere in the body. Chapter 5 describes the use of helical scanning in the setting of musculoskeletal disease. While MRI has become the dominant technique used for musculoskeletal evaluation, CT is making a strong comeback because of helical methodology. This book predominantly deals with diseases of adults. While we believe pediatric radiologists will find an important role for helical CT in the future, there is insufficient literature at the present time on which to base a comprehensive review.

The final section of the book is an appendix containing a technical comparison of current available scanners. This section is written in easy-to-understand terms, so the radiologist can make sense of the specifications and jargon that are commonplace in CT contract negotiations, discussions of service related issues, and vendor's claims regarding the user features of their scanner.

We sincerely hope our readers enjoy this book, find it useful in daily practice, and gain knowledge that ultimately benefits their patients.

Acknowledgments

There are many people who helped and inspired us in so many ways. From our residents and fellows who called to our attention many of the interesting cases in this book to our colleagues who graciously "held down the fort" while we struggled with the nuances of literature, we are in your debt.

The entire group of coauthors thanks Jane Pennington, Ph.D., our editor at McGraw-Hill, for her vision in developing the concept of this book and who, along with Mariapaz Ramos Englis, Tripp Narup and Clare Stanley, streamlined the publication process and brought a high-quality book to market in record time.

Each coauthor has specific individuals to which they would like to express gratitude. Dr. Zeman and Dr. Silverman thank Phil Berman, their research assistant, for enriching the quality of their research and providing many of the 3-D models in their chapters. Yvonne Carew and Katie Corboy, administrative assistants in the Abdominal Imaging Division at Georgetown, also did a terrific job assembling the various chapters and keeping their grumpy and disorganized bosses on target. Radiology colleagues at Georgetown, Drs. Susan Ascher, Cirrelda Cooper, Brian Garra, Rick Patt, and Dave Weltman gave invaluable advice and feedback throughout the whole process of preparing this work. Firas Al-Kawas, Dave Fleischer, and Stan Benjamin of Gastroenterology, along with the gastrointestinal surgeons at Georgetown, Dr. Buras, Dr. Dillon, Dr. Evans, Dr. Nauta, and Dr. Stahl, have taught Dr. Zeman and Dr. Silverman much of what they know about the GI tract. Thanks also go out to Dr. Jeff Posnick, Dr. Mario Gomes, and Dr. Andrew Zeiberg for contributions of case material. Finally, Dr. Zeman and Dr. Silverman are grateful to David Griego, RTR, formerly of Georgetown but now of General Electric Medical Systems, who helped develop many of the Georgetown clinical protocols in this book. Stan Fox, Ph.D., also of General Electric Medical Systems, deserves special mention, as he has had a great influence on many who practice in the CT field, and perhaps more than any one individual in the United States has overseen the maturation and direction of this technology.

Dr. Brink would like to acknowledge the careful mentoring and support of Jay Heiken, M.D., throughout the past several years. His insight into the scientific process and his remarkable understanding of CT have been most helpful in the joint exploration of spiral CT. Dr. Brink would also like to thank Ge Wang, Ph.D., and Michael Vannier, M.D., for their valuable contributions to his understanding of the physical principles of spiral CT. He is also grateful to Arkadiusz Polacin, Ph.D., and Willi Kalender, Ph.D., from Siemens Medical Systems in Erlangen, Germany; Yoram Bressler, Ph.D., from the Coordinated Science Laboratory at the University of Illinois; Francis Schlueter, M.D., Kevin McEnery, M.D., Lane Deyoe, M.D., and John Lim from the Mallinkrodt Institute of Radiology and Washington University School of Medicine.

Dr. Costello acknowledges Ellen Dorrington for her secretarial and editorial assistance, and Elizabeth Scholz, Stanley Dudek, Geraldine O'Connor, and Ann McGinnis for their technical expertise in the CT department at the Deaconess Hospital.

Dr. Davros and Dr. Richmond wish to thank the many individuals who provided them with information regarding scanners and protocols: Stan Fox, Ph.D., and Mark Bowman of General Electric Medical Systems; Jerry Arenson and Esther Medved of Elscint Inc.;

Chris Talbot of Philips Medical Systems; Greg Powell, Ph.D., of Picker International; David Starr, Lisa Reid, and Willi Kalender, Ph.D., of Siemens Medical Systems; and Bryan Westerman of Toshiba Medical Systems.

Dr. Richmond would specifically like to thank the Picker International CT Group who went well beyond his requests for assistance in preparation of his chapter. These individuals include Greg Powell, Ph.D., Dominic Heuscher, Heang Tuy, Greg Cohen, and Sue McDowell. A special acknowledgment is given to Kenneth D. Hopper, M.D., of Penn State University; Lawrence Tanenbaum, M.D., of Edison, New Jersey; Joseph Busch, M.D., of Ogelthorpe, GA; and Marc Kaye, M.D., of the Cleveland Clinic, Florida, for graciously sharing their case material with Dr. Richmond.

Dr. Vieco would like to acknowledge Christina Oliver, RTR, Chief CT Technologist at the Medical Center Hospital of Vermont, for her assistance in the development of the CT angiography protocols in chapter 2. He would also like to thank his family for their patience during this project and his wife Claudia Finkelstein, MDCM, for her many helpful suggestions.

Introduction
Robert K. Zeman

Since its inception and clinical application in the early 1970s, CT scanning has undergone a wide array of refinements. Progressive reduction in scan times, shorter reconstruction times, and improved spatial and contrast resolution have made CT the cross-sectional imaging workhorse for many years. By the mid-1980s many of us felt CT images were as good as they could be; yet there were many conditions that still were difficult to evaluate using conventional CT scanners. A significant number of benign and malignant liver lesions were not identified on conventional scans, staging of pancreatic cancer was not optimal, renovascular and cerebrovascular disease were difficult to assess, and we spent a lot of time chasing pathology such as pulmonary nodules because of misregistration.

We have not yet solved all these problems, but helical/spiral scanning techniques will allow us to take a few more steps down the road of better detection and characterization of disease. A helical acquisition is volumetric in nature; it is acquired during a sustained x-ray exposure which all but eliminates misregistration artifacts because the patient is not breathing in between acquisition of individual sections. The volume of information may be "sliced" with any spacing interval, and the sections may therefore be shifted to optimally depict pathologic processes. If the scan spacing that is selected is less than the collimation, overlapping slices will result. Since reconstruction is performed after the x-ray exposure, generation of overlapping images does not entail additional radiation exposure to the patient compared to conventional scanning. Overlapping sections may be used to produce high-quality three-dimensional (3-D) renderings of the vascular system, bony structures, or even soft-tissues.

Besides its volumetric approach to imaging, the speed and improved throughput of helical scanning have had a dramatic effect on our busy practice. Examination times have been reduced by one-third, with the greatest improvement in efficiency in patients undergoing multiple exams (eg., chest, abdomen, and pelvis CT). Despite many elements of the patient's visit to the CT facility requiring a fixed amount of time (starting an intravenous line, injecting contrast material, review of images, etc.), we have seen a 20 percent increase in our capacity to perform body CT cases, compared to that obtained using a conventional scanner during the same hours of operation. Except for those applications which require very high tube current (milliAmperes, or mA) we scan virtually all our patients helically.

While helical CT offers some real advantages over conventional scanning, it has taken several years to refine the marriage of technical elements that allow for practical day-to-day use of this technology. the four elements necessary for helical scanning are: the slip-ring gantry that allows continuous rotation of the x-ray tube, a high heat capacity x-ray tube, efficient detectors, and a reconstruction algorithm that corrects for table movement during acquisition of the scan. The latter has been progressively improved, so that the 180° interpolation algorithms currently in use produce a section sensitivity profile which closely mimics that of a conventional slice.

Helical scanning will be the dominant cutting edge of CT through the mid-1990s. Despite the many refinements which have occurred, the vendors are aggressively pursuing further hardware and software development to allow more effective helical scanning. Software that allows mixing of helical scans of variable collimation and pitch is already commercially available. Soon software will be available that automatically reduces the milliAmperage during that portion of the exposure when the x-ray beam is traversing the anterio-posterior dimension of the body. This will help reduce heat buildup and allow longer length of exposure for greater cranio-caudal coverage. A software module is now in clinical testing that will allow the scanner to determine the optimal injection delay between the initiation of the contrast injection and the beginning of the scan. This module will analyze vascular or soft-tissue attenuation on very low milliAmpere scans, and trigger the helical scan when attenuation reaches a prescribed level. Hardware advances such as more robust x-ray tubes and use of greater numbers of detectors are also anticipated in the future. Detector arrays arranged as multiple rows may allow greater z-direction coverage per rotation of the tube detector apparatus, and serve to equalize longitudinal resolution with that of the axial plane. Helical technology is now being introduced in mid-tier and even low-priced scanners.

Advances in computing power and workstation design are occurring in tandem with the advances in scanner technology. Helical data sets are excellent for rendering three-dimensional models. Contemporary workstations now take 30 sec or less to generate a model. With sufficient memory, models may be rotated and shown with varying display parameters in near real-time. Digital subtraction CT, image superimposition, and translucent shading of soft-tissue structures is in clinical trials at many sites. Our surgeons already find 3-D views useful for surgical planning. While many facets of the anatomy are displayed with lifelike realism, the anatomy cannot be electronically altered as it would be in the operating suite. In the future, however, surgeons will be able to practice the operation and manipulate the anatomy on virtual-reality or other high-speed graphics platforms. This can be useful not only for surgical planning, but also for training surgeons or linkage to laparoscopic or even robotic devices that will assist the surgeon of the future. It all sounds very futuristic, but these advances will all occur by the year 2000. We will see our diagnostic capability improve, but equally as important, the pivotal role of the radiologist as an anatomic consultant to our colleagues will increase. An understanding of the technical aspects of helical scanning, its strengths and weaknesses, and clinical applications will be essential for the CT radiologist of the 21st century.

Helical/Spiral CT

A Practical Approach

Chapter 1

Helical/Spiral CT: Technical Principles

James A. Brink / William J. Davros

INTRODUCTION

Computed body tomography has been revolutionized by the technical advantages of spiral CT. Established CT applications are improved by the minimization of motion artifacts, the elimination of respiratory misregistration artifacts,[1,2] and the production of overlapping images without additional radiation exposure.[3-5] CT angiography is just one example of the new applications involving multidimensional imaging which have been made possible by these advancements.[6-8] With spiral CT, multiple overlapping transaxial images can be generated from scan data acquired in a single breath-hold. High-quality two- and three-dimensional reformations can be generated from these highly overlapping transaxial images.

Spiral CT scanning involves continuous data acquisition throughout the volume of interest by simultaneously moving the patient through the gantry while the x-ray source rotates.[1,2] The x-ray traces a spiral on the patient's surface resulting in a helix of raw projection data from which planar images are generated (Figure 1-1). Each rotation of the tube generates data specific to an angled plane of section.[9] In order to achieve a true transaxial image, data points above and below the desired plane of section must be interpolated to estimate the data value in the transaxial plane (Figure 1-2). Unlike with conventional CT, the interval (spacing) between reconstructed transaxial images can be chosen retrospectively and arbitrarily. Thus, overlapping images can be generated without an increase in radiation exposure. So long as raw image data is stored in computer memory, transaxial images can be generated with as wide or narrow a reconstruction spacing as desired.

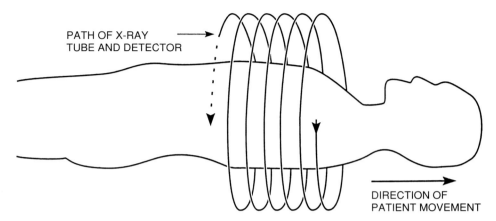

FIGURE 1-1 Schematic drawing of the scanning geometry used in spiral CT. The z-axis parallels the long axis of the patient. *(Courtesy of Kalender et al.[1])*

INTERPOLATION ALGORITHMS

When spiral CT was first released, transaxial spiral CT sections were generated by interpolating scan data points separated by a full 360° rotation of the x-ray tube using a 360° linear interpolation algorithm. This resulted in transaxial images which were nearly identical to conventional scanning. However, longitudinal reformations showed prominent blurring along the direction of table motion (z-axis) as compared to images reformatted from conventional scans.[10] This prompted investigators to develop algorithms which used data closer to the desired plane of section with hopes of improving longitudinal resolution. Interpolation algorithms which used data points separated by about one-half rotation (180°) of the x-ray tube were developed.[2,11] One such algorithm performed simple linear interpolation and another performed higher-order (cubic-spline) interpolation. Regardless of the mathematical technique employed, 180° interpolation resulted in a substantial increase in longitudinal resolution as compared to 360° interpolation, although noise was increased as well (Figure 1-3).

These improvements in interpolation produced two clearcut clinical benefits. First, high resolution multiplanar and three-dimensional imaging were made possible without significant longitudinal blurring. Second, the 180° algorithms permitted scanning at pitch greater than one providing greater coverage with any given spiral scan technique (pitch is equal to the table increment per gantry rotation divided by the collimation). Practically, slice profile broadening prohibits use of pitch values which are greater than two. Results by Polacin, Kalender, and Marchall from phantom studies and mathematical simulations showed the relationship between slice thickness and pitch for 360° linear relative to 180° linear and higher-order (cubic-spline) interpolation algorithms (Figure 1-4).[11] With pitch of two and 360° interpolation, slice thickness (defined in this case as the full width at tenth maximum of the section sensitivity profile) is increased threefold compared to

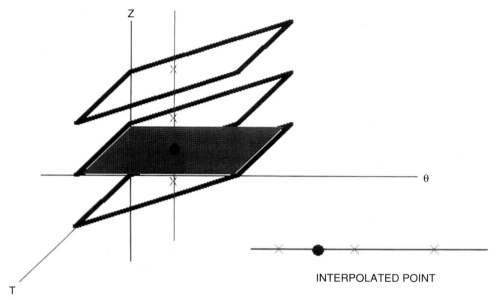

FIGURE 1-2 Schematic of interpolation rationale for helical CT. Data from each rotation of the x-ray tube are specific to an angled plane of section. Data for transaxial sections must be generated by interpolation of data above and below the desired plane of section. Z = longitudinal coordinate of patient cross-section, T = index to position in the detector array, θ = rotation angle with a period of 360°. *(Courtesy of Bresler et al.[9]) (© 1989 IEEE)*

conventional scanning. In contrast, the same parameter is increased by only 50 percent above conventional scanning when 180° interpolation is used.

The 180° interpolation algorithms have some disadvantages as well. The most important of these is an increase in image noise by 12 to 29 percent for the 180° algorithms relative to conventional scanning.[2,11,12] The increase in noise is predictable with linear interpolation, increased by 12 to 13 percent compared to conventional scanning with the same nominal section thickness and dose.[11] Noise is less predictable with higher-order interpolation algorithms but was found empirically to increase by 29 percent with 180° cubic-spline interpolation. Interestingly, noise with 360° linear interpolation is decreased by 17 to 18 percent as compared to conventional scanning due to the relative increase in photon statistics associated with such a broad interpolation range.

Interpolation Artifacts

A second disadvantage of newer interpolation algorithms is an artifact at high contrast transverse interfaces on longitudinal reformations which results in irregular disruption of the interface. We have observed the artifact only with the 180° cubic-spline interpolation method. This "breakup" artifact is shown on the coronal reformation of a fracture

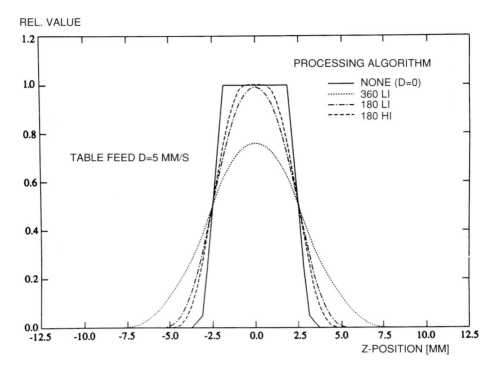

FIGURE 1-3 Section sensitivity profiles for different spiral CT interpolation algorithms (five mm collimation, pitch of one). The profiles for the 180° interpolation algorithms nearly approximate that of the rectangularly shaped profile of conventional scanning. 360 LI = 360° linear interpolation, 180 LI = 180° linear interpolation, 180 HI = 180° higher-order (cubic-spline) interpolation, d = table feed (mm/sec), Rel = relative, z-position = longitudinal position (mm). *(Courtesy of Polacin et al.[11])*

displacement phantom in Figure 1-5.[13] The smooth presenting surface of the phantom (orthogonal to the direction of table travel) is poorly rendered with "breakup" of the edge. The "breakup" artifact may be due to edge ringing or other adverse sequellae of nonlinear (higher-order) interpolation; it has not been seen with either 360° or 180° linear interpolation. Because of this artifact, we have excluded 180° cubic-spline interpolation from our clinical practice, and some manufacturers have excluded it from their equipment.

Another processing artifact unique to spiral CT is the "stairstep" artifact.[14] The artifact is most apparent on inclined surfaces in longitudinally oriented 2-D and 3-D reformations (Figure 1-6). We first observed it in aluminum ramp phantoms used to define the slice profile in conventional CT scanning. When a multiplanar reformation is performed, the ramps should appear as thin, oblique lines. However, with reformations from spiral CT images, they are depicted as steps rather than as straight lines. The longitudinal height of the step is proportional to the table increment and independent of the collimation or reconstruction interval (Figure 1-7). The artifact has been seen with both linear and non-linear (higher-order) interpolation algorithms.

Although the "stairstep" artifact has the same appearance as aliasing due to undersampling, it is a distinct phenomenon that results from the interpolation process. The stairstep appearance is largely due to aliasing when the reconstruction interval is large and the table increment is small (relative to the size of the object). If the reconstruction interval is much less than the collimation resulting in highly-overlapping transaxial images, as is common practice for multiplanar and 3-D imaging, then the interpolation artifact predominates. The artifact results from inconvenient interpolation geometry associated with high contrast interfaces aligned oblique to the direction of table motion.[15] The artifact is most apparent with

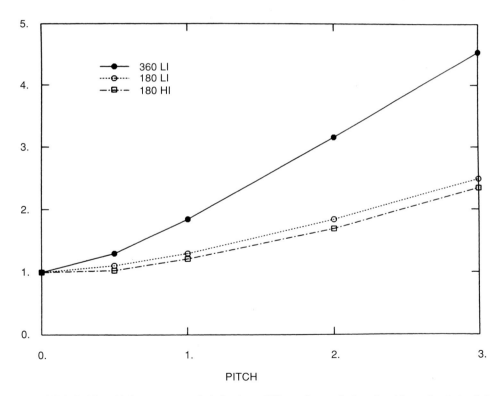

FIGURE 1-4 Slice thickness versus pitch for three different interpolation algorithms. A substantial improvement in slice thickness broadening is seen with 180° interpolation (180 LI, 180 HI) for pitch greater than one as compared to 360° interpolation (360 LI). Graph displays simulated slice thickness (defined here as the full width at tenth maximum of the section sensitivity profile) for spiral CT performed with five mm collimation. Pitch = zero refers to conventional scanning; 360 LI = 360° linear interpolation; 180 LI = 180° linear interpolation; and 180 HI = 180° higher-order (cubic-spline) interpolation. *(Courtesy of Polacin et al.[11])*

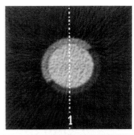
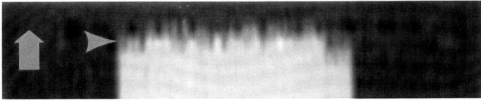

FIGURE 1-5 "Break-up" artifact. Multiplanar reformation of fracture displacement phantom scan acquired with spiral technique (two mm collimation, pitch = 1, 180° cubic-spline interpolation) reveals discontinuity of the phantom surface (arrowhead) orthogonal to the direction of table travel (arrow). The artifact was seen when 180° higher-order (cubic-spline) interpolation was used but not with 360° linear or 180° linear interpolation. *(Courtesy of Brink et al.[16])*

narrow structures of high contrast which are imaged with high zoom. The artifact is also worse with oblique surfaces which are nearly parallel to the transverse (xy) plane as opposed to oblique surfaces which are nearly parallel to the direction of table motion (z-axis).

OPERATOR-DEFINED PARAMETERS

More input from both the physician and technologist is required to perform a spiral CT scan than a conventional scan. First, the operator must decide on the scan timing parameters, considering both the patient's tolerance for breath-holding and the scanner's capabilities. In addition to the collimation, one must specify a measure of the table feed. Some manufacturers refer to this parameter as the table increment per gantry rotation. Other manufacturers simply refer to it as the table speed, especially if only a one sec gantry rotation period is available. An increasingly popular way to specify table feed is as a multiple of the collimation. This is called pitch or pitch ratio.* The operator must also choose the spacing at which transaxial images will be reconstructed.

---

*pitch = (table increment per gantry rotation) / (collimation)

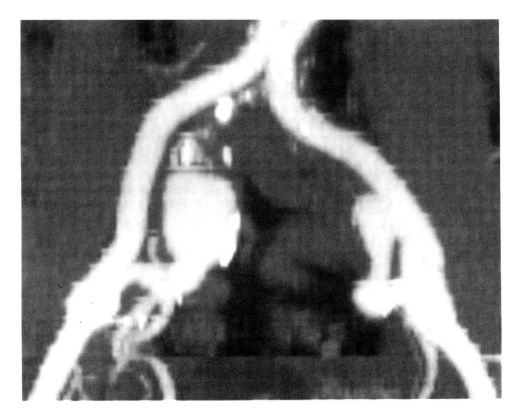

FIGURE 1-6 "Stairstep" artifact. Coronal maximum intensity projection from spiral CT (three mm collimation, five mm table increment, one mm reconstruction interval) of the iliac arteries. The "stairstep" artifact is seen as discontinuities along arteries oriented oblique to the direction of patient travel. The artifact is more pronounced when the artery is nearly parallel to the transverse plane and is less pronounced when the artery is nearly parallel to the direction of patient travel. *(Courtesy of Brink et al.[16])*

Scan Timing

The scan timing parameters are dependent upon the patient's ability to hold his or her breath, as well as specifications of the CT scanner.[16] If a patient is unable to hold his or her breath beyond a certain duration, then one does not wish to exceed that value in performance of a spiral scan. Some manufacturers have the capability of performing only one preprogrammed spiral scan. Others permit the performance of multiple preprogrammed spiral scans such that two or three separate spiral scans can be performed with a short breathing interval between the scans (Figure 1-8). This is advantageous in patients who are unable to hold their breath for a prolonged period, and essential if combined exams (i.e., thorax and abdomen) are to be performed.

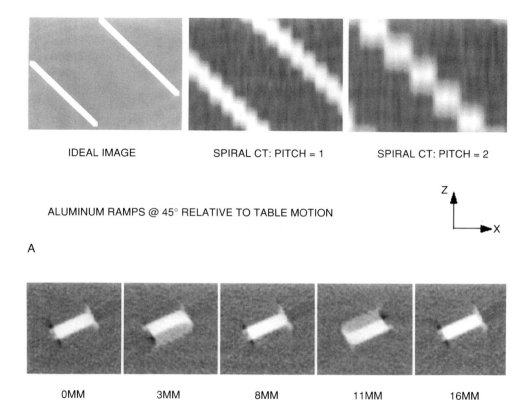

FIGURE 1-7 "Stairstep" artifact. (A) Longitudinal reformations from spiral CT (eight mm collimation, eight and 16 mm table increment (middle and right, respectively), one mm reconstruction interval) of thin aluminum plates oriented oblique to the direction of patient travel. These should appear as straight lines in ideal reformations (left), but appear as discontinuous surfaces or "stairsteps" (middle, right). The height of the "stairstep" is proportional to the table incrementation. (B) Source transaxial images from scan performed with 16 mm table increment reveal asymmetry to the depiction of the aluminum plates in cross-section which is dependent upon table position. The blur about the leading and trailing edges of the phantom is symmetric at zero, eight, and 16 mm. The blur is skewed toward the leading edge of the aluminum plate at three mm and is skewed toward the trailing edge at 11 mm. Thus, the spatial period of this artifact is equal to the table increment. The artifact results from inconvenient interpolation geometry associated with high contrast interfaces which are obliquely aligned to the direction of patient travel. *(Courtesy of Brink et al.[16])*

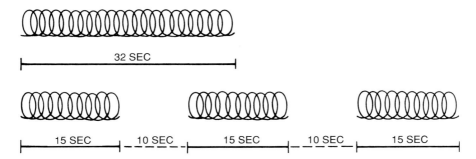

FIGURE 1-8 Single versus multiple helical scans. Some manufacturers permit the performance of only one preprogrammed helical scan. Others permit the performance of multiple sequential helical scans separated by short breathing intervals, allowing patients with diminished breath-holding capacity to undergo spiral scanning. *(Courtesy of Brink et al.[16])*

Many scanners require a reduction in tube current with prolonged spiral scanning resulting in increased image noise, which is already increased by the use of 180° interpolation (see *Interpolation Algorithms*). In such instances, a prolonged scan may not be advantageous, especially if one is scanning a dense body part such as the abdomen or pelvis or scanning with thin (two to three mm) collimation for spiral CT angiography. Dividing the volume into smaller subvolumes which are scanned separately and interposed with a short breathing interval may provide for sufficient tube cooling to permit scanning at a higher tube current. Strategies for dealing with tube current and coverage limitations will be specifically addressed in each of the subsequent clinical chapters.

Collimation and Table Incrementation

The choice of collimation is based primarily on the organ of interest. This decision is made for conventional and spiral scanning as follows:

a. two to three mm collimation is employed for small structures such as renal arteries and lung nodules
b. five mm collimation is used routinely in the neck
c. seven to 10 mm collimation is typically used in the chest.
d. five to eight mm collimation is usually used in the abdomen

The table increment is generally set equal to the collimation (pitch = 1). However, one may double the table increment relative to the collimation (pitch = 2) with a minor penalty in longitudinal resolution so long as 180° interpolation is used (see *Interpolation Algorithms*, Figure 1-4).

Posting a table of longitudinal coverage obtained with different combinations of available collimation settings and table feed settings for a given scanner is helpful to remind physicians and technologists of available options in choosing spiral scan parameters (Table 1-1). The longitudinal coverage is computed by multiplying the table speed by the spiral scan duration.

Generally, one would like to minimize the collimation to cover the volume of interest accepting a pitch up to two, providing 180° interpolation is employed. Thus, if one needs to scan a volume which is 15 cm in length with a 30-sec scan on a scanner that has a 1-sec gantry rotation period, one must use a table speed of five mm/sec. Depending on the available collimation settings of a given scanner, one may then choose either five mm collimation with a pitch of one, or three mm collimation with a pitch of 1.67. Both of these combinations of collimation and pitch would achieve the same coverage. For applications which require high spatial resolution such as CT angiography, three mm collimation is preferable because the effective slice thickness with three mm collimation and a pitch of 1.67 is less than with five mm collimation and a pitch of one. However, one must be certain that noise is not prohibitive with the smaller collimation value given increases in noise which may be present due to 180° interpolation, or due to a necessary reduction in tube current associated with prolonged spiral scanning on some scanners (see *Scan Timing*).

Reconstruction Spacing

Several factors determine the choice of the reconstruction interval or spacing. There is a tradeoff between practical issues such as processing time, the number of images to review, and image storage requirements versus the increased longitudinal resolution which one may achieve with highly overlapping transaxial images. Longitudinal resolution is dependent upon the detector collimation, table feed, and reconstuction interval. The table feed tends to broaden the slice profile with spiral CT compared to conventional CT (see *Interpolation Algorithms*, Figure 1-3) and decreases longitudinal resolution. Conversely, the reconstruction interval may be decreased with spiral CT without a penalty in x-ray dose resulting in an increase in longitudinal resolution. This is unlike conventional CT where such a benefit comes only with an increase in x-ray dose.

In clinical practice, Urban and colleagues[5] showed a 10 percent improvement in the detection of small lesions within the liver with spiral CT when a 50 percent overlap was used as compared to no overlap. Their confidence was also increased when a 50 percent overlap was used as 33 percent more lesions were identified as "definite" and the number of "probable" or "possible" lesions decreased by 23 percent and 44 percent, respectively. This is because the conspicuousness of a small lesion centered between two contiguous sections is decreased by volume averaging (Figure 1-9). When the reconstruction interval is chosen to be one-half of the collimation (50 percent overlap), the same lesion may fall within the center of an overlapping slice and its relative conspicuousness is increased.

If 50 percent overlap improves detection of small lesions, would greater overlap (e.g., 80 percent or 90 percent) provide additional benefit? This question was addressed in

TABLE 1-1 Longitudinal coverage (cm) using varied combinations of collimation, table speed, and pitch[a] for 30 sec exposure

Collim. (mm)	2 mm/ sec	3 mm/ sec	4 mm/ sec	5 mm/ sec	6 mm/ sec	7 mm/ sec	8 mm/ sec	9 mm/ sec	10 mm/ sec	11 mm/ sec	12.6 mm/ sec	13 mm/ sec	14 mm/ sec	15 mm/ sec	16 mm/ sec
2 mm	6 cm (1.0)	9 cm (1.5)	12 cm (2.0)												
3 mm		9 cm (1.0)	12 cm (1.33)	15 cm (1.67)	18 cm (2.0)										
4 mm			12 cm (1.0)	15 cm (1.25)	18 cm (1.5)	21 cm (1.75)	24 cm (2.0)								
5 mm				15 cm (1.0)	18 cm (1.2)	21 cm (1.4)	24 cm (1.6)	27 cm (1.8)	30 cm (2.0)						
7 mm						21 cm (1.0)	24 cm (1.14)	27 cm (1.29)	30 cm (1.43)	33 cm (1.57)	36 cm (1.71)	39 cm (1.86)	42 cm (2.0)		
8 mm							24 cm (1.0)	27 cm (1.12)	30 cm (1.25)	33 cm (1.37)	36 cm (1.5)	39 cm (1.62)	42 cm (1.75)	45 cm (1.87)	48 cm (2.0)

[a] Some devices allow the user to specify table speed while others allow programming of pitch. The pitch is given in parentheses for each of the table speed/collimation combinations up to a pitch of 2.0. The table assumes a 30 sec exposure with 360° tube rotation requiring 1 sec.

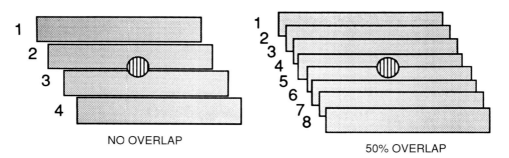

FIGURE 1-9 Value of overlapping sections. A small lesion may have low conspicuousness if centered at the periphery of two contiguous sections (scans number two and three left). However, with 50 percent overlap (right), the lesion will fall within the center of an overlapping image (scan number four) and will be more conspicuous than on the nonoverlapping contiguous images. By creating sections with 50 percent overlap, the number of scans will double.

theoretical studies of the influence of reconstruction interval on longitudinal resolution.*[17,18] To illustrate these principles by means of example, consider three scans performed with five mm collimation: conventional CT, spiral CT with pitch of one, and spiral CT with pitch of two (Figure 1-10). For reconstruction intervals exceeding the collimation, longitudinal resolution is equal to the reconstruction interval. When images overlap by 20 percent (slice interval of 4 mm), longitudinal resolution is still given by the reconstruction interval. Decreasing the reconstruction interval to smaller values with greater degrees of overlap provides no improvement in longitudinal resolution for spiral CT with pitch of two. However, this plateau does not occur until 40 percent overlap (three mm reconstruction interval) for spiral CT with pitch of one. With conventional scanning, longitudinal resolution is slightly improved beyond spiral CT with pitch of one; its plateau occurs at 60 percent overlap (two mm slice interval). However, for a given x-ray dose, spiral CT allows substantially better longitudinal resolution than conventional CT due to its inherent retrospecive reconstruction capability. Based on these simulations, we recommend reconstructing one to two slices per table increment for routine diagnosis and three to five slices per table increment for multidimensional imaging.

Recently, these theoretical predictions were validated empirically by Kalender et al. using spheres of 260 Hu attenuation and five mm diameter as test objects.[19] Based on

---

* In these studies, the section sensitivity profiles (SSPs) and transfer functions were derived for conventional and spiral CT. For spiral CT with 180° linear interpolation, the SSP was computed as the convolution of the detector response, table motion, and low-pass filtering functions. Since the bandwidth of the transfer function is inversely proportional to the sharpness of the SSP, longitudinal resolution was approximated as one-half the reciprocal of the one-tenth-cutoff frequency of the transfer function.

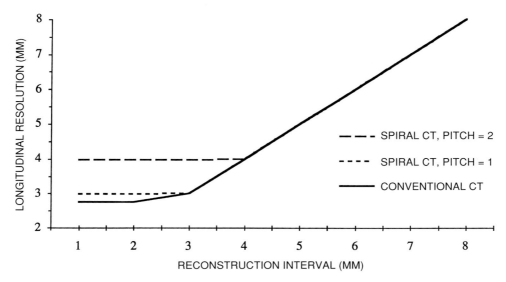

FIGURE 1-10 Longitudinal resolution versus reconstruction interval for scans performed with five mm collimation (conventional scanning, spiral CT with pitch of one, and spiral CT with pitch of two). For reconstruction intervals greater than the collimation, longitudinal resolution is given by the reconstruction interval and the curves overlap. A reconstruction interval limit of four mm (20 percent overlap) is evident for spiral CT with pitch of two, below which longitudinal resolution is not improved. A similar lower limit spiral CT with pitch of one is present at three mm reconstruction interval (40 percent overlap), below which longitudinal resolution is not improved. Finally, the plateau for longitudinal resolution with conventional CT occurs at two mm slice interval (60 percent overlap) and is marginally better than with spiral CT with pitch of one. Graph plots simulated results for longitudinal resolution, measured as one-half of the reciprocal of the one-tenth-cutoff frequency of the transfer function. Spiral scan data are presumed to undergo processing with 180° linear interpolation. Percent overlap is based on nominal rather than effective slice thicknesses. *(Adapted from Brink* [16] *and Wang* [17,18] *et al.)*

these experiments, the authors conclude that at least two images should be reconstructed per table increment, and that the theoretical maximum longitudinal resolution is closely approached when one reconstructs four to five slices per table increment.

PRACTICAL CONSIDERATIONS IN CHOOSING EQUIPMENT

There are significant design differences among the helical/spiral scanners currently in use. These devices differ in their hardware, approach to scanning, and user features. Detailed specifications gleaned from the manufacturers' technical and product sheets and an explanation of the reported parameters are contained in appendix 1 at the end of the book. The scanners which are available do have some common elements. These along with important user features will be presented in this section.

X-ray Generators and Tubes

Helical scanning significantly challenges the x-ray generators and tubes in use for CT. The power requirements for tubes and generators increase proportionately as the gantry rotation period is reduced for a constant milliAmperes-sec (mAs). In helical CT using a gantry rotation period of one sec, peak power levels of 40 kW or higher are needed. This is approximately twice the maximum power level of many conventional scanners. The generator and tube must be appropriately matched. The tube must be capable of running at high power without overheating.

Achieving a specific absolute power level has not been the sole limiting factor in tube design for helical CT. Buildup of anode heat has actually been a far greater obstacle. This is especially so in helical CT of the abdomen because scanning the abdomen requires higher milliAmperes-sec than scanning other body parts. The range in total (bulk) heat capacity of commercially available tubes for helical CT is 2.0 to 5.2 million heat units with anode cooling rates up to 0.9 million heat units/minute. Tube life appears comparable to that of conventional scanners for most vendors (approximately 50,000 slices).

Although anode cooling is important, focal track cooling is even more important. The focal track refers to the site where electrons impinge on the tungsten target portion of the anode. The target is attached to and surrounded by an underlying graphite base. Unlike conventional CT, helical CT rapidly heats the focal track because of its sustained exposures. The track must handle large absolute amounts of heat, but also effectively allow heat to dissipate into the remainder of the anode. The physical composition of this track and its ability to cool prove to be far more important than the specific manufacturers' claims regarding the absolute bulk thermal state of the tube or the cooling rate of the anode as a whole. Do not be taken in by claims that bigger is better. Tubes, however, with a heat capacity of less than three million heat units are not conducive to scanning the abdomen or extended helical/spiral coverage.

The tube cooling algorithm is a computer model used to predict the heat status of the tube, anode, and focal track. The algorithm sets the milliAmpere ceiling for a specific length of helical exposure and the interval that must elapse for tube cooling between helical exposures. The vendors all differ on how liberal this algorithm is in allowing the user to "push" the tube and focal track to its maximum heat tolerance. The radiologist buying equipment must carefully review the allowable combinations of scan parameters (milliAmperes, length of helical exposure, and kiloVolt peak). While most radiologists will not ask the milliRoentgen/milliAmpere output of the tube (radiation dose in milliRoentgens produced per milliAmpere setting), their "radiologic" eye will tell them if the image looks photopenic ("noisy" or "grainy") in the context of what he or she considers acceptable clinical image quality.

The Slip-Ring Gantry

Slip-ring gantries contain sets of rings and electrical components that rotate, and sliding contacts or brushes that are stationary. There are no electrical cables connecting the gantry components to the ground because these would hinder continuous rotation. In slip-ring CT scanners there usually are multiple parallel slip-rings with one supplying high voltage to the tube and generator, another transporting digital data to and from the detectors, and a third providing relatively low voltage for operation of control systems.

The various commercially available systems differ significantly in how voltage is delivered to the x-ray tube. With high voltage slip-rings (Toshiba 900S, Buffalo Grove, IL) all the high voltage is developed on the ground and passed across the rings to the tube. In this design, the rings are enclosed in a rotating sealed chamber that contains either inert gas or dielectric oil as an insulator. In hybrid slip-ring devices, part of the voltage step up takes place on the ground (to about 10,000 V) and the rest on the rotating portion of the gantry (Siemens Somatom Plus and Plus-S, Iselin, NJ). In these devices, the entire gantry is also sealed. In the low voltage slip-ring devices (General Electric HiSpeed, Milwaukee, WI) relatively low (540 V) direct current voltage is passed across the slipring; high voltage for powering the x-ray tube is actually generated on the rotating portion of the gantry. This design permits an open, air-cooled gantry with reduced space requirements. The challenge of the low-voltage approach has been to develop generators that are powerful enough to step up voltage from 540 V to 140 kV yet are sufficiently compact and lightweight to be rotated within the gantry (Figure 1-11).

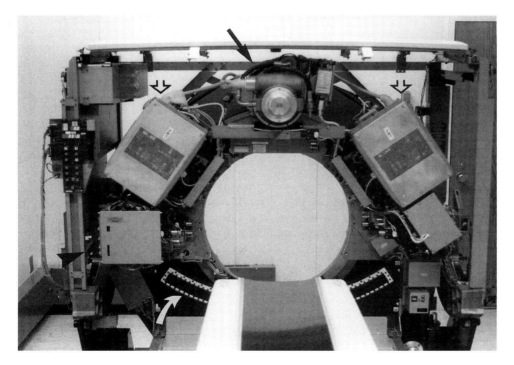

FIGURE 1-11 Gantry of low voltage slip-ring device helical scanner. In a low voltage slip-ring scanner, x-ray tube (solid arrow), transformers (open arrows), generator (arrowhead), and detectors (curved arrow) are all mounted on the rotating portion of gantry. *(Courtesy of Zeman et al.[26])*

Gantry Geometry

All vendors except Picker use rotate-rotate (third generation) geometry for their helical/spiral scanners. Picker uses rotate-fixed (fourth generation) geometry. *From a clinical perspective, we do not believe that there is any inherent advantage of fourth generation geometry over third generation geometry, or vice versa.* While this could be demonstrated with an extensive point-counterpoint argument, we feel the geometry is only important in the context of a total system. In fourth generation geometry scanners (even before the advent of helical scanning), large numbers of views are obtained and averaged to generate ray densities similar to third generation scanners. Spatial resolution would suffer if this high sampling rate was not used. The increased sampling results in increased quantum and electronic noise, but this does not appear to significantly degrade clinical images. Tubes, generators, detectors, and reconstruction algorithms appear far more important than the geometry.

Detector Technology

Refinements in detector technology not only have made it possible to reduce the dose of radiation to the patient, but also support faster, higher-quality image acquisition with less x-ray production. Since the limitation of contemporary x-ray tubes is buildup of heat during sustained production of x-rays, improved use of the photons that are produced can reduce the milliAmpere-sec necessary for image production and therefore the heat buildup associated with that milliAmpere per sec. In conventional CT, the role of the detector in sparing the x-ray tube is not as significant, because the tube turns on and off, and can cool down between each individual slice. The role of improved detector efficiency is far more critical in "saving" the tube during continuous operation such as occurs in helical CT.

X-ray detectors are used in CT scanners to count the number of x-rays that are transmitted through an object. This value is used in conjunction with the number of x-rays incident on an object to compute the linear attenuation coefficient along a path traversed by the x-ray beam. Both ultimately contribute to the data used to reconstruct the image. There are three important detector features to consider when comparing CT scanners: the type of detectors used, the number of detectors, and the concentration of detectors per degree of arc which is irradiated.

The two general types of detectors currently used in helical CT scanners are solid state detectors (SS) and gas-filled ionization detectors. Solid state detectors, as their name implies, are made of solid materials that give off light when they are struck by x-rays. Early solid state detectors were NaI(Tl) and CsI. Later these were replaced with ceramic compounds doped with rare earth elements. In order to collect the light signal from solid state detectors, photomultiplier tubes or photodiodes are used. These two devices convert the light signal to an electrical signal. The electrical signal acquired from solid state detectors is the amount of charge collected over a fixed time interval. Solid state detectors have the advantage of being small. They also have high x-ray-to-electrical signal conversion efficiencies (75 to 85 percent depending on how measured). If there is one weakness of solid state detectors it is the difficulty in manufacturing them. Companies that use solid state detectors include Elscint (Hackensack, NJ), General Electric Medical Systems, Picker International (Highland Heights, OH), and Toshiba America Medical Systems (Tustin, CA).

Gas-filled ionization chambers used today are filled exclusively with the inert gas Xenon. When an x-ray enters a Xenon-filled chamber it may ionize Xe atoms. If an atom is ionized, freed electrons will drift towards a positively charged collecting anode and the positively charged atom will drift towards the negatively charged outer walls of the chamber to be neutralized. The electrical signal acquired from a Xe gas detector is the amount of charge collected over a fixed time interval; this is called integral mode. They tend to be less efficient at producing an output signal for a given input signal (40 to 60 percent). Their main advantage is that they are easy to manufacture, require no exotic materials, are inexpensive relative to solid state detectors, and have a fast response time. The two vendors that use gas-filled ionization chambers on their premium line helical CT scanners are Philips Medical Systems (Shelton, CT) and Siemens Medical Systems.

The absolute number of detectors a helical CT scanner possesses is a measure of its immunity to produce artifacts from detector failure. It also is a measure of the scanner's complexity. Among scanners of the rotate-rotate geometry, Toshiba Medical Systems leads in the number of detectors in a single bank with 896 solid state detectors spread over an arc of 49°. Elscint uses 1052 solid state detectors in a unique two-bank detector array, each bank having 526 detectors over an arc of 43°. Picker International, using the rotate-fixed geometry, leads the industry with a total of 4800 SS detectors in their PQ-2000 scanner.

Perhaps more important than the absolute number of detectors is the concentration of detectors over the fan beam arc. The number of detectors per degree of arc subtended by the x-ray fan beam is a measure of the scanner's ability to acquire independent views through an object, provided that signal can be extracted from detectors quickly. The more views a scanner gets of an object the better, in theory, it can reconstruct the high contrast fine structure of that object. If a vendor lacks a high density of detectors per degree of arc, this can be compensated for to some degree by sampling the signal more often as the x-ray-tube detector bank rotates about the object of interest. All vendors range between 42 and 49 detector bank degrees of arc with the number of detectors per degree ranging from 12 to 18.3 (see appendix). In fact, even with fourth generation geometry, (e.g., 4800 detectors spread over 360°), about one-sixth are active assuming a 45 to 50° fan beam. This is roughly 800, which is quite comparable to the number of active detectors during a third generation geometry exposure.

Physicists judge detectors on three basic criteria: efficiency, response time, and temporal stability. While solid state detectors appear to be the big winner in each of these categories, it is important for the radiologist to assess image quality on routine images. Image quality is a combination of detector properties, gantry geometry, and scanning parameters such as milliAmperes, collimation, pitch, etc. Whenever reviewing vendor's images, ask for the parameters. Visualize how you would use the machine. The user features may prove to be as important as image quality.

Equipment Helical/Spiral Scanning Capability

User features that affect scanning capability are constantly evolving. The greatest difficulty the radiologist faces in choosing a new helical/spiral scanner is sorting out those features that currently exist, those that will soon exist, and those that someday may (or may not) exist. We fared no better in sorting out features, but to the best of our ability, these are presented in appendix 1. When buying a scanner, viewing its routine operation at a high volume site is critical to envision the way it may ultimately be used in your practice. Throughout the clinical sections in this book, many pearls are presented that will help the radiologist work around some of the limitations that may be encountered on specific devices.

We find that the greatest limitations that must be contended with during helical/spiral scanning is lack of milliAmperes, inadequate coverage while maintaining a 1:1 pitch ratio, and needless delays between back-to-back helical scans or helical scans followed by non-helical sections. The vendors have varied in their success in addressing these problems, but by the time of publication, we suspect that many of the obstacles to effective helical scanning will no longer be an issue. More robust tubes, higher milliAmpere capability, and elimination of software resets or reentering scanning protocols between groups of scans are on the way for most vendors.

MULTIDIMENSIONAL IMAGING

Multidimensional Imaging Techniques

A variety of two- and three-dimensional techniques are available for displaying spiral CT image data in nontransaxial planes. Among multiplanar reformations (MPRs), high quality coronal and sagittal reformations are readily generated from transaxial spiral CT images acquired in a single breath-hold and reconstructed with a high degree of overlap (three to five images per table increment). In addition, obliquely-oriented images may be generated in the paraxial, paracoronal, and parasagittal planes. Some reconstruction software packages offer the possibility of generating two-dimensional reformations oriented in a curved plane. In such instances, the operator prescribes a curved line on a reference image using a trackball or mouse to define the plane of image reformation. Such reformations are useful for displaying anatomy which may curve or spiral through multiple imaging planes (such as an aortic dissection). However, because of the subjective and arbitrary process used to define the imaging plane, curved-planar reformations should be interpreted with caution.

Among three-dimensional imaging techniques, the maximum intensity projection (MIP) and the shaded-surface display (SSD) are the most widely used.[20,24] Each technique has specific advantages and disadvantages (Figure 1-12). In CT angiography, the maximum intensity projection provides good separation of the enhanced stenotic lumen from calcified plaque along the vessel wall since absolute attenuation information is preserved

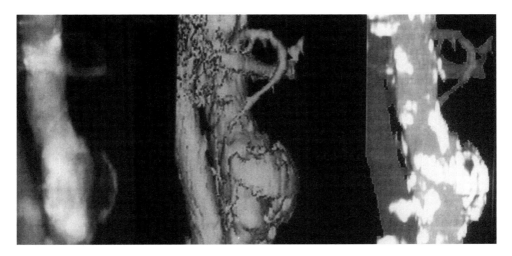

FIGURE 1-12 Three-dimentional reformations. Ray-sum projection (left), shaded-surface display (SSD, center), and maximum intensity projection (MIP, right) from spiral CT scan of a fusiform abdominal aortic aneurysm. The MIP provides good separation of the enhanced aorta from the calcified plaque in the vessel wall. The SSD renders both structures with the same intensity and risks underestimation of stenoses that are due to calcified plaque. Conversely, the ray-sum and SSD provide better depiction of overlapping vessels than the MIP.

within the image. However, it provides poor depiction of overlapping vessels—areas of overlap are not depicted as a focal area of increased opacity. This problem may be minimized by generating a series of MIPs that rotate about a major anatomic axis so that vessels which overlap en face can be viewed in tangent. Conversely, the shaded-surface display does not permit separation of calcified plaque from the enhanced stenotic lumen as both structures are set to "white" if they are above the attenuation threshold set by the operator. However, the SSD provides better depiction of overlapping vessels than the MIP due to the perception of depth associated with the SSD.[8,21,22]. Another technique called the ray-sum projection depicts the additive pixel values along the observer's line of sight. It also is excellent for displaying overlapping vessels.

For both two- and three-dimensional reformations, the first processing step interpolates the image data longitudinally.[20] Under most clinical circumstances, even with a small reconstruction interval and highly overlapping transaxial images, the voxels are anisotropic (their height along the z-axis is greater that their dimensions in the transverse plane). A longitudinal interpolation is performed to obtain isotropic voxels (equal in all three dimensions) (Figure 1-13). Once this is done, two-dimensional multiplanar reformations can be readily generated by mapping selected parts of the matrix of interpolated image data onto reformatted gray-scale image planes.

Both maximum-intensity projections and shaded-surface display images require additional preprocessing for best results. The matrix of interpolated image data must be edited

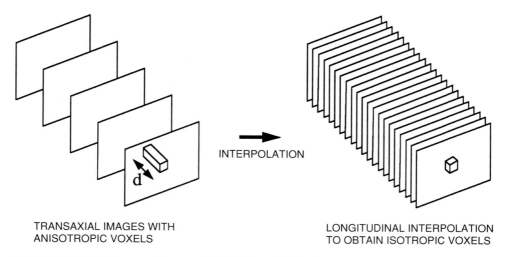

FIGURE 1-13 Initial processing step for both 2-D and 3-D reformations. Following reconstruction of the spiral CT data into transaxial images, the voxels are usually anisotropic (their z-axis dimension is greater than their dimensions in the transverse plane). The transaxial image data undergo longitudinal interpolation to generate multiple intervening slices with isotropic voxels (equal in all three dimensions).

to remove unwanted structures. For spiral CT angiography, bone is generally removed from the imaging volume to increase the subject contrast of enhanced blood vessels and to avoid confusion of calcified plaque with bone. For maximum intensity projections, inclusion of soft-tissue within the edited volume may have additional disadvantages (see *Technical Optimization for Multidimensional Imaging*).

Unwanted structures may be removed by a variety of techniques. The most straightforward of these is the manual trace technique. Here, the operator defines a region-of-interest (ROI) which circumscribes the structures that one would like to include in the edited volume. All structures outside of the ROI are excluded. Initial implementations of the manual trace technique were performed on a slice-by-slice basis and were quite time consuming. Current versions permit one to divide the imaging volume into several slabs or partitions. The operator prescribes the ROI on a transaxial reference MIP for each slab and the ROI is propagated to all slices within the slab. This decreases the time requirement for the manual trace technique by an order of magnitude. Recently, 3-D connectivity-based editing techniques have emerged which permit an ROI to "grow" from seed points placed within the imaging volume. With these techniques, one may place seed points in the lumbar spine and "grow" a 3-D ROI to remove the spine. However, difficulites can be expected with a diffusely calcified aorta which is in contact with the spine for CT aortography. The ROI may "grow" to include the aorta with the spine for removal from the imaging volume.

Maximum intensity projections are generated by passing imaginary rays through the matrix of interpolated image data and mapping the maximum attenuation value along each ray to a grayscale image (Figure 1-14). These images can be oriented in major anatomic planes (coronal, sagittal, transaxial), or they can be oriented in oblique planes, rotating about the major anatomic axes. Such maximum intensity projections can be viewed in cine display fashion and will give the appearance of continuous rotation of the object of interest if they are generated at fine degrees of rotation. Such a family of maximum intensity projections is commonly named according to the axis about which they rotate. For example, a set of maximum intensity projections is commonly generated at 6° increments from the coronal to the sagittal plane rotating about the z-axis (named MIPz), or from the transaxial to the coronal plane rotating about the x-axis (named MIPx).[21,25] Ray-sum views may be similarly displayed and allow overlapping structures to clearly be seen throughout the 360° rotation of a model. Like maximum intensity projection views, they may be performed in the absence of, or following designation of a threshold value.

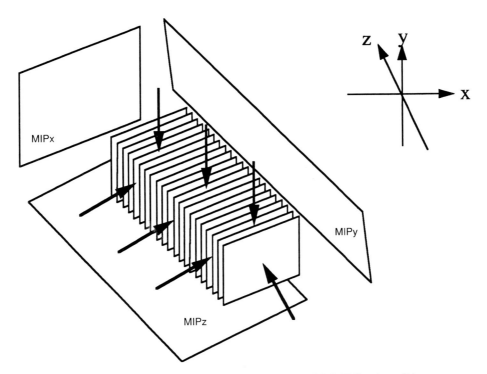

FIGURE 1-14 Generation of maximum intensity projections (MIPs). Following editing to remove unwanted structures, imaginary rays are passed through the matrix of interpolated image data. The maximum attenuation value along each ray is mapped to a grayscale image. A set of MIPs which rotate about major anatomic axes is commonly displayed in a cine fashion to give the appearance of continuous rotation of the object of interest. MIP sets are commonly named according to the axis about which they rotate (MIPx = MIPs which rotate about the x-axis, MIPy = MIPs which rotate about the y-axis, MIPz = MIPs which rotate about the z-axis).

Shaded-surface display images are almost always generated by setting an arbitrary threshold; voxels in the matrix of interpolated image data with attenuation values greater than the threshold are set to "white." All others with lesser attenuation values are set to black.[20,23,24] The matrix of thresholded image data is then rendered as a three-dimensional image with depth perception given by shading techniques. The orientation of the image is given by an imaginary light source which can be positioned arbitrarily permitting one to view the three-dimensional model from any perspective.

Technical Optimization for Multidimensional Imaging

The technique that one chooses for spiral CT greatly influences the success of multidimensional imaging. For spiral CT angiography, the way that clinical scans are performed (collimation, table increment) and postprocessed (reconstruction interval, volume editing technique, and rendering technique) impacts on the depiction of small vessels. Longitudinal resolution is maximized when collimation, table increment, and reconstruction interval are minimized. However, decreasing the collimation results in increased pixel noise. Decreasing the table increment limits scan coverage when other parameters are held constant, and decreasing the reconstruction interval increases image processing time (see *Operator Defined Parameters*).

The impact of these technical parameters on the success of multidimensional imaging is well illustrated in the use of spiral CT for the diagnosis of renal arterial stenosis. Clinical studies have shown frequent overestimation of renal arterial stenoses.[21,22] Although Rubin et al.[21] detected significant renal arterial stenoses on MIPs generated from spiral CT scans (three mm collimation, pitch of one to two, and two mm reconstruction interval) with 92 percent sensitivity and 83 percent specificity, five out of seven (71 percent) severe stenoses (90 to 99 percent diameter reduction) appeared occluded; patency was inferred from opacification of the vessel distal to the stenosis. Similarly, nine out of seventeen (53 percent) moderate stenoses (50 to 69 percent diameter reduction) diagnosed at conventional arteriography were misdiagnosed as hemodynamically significant (greater than or equal to 70 percent diameter reduction) with spiral CT MIPs in this study. Galanski et al.[22] also found that all severe stenoses appeared as pseudo-occlusions. Conversely, both true renal artery occlusions in their series had good collateral perfusion and were misdiagnosed as severe stenoses. Both of these studies also reported a few cases in which the severity of the stenosis was underestimated.

Underestimation of stenosis is likely to occur with cross-sectional imaging techniques because the diameter of the blood vessel is overestimated due to volume averaging. However, the degree of overestimation is greater for stenotic vessel segments than for normal vessel segments which leads to a decrease in the apparent percent stenosis. Overestimation of stenosis is likely to occur when low subject contrast is present between the vessel and background tissue, either by reduction of vessel attenuation or elevation of background attenuation.[25]

Vessel attenuation is reduced when the vessel diameter is less than the effective slice thickness (Figure 1-15, 1-16). Background attenuation is elevated by inclusion of soft tissue

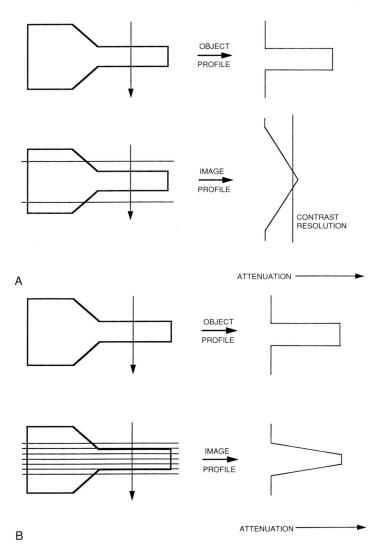

FIGURE 1-15 Impact of slice thickness (relative to object diameter) on attenuation profile from longitudinal reformation. Diagram models imaging response of a stenotic vessel on longitudinal 2-D or 3-D reformations. When the slice thickness is greater than the vessel diameter (A), convolution of the actual profile with the slice profile results in an image profile which is reduced in height proportional to the ratio (vessel diameter/slice thickness). When the slice thickness is less than or equal to the vessel diameter (B), the height of the image profile is not reduced. In both cases, the profile is widened by twice the slice thickness. In (A), the vessel may not be resolved, particularly if the baseline attenuation is elevated (as with inclusion of soft tissue in the edited volume, Figure 1-16. (Diagrams are based on idealized object and slice profiles and are adapted from Brink et al.[25])

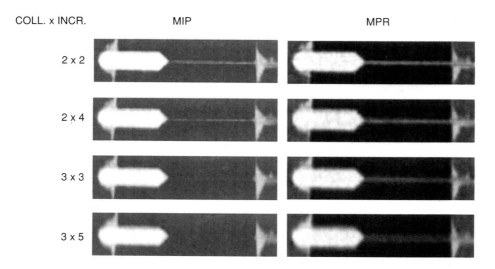

FIGURE 1-16 Depiction of an 85 percent stenosis (1.7 mm diameter stenosis) in an 11.1 mm diameter, transversely oriented phantom vessel with different coronal test images and scan techniques. (Left) Coronal MIP images for various scan techniques using two and three mm collimation and two to five mm table increments. The stenotic lumen becomes indistinguishable from the water (soft-tissue) attenuation background for scans performed with three mm collimation. (Right) Coronal MPRs for the same combinations of collimation and table increment. Increased blurring of the stenotic lumen is apparent with increasing collimation and table increment; however, the blurred lumen is still recognizable against the fat attenuation background. The same phenomenon was also present for MIP images which were generated after editing the image volume to remove water (soft-tissue) which surrounded the vessel and adjacent fat. The difference between left and right represents different styles of editing the image volume. The MIP generated from unedited image data (Left) illustrates the effect of including soft-tissue such as the psoas muscle within the edited volume. The MPR image (Right) illustrates the effect of limiting the edited volume to strictly the vessel and surrounding fat. Thus, care should be taken to exclude soft-tissue from the edited volume to avoid overcalling stenoses as occlusions. *(Adapted from Brink et al.[25])*

such as the psoas muscle in the edited volume prior to 3-D rendering. Under these conditions, a stenotic vessel may appear occluded if it falls below the low contrast resolution of the imaging system (Figure 1-16).[25] These effects are substantially greater in longitudinal 2-D and 3-D reformations than in the transverse plane because longitudinal resolution is considerably worse than in-plane resolution.[10] Care must be taken to maximize longitudinal resolution by carefully controlling the collimation, table increment, and reconstruction interval. Care must also be taken to exclude soft tissue from the edited volume to avoid overcalling stenoses as occlusions on maximum intensity projections.

CONCLUSION

Spiral CT scanning requires knowledge of several technical parameters that are not present with conventional CT scanning. One needs to carefully select the collimation, table increment, reconstruction interval, and in some instances, the interpolation algorithm. Minimizing these numeric parameters maximizes longitudinal resolution but with various tradeoffs. Decreasing the collimation decreases the effective slice thickness but increases pixel noise. Limiting the table increment to pitch of one limits the broadening of the effective slice thickness associated with the spiral technique but also limits the coverage which can be achieved with a given spiral scan. Generally, one strives to minimize the collimation to cover the volume of interest accepting a pitch up to two provided 180° interpolation is used. The reconstruction interval is also minimized to maximize longitudinal resolution but with tradeoffs of increased image processing time, data storage requirements, and physician time for image review. For routine diagnosis, we recommend reconstruction of one to two slices per table increment, and for multiplanar and 3-D imaging, we recommend reconstruction of three to five slices per table increment. The scan timing is dictated by both patient and machine considerations.

REFERENCES

1. Kalender WA, Sissler W, Klotz E, Vock P. Spiral volumetric CT with single-breath-hold technique, continuous transport, and continuous scanner rotation. *Radiology* 1990; **176:**181–183.
2. Crawford CR, King K. Computed tomography scanning with simultaneous patient translation. *Med Phys* 1990; **17:**967–982.
3. Iock P, Soucek M, Daepp M, Kalender WA. Lung: spiral volumetric CT with single-breath-hold technique. *Radiology* 1990; **176:**864–867.
4. Costello P, Anderson W, Blume D. Pulmonary nodule: evaluation with spiral volumetric CT. *Radiology* 1991; **179:**875–876.
5. Urban BA, Fishman EK, Kuhlman JE, Kowashima A, Hennessey JG, Siegelman SS. Detection of focal hepatic lesions with spiral CT: comparison of 4- and 8-mm interscan spacing. *AJR* 1993; **160:**783–785.
6. Heiken JP, Brink JA, Vannier MW. Spiral (helical) CT. *Radiology* 1993; **189:**647–656.
7. Fishman EK, Wyatt SH, Ney DR, Kuhlman JE, Siegelman SS. Spiral CT of the pancreas with multiplanar display. *AJR* 1992; **159:**1209–1215.
8. Rubin GD, Dake MD, Napel SA, McDonnell CH, Jeffrey RB. Three-dimensional spiral CT angiography of the abdomen: initial clinical experience. *Radiology* 1993; **186:**147–152.
9. Bresler Y, Skraba CZ. Optimal interpolation in helical scan computed tomography. *Proc ICASSP* 1989; **3:**1472–1475.
10. Brink JA, Heiken JP, Balfe DM, Sagel SS, DiCroce J, Vannier MW. Spiral CT: decreased spatial resolution in vivo due to broadening of section-sensitivity profile. *Radiology* 1992; **185:**469–474.
11. Polacin A, Kalender WA, Marchal G. Evaluation of section sensitivity profiles and image noise in spiral CT. *Radiology* 1992; **185:**29–35.
12. Wang G, Vannier MW. Helical CT image noise—analytical results. *Med Phys* 1993; **20:**1635–1640.
13. McEnery KW, Wilson AJ, Murphy WA. Comparison of spiral CT versus conventional CT multiplanar reconstructions of a frature displacement phantom. *Invest Radiol* 1994; **29:**665–670.

14. Wang G, Vannier MW. Stairstep artifacts in three-dimensional helical CT. *Radiology* 1994; **191:**79–83.
15. Polacin A, Kalender WA, Brink JA, Vannier MW. Measurement of slice sensitivity profiles in spiral CT. *Med Phys* 1994; **21:**133–140.
16. Brink JA, Heiken JP, Wang G, McEnery KW, Schlueter FJ, Vannier MW. Spiral (helical) CT: principles and technical considerations. *Radiographics* 1994; **14:**887–893.
17. Wang G, Vannier MW. Longitudinal resolution in volumetric x-ray CT—analytic comparison between conventional and helical CT. *Med Phys* 1994; **21:**429–433.
18. Wang G, Brink JA, Vannier MW. Theoretical FWTM values in helical CT. *Med Phys,* in press.
19. Kalender WA, Polacin A, Suss C. A comparison of conventional and spiral CT: an experimental study on the detection of spherical lesions. *J Comp Avial Tomography* 1994; **18:**167–176.
20. Fishman EK, Magid D, Ney DR, Chaney EL, Pizer SM, et al. Three-dimensional imaging. *Radiology* 1991; **181:**321–337.
21. Rubin GD, Dake MD, Napel S, Jeffrey RB, McDonnell CH, et al. Spiral CT of renal artery stenosis: comparison of three-dimensional rendering techniques. *Radiology* 1994; **190:**181–189.
22. Galanski M, Prokop M, Chavan A, Schaefer CM, Jandeleit K, et al. Renal arterial stenoses: spiral CT angiography. *Radiology* 1993; **189:**185–192.
23. Vannier MW, Marsh JL, Warren JO. Three-dimensional CT reconstruction images for craniofacial surgical planning and evaluation. *Radiology* 1984; **150:**179-184.
24. Magnusson M, Lenz R, Danielsson PE. Evaluation of methods for shaded surface display of CT volumes. Computerized Medical Imaging and Graphics 1991; **15**(4):247–256.
25. Brink JA, Lim JT, Wang G, Heiken JP, Deyoe LA, Vannier MW. Technical optimization of spiral CT for depiction of renal artery stenosis: in vitro analysis. *Radiology,* in press.
26. Zeman RK, Fox SH, Silverman PM, et al. Helical (spiral) CT of the abdomen. *AJR* 1993; **160:**719–725.

Chapter 2

Head, Neck, and Spine

Pedro T. Vieco

INTRODUCTION

The purpose of this chapter is to introduce the reader to applications, technique, interpretation, advantages, and disadvantages of helical CT imaging in the head and neck. Emphasis will be placed on CT angiography (CTA) as this probably is the most significant step forward that helical scanning has provided, and a powerful tool for the neuroradiologist. Most CTA research has concentrated on the carotid bifurcation and the circle of Willis, and it is now apparent that a variety of pathologies may be successfully imaged with this technique. An overview of applications in more traditional imaging of the neck and spine will also be provided.

ADVANTAGES AND DISADVANTAGES OF HELICAL CT

Since the advent of CT scanning, efforts have been made to increase scan speed.[1] With the more primitive early scanners, prolonged scan times made CT only applicable in areas of the body where physiologic motion was minimal. Historically, motion produced so much artifact that examination of the abdomen, for example, was limited or not possible. Over the years, technologic advances have steadily reduced examination times. Most recently, the development of helical CT scanning has reduced it further. Continuous tube rotation and x-ray exposure coupled with constant table speed has allowed for large volumes of tissue to be imaged in very short time periods. While tube heat buildup poses a problem in scanning the spine, this has not proved insurmountable for head and neck imaging. Reconstruction artifacts associated with helical methodology, however, have prevented its widespread use for routine head studies.

Aside from the obvious advantages associated with rapid scanning, namely increased patient throughput and the ability to rapidly scan clinically tenuous patients, it became clear that helical CT also offered additional properties not present in conventional, step-by-step axial CT scanning.[2] Because helical CT data aquisition is a continous rather than a stepwise process, three-dimensional rendering with this technique is free of many of the artifacts inherent in conventional CT. It also became clear that the high-speed capabilities of helical scanning were rapid enough to "capture" boluses of intravenous contrast as they passed through volumes of interest in the arterial phase. Used in combination, computer generated models of arterial and venous anatomy can be made.[3-10] The contrast enhancement and imaging techniques (Tables 2-1, 2-2) dramatically differ from those used in conventional CT, and will be presented in detail later in this chapter. Although CT angiography research is in its infancy, the initial results are promising when compared to current invasive and noninvasive techniques.

TABLE 2-1 Protocol for CT angiography of the carotid bifurcation

Scan Mode	Helical
Gantry Angulation	None
Scan Parameters[a]	120 kVp, 280 mA, 1 sec scan
Field of view	15 cm
Pitch	1:1
Collimation[b]	3 mm
Number of axial images[c]	60 (may be less)
Area of interest	C6–7 to skull base
Patient instructions	Quiet breathing, no swallowing
Contrast	Nonionic, 300 mgI/mL
Amount	75 mL
Route	Intravenous via antecubital vein
Rate	2 mL/sec
Scan delay[d]	25 sec
Reconstruction Algorithm	Standard
Images Used For Rendering	Overlapping—1 mm spacing
Threshold for 3-D Rendering	100 Hounsfield units
3-D Display Modes	Shaded-surface, MIP

[a]Scan parameters will vary with different devices. Lowering of mA may reduce source image quality
[b]Alternative is to use two mm collimation at pitch ratio of 1.5:1
[c]If duration of helix is limited, carefully position at level of bifurcation using noncontrast localizing scans
[d]Scan delay may vary. Alternative is to perform test injection

TABLE 2-2 Protocol for CT angiography of the circle of Willis

Scan Mode	Helical
Gantry Angulation	None
Scan Parameters[a]	120 kVp, 280 mA, 1 sec
Field of view	12–13 cm
Pitch	1:1
Collimation	1 mm
Number of axial images[b]	60 (may be less)
Area of interest	Foramen magnum to midskull
Patient instructions	Quiet breathing, no swallowing
Contrast	Nonionic, 300 mgI/mL
Amount	100 mL
Route	Intravenous via antecubital vein
Rate	2 mL/sec
Scan delay	20 sec
Reconstruction Algorithm	Standard
Images Used For Rendering	nonoverlapping—1 mm spacing[c]
Threshold for 3-D Rendering	100 Hounsfield units
3-D Display Modes	Shaded-surface, MIP

[a] Scan parameters will vary with different devices. Lowering of mA may reduce source image quality
[b] If duration of helix is limited, carefully position at level of circle of Willis using noncontrast localizing scans. Minimum of 40 sec exposure is necessary to assure adequate coverage
[c] Overlapping .5 mm if available

CT ANGIOGRAPHY OF THE CAROTID BIFURCATION

The history of CT evaluation of the carotid bifurcation is surprisingly long. As early as 1982, Riles et al.[11] described rapid scanning techniques in suspected occlusion of the internal carotid artery. In this report, the authors were able to establish patency of this vessel contradicting the findings of catheter angiography. Then in 1984, Heinz et al.[12,13] described a small series of patients studied with thin-section CT after bolus infusion. They were able to detect atheromas and ulcers, and were the first to use computer-aided reconstructions in this area.

The premise of CT angiography is quite simple: The scan must be acquired through an area of interest with sufficient speed so as to capture the data in the desired vascular phase. Most, if not all, of the recent efforts in this regard have concentrated on arterial anatomy in an attempt to obviate invasive conventional angiography. This is done by administering an intravenous bolus of contrast to the patient and delaying the onset of scanning until the expected time of arterial opacification in the area of interest. The data set from the axial source images can then be reconstructed by a variety of different techniques, usually in an attempt to develop a three-dimensional model of the vasculature. The appeal of CT angiography is the ability to construct an accurate three-dimensional model that can be viewed from an infinite number of vantage points. This is done on modern scanners in about a minute of scan time, and is minimally invasive.

Indications, Scanning Technique, and 3-D Rendering Methodology

The major indication for carotid CTA is evaluation of patients with suspected carotid artery stenosis.[5,7,8,10] The protocol used for CT angiography of the carotid bifurcation at our institution is summarized in Table 2-1. Three millimeter collimation is used in order to completely cover the region of the bifurcation in a timely fashion. This allows for a maximum length of 18 cm of tissue in the z-axis. With the extended helical capability on the GE HiSpeed, 60 sections may be performed. This is more than adequate in most cases. For scanners limited to shorter exposures, noncontrast sections should be performed to localize the bifurcation, and the subsequent helical study should be limited just to that area. The starting point is chosen empirically; most bifurcations will be above the C6-7 level.[5] Starting lower in the neck would provide a margin of safety so that a low bifurcation would not be missed. It is impossible for most patients to hold their breath for 60 seconds, but quiet breathing without swallowing provides satisfactory images.

We prefer the use of nonionic contrast to reduce nausea which may introduce motion artifact and render the study useless or inaccurate. A 300 mgI/mL concentration is used. Contrast is injected at a rate of 2 mL/sec for a total of 75 mL. Parameters that will affect contrast delivery to the area of interest are quite complex and vary from patient to patient.[14] The delay between initiation of the contrast injection and scanning shown in Table 2-1 has worked well in the variety of patients we have studied. It is probably better to scan slightly later than optimal (risking increased venous anatomy in the reconstruction), than to scan too early. In my experience, it is usually too late to re-scan once it is discovered that the arterial bolus has been missed. In some centers, a small test bolus (20 mL) of IV contrast is given prior to performing the helical scan. Repeated nonhelical scans at the level of the carotid bifurcation are performed at one- to two-sec intervals to determine the optimal scan timing.[8] In this way a histogram of density versus time can be made over the carotid artery. The scan delay could then be customized for each patient, with scanning to start at the upslope of the curve prior to the attenuation peak. While this approach is usually not necessary, it does result in a high-quality exam.

The overlapping sections (which have been reconstructed at one mm intervals) will be downloaded to a 3-D workstation. For our work we have used the GE Windows advantage, but other workstations produce similar images. Traditional volume rendering is performed. A threshold (minimum attenuation value of pixels to be included in the model) is adjusted from case to case, but a value of 100 Hounsfield units will usually exclude all soft-tissue from the model. At this threshold, bone and calcification will be included in the volume of interest and can be removed with a variety of techniques (such as electronic scalpel lines) depending on the software used. Limiting the model to a subset volume of interest that includes only pertinent anatomy will decrease both computer memory and time requirements for model generation. However, this capability is not uniformly present in software packages that are commercially available. Once the model is postprocessed, a three-dimensional model of the isolated bifurcation will result, and can be viewed from any angle using a trackball or other similar device.

Initial Experience with CT Angiography Versus Other Techniques

The three-dimensional model convincingly demonstrates normal anatomy as well as moderate and severe stenosis (Figures 2-1–2-3). Our CTA results have shown excellent correlation with digital subtraction angiography (DSA). Recent literature regarding CT angiography of the carotid bifurcation has, with one exception, been encouraging (Table 2-3).[5,7,8,10] Agreement with comparative modalities have been as high as 92 percent for angiography and 97 percent for ultrasound.[7] Importantly, two studies have reported complete correlation in those patients with severe (greater than 70 percent) stenosis.[5,7] The North American Symptomatic Carotid Endarterectomy Trial (NASCET) has shown that symptomatic patients in this group conclusively benefit from surgery.[15] Any imaging modality that hopes to take the place of catheter angiography must be able to accurately distinguish this subgroup, as well as distinguish severe stenosis from complete occlusion.[16] CT angiography has fared well in this regard as well, with no false positives or negatives reported in three of four studies.[5,7,10] One study reported unacceptably high disagreement between CT and catheter angiography in the severe stenosis category, and a high false positive rate for occlusion.[8] Four mildly stenotic or normal carotid bifurcations were incorrectly judged to be completely occluded by CT angiography in this study. No attempt was made to explain this marked discrepancy. However, this study differs from the others in several important respects which may have affected the results: It has the smallest sample size, collimation and reconstruction slice thickness were the largest of any of the other studies, no attempt was made to eliminate calcification from the models, contrast volume delivered per patient was the smallest, source images were not evaluated, and the images were reviewed by a single examiner.

Advantages, Limitations, and Pitfalls of Carotid CTA

While we are enthusiastic about the future role of carotid CTA, there are potential limitations of which the radiologist must be aware. A major problem in the analysis of CT

(Text continues on page 40)

TABLE 2-3 Accuracy of CT angiography of the carotid bifurcation

Study	Number of patients/ bifurcations	Correlation %, modality	Patients with severe stenosis by CT and angio, (%)
Schwartz et al.,[7] 1992	20/40	92, angiography 97, ultrasound	20/20 (100)
Marks et al.,[5] 1992	14/28	89, angiography	7/7 (100)
Dillon et al.,[10] 1993	27/50	82, angiography	14/17 (82)
Castillo,[8] 1993	10/20	50, angiography	3/6 (50)

Summary of recent literature evaluating CT angiography of the carotid bifurcation. For explanation, see text.

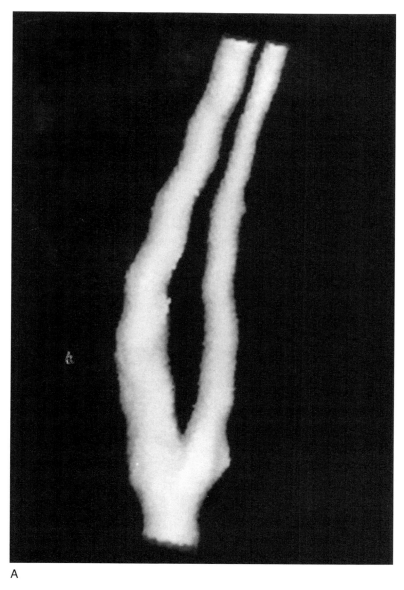

A

FIGURE 2-1A Normal CT angiograms in the same patient of the carotid bifurcations bilaterally. Separate reconstructions of the right (A) and left (C) carotid have been made and viewed in a shaded-surface display format. Digital subtraction angiograms of the right (B) and left (D) carotids for comparison. This patient was studied for left hemisphere ischemic symptoms and was found to have isolated middle cerebral atherosclerotic disease (not shown).

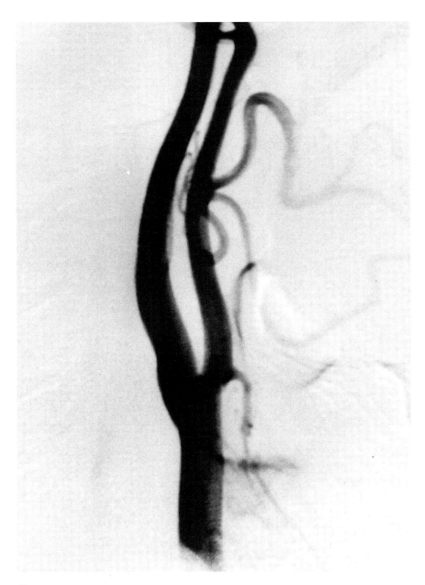

FIGURE 2-1B *(continued)*

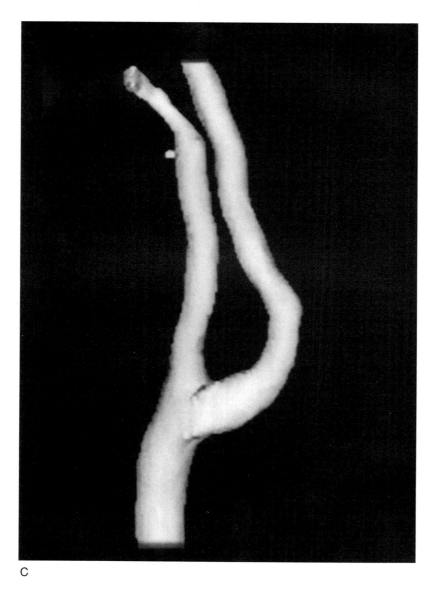

FIGURE 2-1C *(continued)*

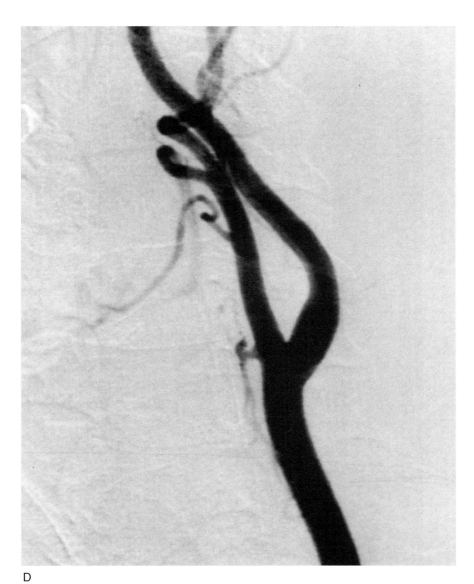

FIGURE 2-1D *(continued)*

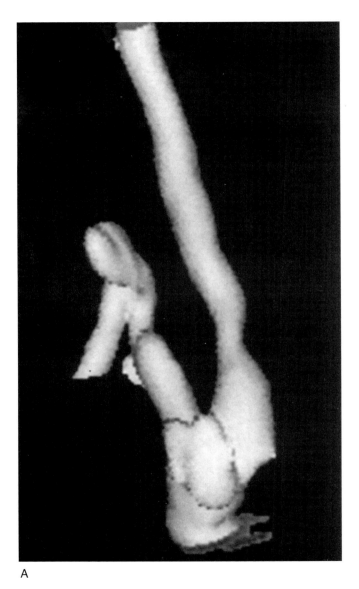

FIGURE 2-2A The CT angiogram (A) of the right carotid bifurcation showed moderate stenosis in the shaded-surface display format.

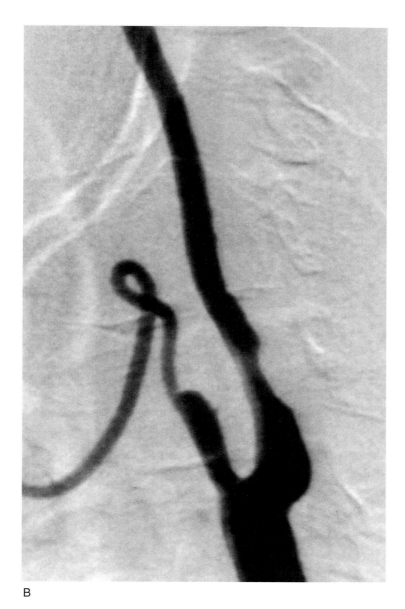

FIGURE 2-2B (B) Moderate stenosis was confirmed by catheter angiography.

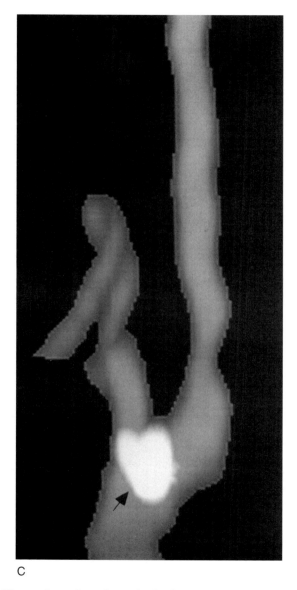

FIGURE 2-2C (C) The maximum intensity projection image (same view as A, above) can distinguish calcification (arrow) from contrast in the vessel lumen.

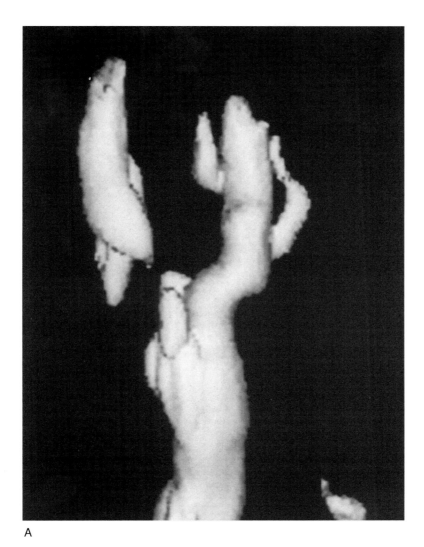

A

FIGURE 2-3A Severe stenosis of the right internal carotid artery demonstrated by both CT angiography (A) and catheter angiography (B).

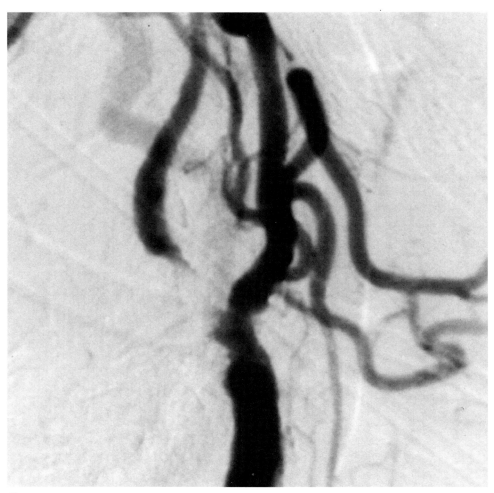

B

FIGURE 2-3B *(continued)*

angiograms results when there is calcification at the bifurcation. In the shaded display format, calcification and intraluminal contrast will be indistinguishable, as both will usually have attenuation values above the threshold setting (Figures 2-4 A, B, C). This could lead to underestimation of the degree of stenosis in these cases. Some authors have applied various additional postprocessing techniques in an attempt to specifically exclude carotid calcifications,[5,7] or have advocated using a maximum intensity projection display for analysis.[5] Both have been quite successful in eliminating this problem in most cases.

Another practical approach may be to review the source images.[5] If significant calcification is present, the shaded-surface display will be misleading and clarification is necessary. Alternatively, direct measurements from the source images can be made to include only lumen and exclude calcifications at areas of maximal narrowing (Figure 2-4 D, E).

There are some other limitations to CT angiography when compared to other current techniques. First, there is an intravenous contrast requirement with a small but finite morbidity and mortality.[17] A cooperative patient is required, as any motion can introduce artifact and give inaccurate results. In addition, it does take a significant amount of physician or technologist time to prepare the model for final analysis. Cases will vary, but 20 to 30 minutes may be necessary to sufficiently remove nonpertinent anatomy from the model and to take measurements. Very often the carotid bifurcation is closely applied to the jugular vein. Even with short scan times and small postinjection delays, some venous anatomy will appear on the reconstruction. This has the potential to conceal significant pathology if postprocessing techniques cannot adequately remove the jugular vein from the model. In the vast majority of cases, however, careful use of electronic scalpel lines can effectively isolate the carotid. In any case, review of source images will be helpful in this regard.

CT angiography is presently limited in that the intracranial circulation cannot be simultaneously evaluated for other lesions that may effect treatment, unlike conventional angiography.[16] Vessel resolution, likewise, does not yet approach conventional angiography. Beam-hardening artifact from dental work can significantly degrade models high in the neck, although this has not affected the carotid bifurcation in my experience. As in all modalities, there will be interobserver variablility in terms of both interpretation and postprocessing of the models. While standardized, technologist-generated views of these models can be made, I advise the radiologist to take as active a role as possible. Full and careful review of source images, while sometimes tedious, can provide essential information that can be lost on postprocessed images.

CT angiography has many desirable qualities as well. Data aquisition is very rapid, taking a minute or less. The potential for scanning sick or claustophobic patients is therefore improved. Current MR angiography (MRA) protocols do not approach this speed,[18] and CT angiography is not affected by turbulent flow which can overestimate stenosis measurements with MRA.[19] Similarly, limitations on patient selection imposed by MR imaging (such as cardiac pacemakers, etc.) are not present with CT angiography. Although present experience is limited, data on sensitivity and specificity is encouraging, particularly in the diagnosis of severe (surgical) stenosis as discussed above. Conventional angiography is relatively slow, invasive, and provides a limited number of views for analysis. With CT angiography, the bifurcation can be viewed from any angle and in cross-section, making the likelihood of true stenosis measurements made intuitively more likely. Aside from three-dimensional renderings, helical data is particularly suited for multiplanar reconstructions. We have used such capability in the diagnosis of bilateral vertebral artery dissection (Figure 2-5). Subjectively, the images generated are esthetically pleasing and easy to understand.

(Text continues on page 48)

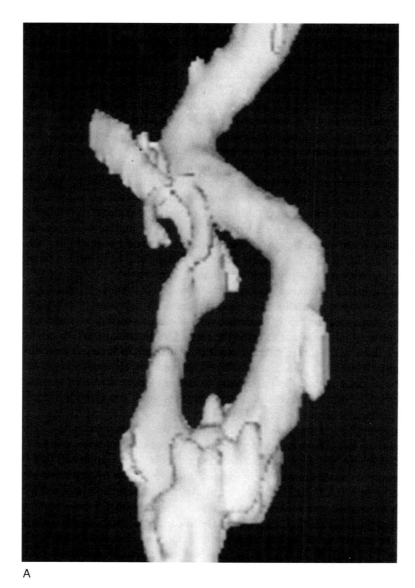

FIGURE 2-4A The shaded-surface display CT angiogram (A) can underestimate stenosis when significant calcification is present.

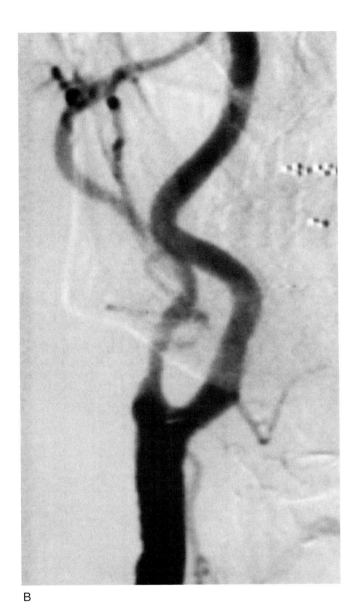

FIGURE 2-4B DSA, common carotid injection, for comparison.

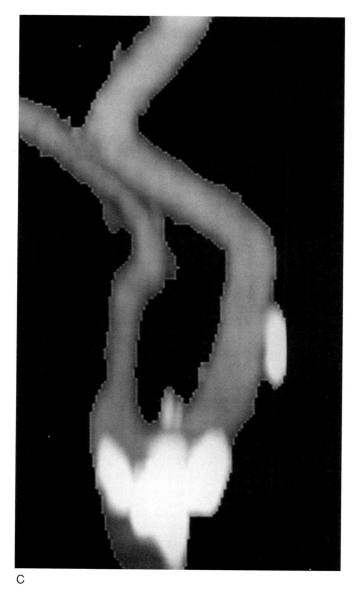

C

FIGURE 2-4C The maximum intensity projection format (C) allows differentiation between calcification and intraluminal contrast. In this patient calcification is quite extensive, making accurate measurements of luminal diameter impossible.

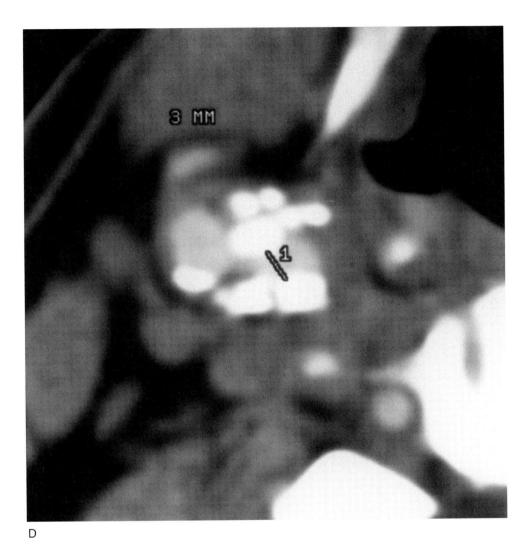

D

FIGURE 2-4D In these cases, direct measurements of lumen diameter can be made directly from the axial source images at the site of maximal narrowing (D) and at the more normal appearing cervical internal carotid higher in the neck (E).

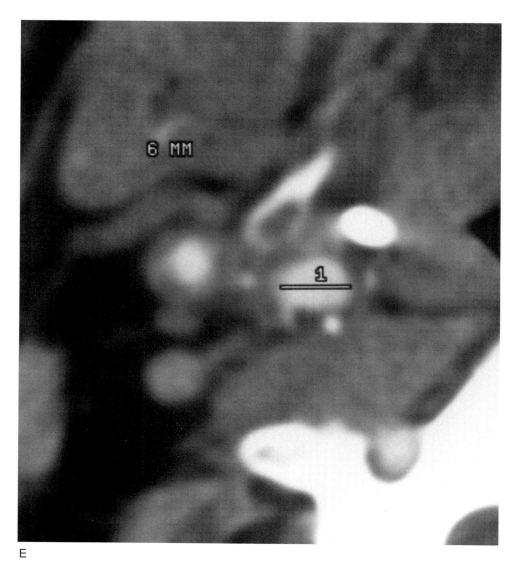

FIGURE 2-4E *(continued)*

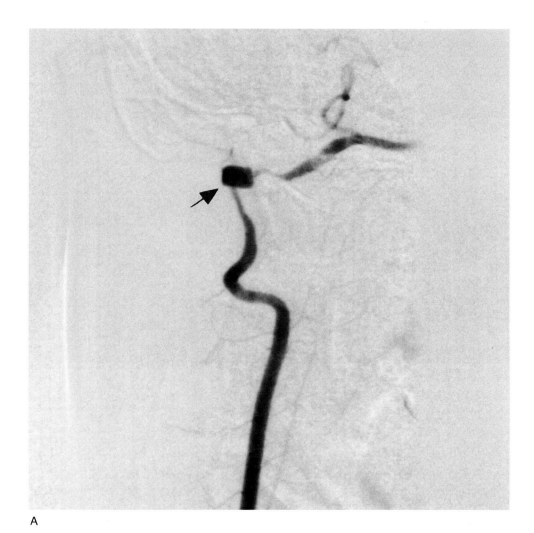

A

FIGURE 2-5A Bilateral verterbral artery dissection demonstrated by DSA and helical CT. The protocal used was as in Table 2-1. This young woman had the sudden onset of a lateral medullary syndrome after a hyperextension neck injury. (A) DSA, right vertebral artery injection showing narrowing of the vertebral artery as well as pseudoaneurysm formation (arrow).

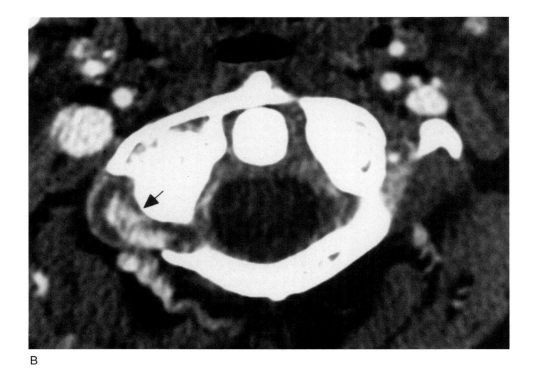
B

FIGURE 2-5B Helical CT image, axial plane, after bolus infusion. The focal expansion of the vessel lumen is well demonstrated (arrow).

There is, therefore, great enthusiasm and acceptance for carotid CTA from clinical collegues at our institution. It is certain that as interest in this field grows, further advances in both hardware and software will be made. It will perhaps soon be possible to evaluate both the extra- and intracranial circulations with a single bolus of intravenous contrast. Further work is necessary to see if CT angiography can supplant and/or augment currently accepted imaging strategies for screening and definitive diagnosis.

CT ANGIOGRAPHY OF THE INTRACRANIAL CIRCULATION

The visualization of aneurysms and other vascular pathology by CT scanning is not a new concept.[20–22] The application of computer-assisted three-dimensional modeling of vascular anatomy with CT scanning is a more recent development.[23,24] All commonly encountered

(Text continues on page 50)

Chapter 2 Head, Neck, and Spine   49

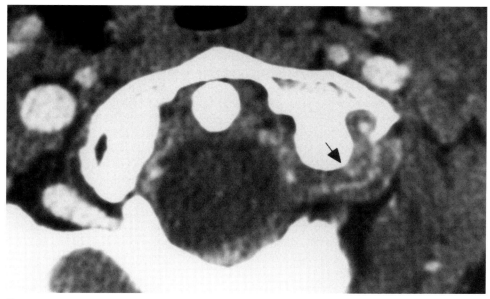

C

FIGURE 2-5C Same as B, slightly more caudal. The left vertebral artery has a narrowed lumen and a thickened wall as it enters the foramen magnum (arrow). Dissection of this vessel was confirmed by DSA (not shown).

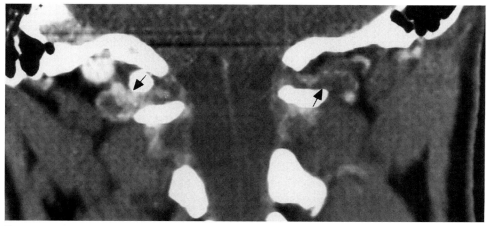

D

FIGURE 2-5D Coronal reconstruction image shows the pseudoaneurysm (arrow, patient's right) and the dissected left vertebral (arrow, patient's left).

types of vascular abnormalities have well-described CT and MR characteristics. The short acquisition times of helical scanning have allowed the "capture" of an intravenous bolus as it passes through the arterial circulation. This, coupled with the superior three-dimensional qualities of helically acquired images, allows for highly detailed models of small vascular structures such as the circle of Willis and the remainder of the intracranial circulation. Abnormalities that have been demonstrated with catheter angiogram correlation include berry aneurysms (in the setting of acute subarachnoid hemorrhage and for screening), complications of subarachnoid hemorrhage, intracranial occlusive disease, and arteriovenous malformations. CT angiography in these areas may provide a rapid, minimally invasive technique to give critically needed information in patients who are often clinically tenuous. Catheter angiography could conceivably be avoided, at least in selected cases. The advantages and pitfalls of the use of CT angiography in these indications will be addressed below.

A diagram reviewing the anatomy of the circle of Willis, its vascular segments, and the vertebrobasilar system is shown in Figure 2-6. The reader should be reminded that the balanced and symmetric appearance which is demonstrated is the exception rather than the rule. Variation, atresia, or hypoplasia of a portion of the vascular ring will be present in roughly 80 percent of adults.[25]

Circle of Willis: Indications, Scanning Technique, and 3-D Rendering Methodology

The major indication for CTA of the circle of Willis is subarachnoid or intracranial hemorrhage. The patients are usually critically ill and clinically unstable. The timely diagnosis of the etiology of bleeding is essential for planning early surgery or other intervention.

The technique used for CT angiography of the circle of Willis at our institution is given in Table 2-2. Several comments are in order when comparing this protocol to that of the carotid bifurcation (Table 2-1). The field of view has been decreased slightly to 12 to 13 cm as this will easily encompass the skull base while reducing the amount of nonpertinent anatomy that would require additional postprocessing for removal after model generation. Pitch remains constant at 1:1, however the collimation has been reduced to one mm. With 60 slice capability, this represents adequate z-axis coverage, from about the foramen magnum to the mid-Sylvian fissure in most patients. By narrowing the collimation and limiting the z-axis covered to only what is critical, partial volume averaging can be reduced. Conscious patients are asked to breathe quietly and to refrain from swallowing during the acquisition (60 sec). Unconscious patients are placed in a head-holder for the scan.

Contrast considerations again center on reducing patient discomfort which could cause unwanted motion, therefore nonionic contrast is used. We use slightly more contrast (100 mL) as compared to the carotid study, but the rate has remained the same. The volume and rate of contrast injection was empirically chosen, but subsequently confirmed as optimal in the setting of CT angiographic evaluation of patients with acute subarachnoid hemorrhage (see below). In these patients, the room for error is nil and it is thought better

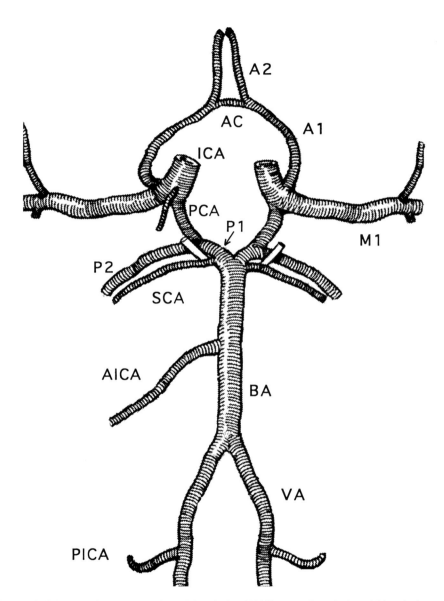

FIGURE 2-6 Schematic representation of the circle of Willis, seen from below. Abbreviations: A2 = A2 segment anterior cerebral artery (ACA), A1 = A1 segment of ACA, AC = anterior communicator, ICA = internal carotid artery, M1 = M1 segment middle cerebral artery, P1 = P1 segment posterior cerebral artery (PCA), P2 = P2 segment of PCA, SCA = superior cerebellar artery, BA = basilar artery, AICA = anterior inferior cerebellar artery, VA = vertebral artery, PICA = posterior inferior cerebellar artery.

to err on the side of administering too much rather than too little contrast for visualization of potential aneurysms. Scan delays of 20 sec from the onset of contrast injection seem to work well in the patients we have studied.

The model is made directly from the axial source images rather than retrospective images as in the carotid studies. Our current version of software does not allow for overlapping images to be generated at spacing of less than one mm (the thickness of the actual collimation used). Therefore, no increased z-axis resolution is to be expected on the model by retrospective imaging. Other sites using the HiSpeed scanner with newer software reconstruct overlapping scans at one-half mm spacing. This should be advantageous, and result in even better-appearing models than those built without overlapping reconstruction. Preliminary evaluation of the model is done in a shaded-surface display format, although maximum intensity projection (MIP) displays can also be examined. Axial source images are also reviewed for every case to confirm or disprove suspected abnormalities. Model generation times are on the order of one to two minutes, and are therefore suitable for the evaluation of critically ill patients. Several minutes are required to reconstruct the source images after they are acquired, a step necessary prior to model generation. The total time required from the onset of the acquisition to a completed model is approximately five minutes.

Once the model is generated, review can take place. We routinely examine these studies using a shaded-surface display. With this type of model, structures appear as surfaces of solid objects as if illuminated from a point source. Using a trackball or other similar device, the model is slowly rotated in space. Actively rotating the vessels in real-time on an interactive display appears to be helpful in seeing small aneurysms at vascular branch points. We have found that scrupulous exclusion on nonpertinent anatomy (such as the bone of the skull base) can be tedious and is frequently unnecessary. The removal of the deep venous system, pineal calcifications, and occiput will nearly always be necessary for unobscured views of the posterior fossa.

Circle of Willis: Model Interpretation and Experience in Patients with Acute Subarachnoid Hemorrhage

Vascular resolution in the posterior fossa has been excellent, presumably because the thin collimation used reduces beam-hardening artifact. For an aneurysm search, particular attention is paid to common sites of aneurysm location, such as the anterior/posterior communicators and the MCA trifurcation. These areas can be selectively magnified and rotated from different viewing angles as needed. The circle of Willis can be clearly seen in virtually all patients; most branches will be identified extending peripherally at least two to three cm from their origin (Figures 2-7, 2-8).

The major use of CT angiography at our institution has been for the evaluation of patients with acute subarachnoid hemorrhage (SAH). In this clinical setting, patients are initially evaluated by unenhanced CT scanning or lumbar puncture. The currently

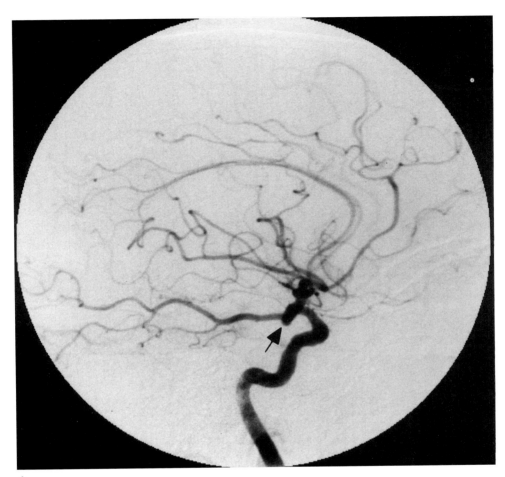

A

FIGURE 7A Small supraclinoid internal carotid artery aneurysm seen by CT angiography and DSA. This is one case in which CT angiography was judged subjectively better than DSA for aneurysm characterization due to the ability to examine the model from any angle.[31] The right internal carotid artery injection DSA, lateral view, (A), demonstrates the small aneurysm (arrow). The neck, however, is partially obscured by the posterior communicating artery. PA and oblique views (not shown) could not separate the two structures.

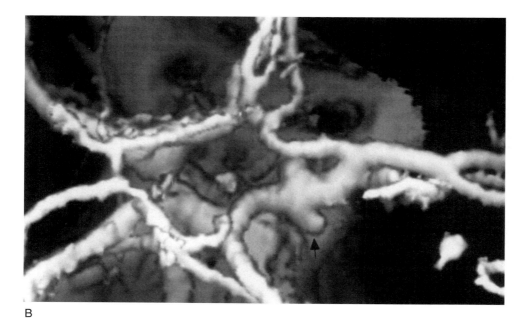

FIGURE 2-7B CT angiogram, shaded-surface display, seen from above, behind, and slightly to the patient's right. The small aneurysm is clearly visible arising from the supraclinoid internal carotid (arrow). Without further angiography, this patient's aneurysm was successfully clipped.

accepted approach to the patient with acute SAH is emergent catheter angiography to detect or exclude berry aneurysm.[26] Before discussing the results of CTA, it is important to recognize that there are many clinically significant questions that catheter angiography may answer in the patient with SAH. In order to be a viable screening technique in this setting, CTA must be able to answer many of these same questions.

Surgically important information obtained from conventional catheter angiography includes presence/absence of additional aneurysms, size, characteristics of the aneurysm neck, the direction of pointing of the aneurysm, the presence of vasospasm, and the patency of adjacent segments of the circle of Willis. In the cases where multiple aneurysms are present, some determination must be made as to which one was the source of bleeding. The pattern of hemorrhage as seen on the noncontrast CT scan can influence the angiographic approach.[27] For example, subarachnoid blood confined to the cistern of the lamina terminalis is very likely to have come from a ruptured anterior communicator. In addition, blood confined to the perimesencephalic cistern is often associated with negative catheter studies for aneurysm.[28]

Catheter angiography is known to be highly accurate in the detection of aneurysms, and is considered the gold standard in this clinical setting. Once a source of bleeding is identified,

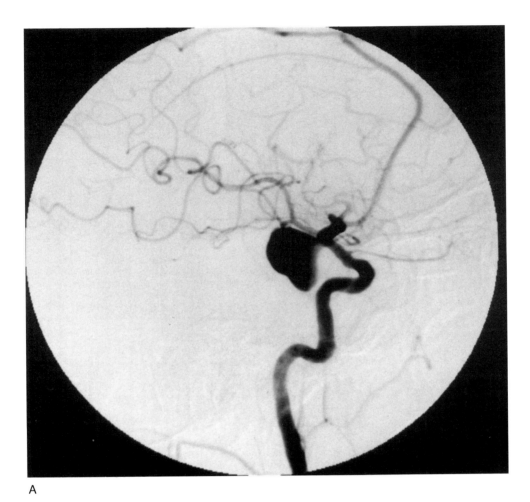

A

FIGURE 2-8A Large posterior communicating artery aneurysm seen with CT angiography and DSA. (A) DSA, right internal carotid artery injection, lateral view which confirms the aneurysm.

usually the patient has surgery as early as is clinically feasible. Approximately 85 percent of patients will have a berry aneurysm as a source of hemorrhage.[26] A small percentage of patients will have an arteriovenous malformation or other vascular anomaly. About 15 percent of patients will have high-quality catheter angiography and no source of bleeding will be found. Repeat angiography in these patients will usually not demonstrate a cause which was missed on the initial examination.[26]

After aneurysm clipping, repeat angiography to confirm adequate clip placement is not usually routinely done. Exceptions to this practice will occur when placement of the clip

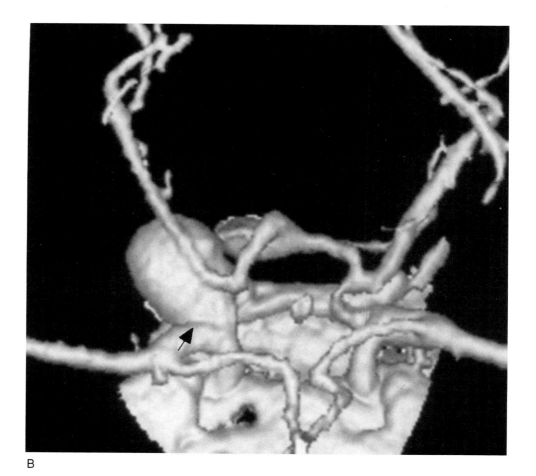

B

FIGURE 2-8B CT angiogram, shaded-surface display, viewed from above and in front demonstrates the large aneurysm seen to involve the posterior communicator (arrow).

was particularly difficult. In these cases, multiple unusual projections may have to be done in order that the residual neck of the aneurysm is not obscured by the clip.[26] Repeat angiography may also be necessary for the diagnosis of vasospasm after clip placement. It is recommended that MR evaluation in patients with aneurysm clips be avoided if at all possible.[29] This is in light of a recent report of a patient death when scanning after clip placement was done, even after a careful attempt to document the type of clip present was made.[30]

Preliminary work with CT angiography suggests that much of the information that previously could be supplied by catheter angiography alone could be given by CT angiography

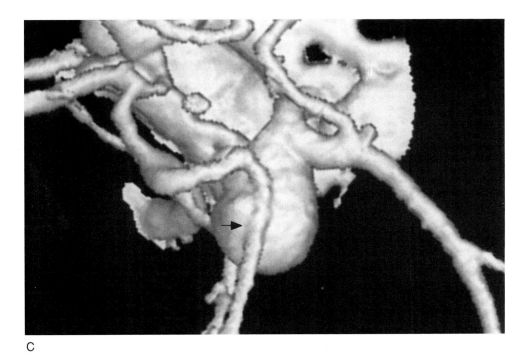

C

FIGURE 2-8C CT angiogram, shaded-surface display, viewed from above, behind, and to the patient's right. Note the relationship to the posterior cerebral artery (arrow) which is draped over the aneurysm. This relationship was not fully appreciated on DSA as the posterior cerebral artery does not fill on the internal carotid injection, nor did the aneurysm fill on the vertebral artery injection (not shown). This is another case where CT angiography was thought superior to DSA in depicting surrounding anatomy.[31] This is by virtue of simultaneous filling of all segments of the circle of Willis.

in the clinical setting of SAH. If this is the case, this would be a significant step forward in the care of these patients. The time required to establish the diagnosis, as well as complications of catheter angiography could both be decreased.

Since CT angiography offers the possibility of rapid, noninvasive detection of aneurysms, Vieco et al.[31] compared a series of patients with acute SAH with CT angiography and DSA. Fifteen consecutive patients with SAH documented by unenhanced CT and/or spinal tap were studied by both techniques. In all cases, patients presented to the emergency room with a clinical history which warranted unenhanced CT scanning or lumbar puncture to exclude recent SAH. Once the diagnosis was confirmed, CT angiography was done, in most cases without removing the patient from the scanner. All patients had CT angiography and DSA performed within four hours; in all cases the CT angiogram was performed first. The technique employed for CT angiography was the same as in Table 2-2. However, several patients were studied with only 30 helical images as this was the maximum available prior to our current 60 slice capability. In these cases scanning was started at the level of the sellar floor; therefore the posterior fossa was not fully evaluated in these patients. Catheter angiography (DSA) was done using a 1024 × 1024 matrix with selective internal or vertebral injections. At least two views were done for each injection; oblique views to better visualize the anterior communicator were also done in each case. The CT angiograms and the DSA studies were reviewed together for vascular segments of the circle of Willis detected, presence of aneurysms, aneurysm size, aneurysm location, and aneurysm relationship to surrounding anatomy. Some of the findings are summarized in Tables 2-4–2-7.

CT angiography was able to detect nearly all vascular segments present on the corresponding DSA study (Table 2-4). The discrepancies were found in the identification of one atretic A1 segment of the anterior cerebral artery and three atretic posterior communicating arteries in separate patients. These observations were made in review of the shaded-surface display models. Vessels of these very small diameters may be mathematically excluded from the model when it is generated. Such anatomy is below the resolving capability of this technique of model generation at the present time. When the source images were reviewed, however, all of these segments were found to be present as in the DSA. Numbers of aneurysms detected with DSA were the same as with CT angiography (Table 2-5). A variety of aneurysm locations were present; the anatomic sites found were identical for both techniques (Table 2-6). Aneurysm size measurements also correlated well (Table 2-7).

Aside from these parameters, a subjective judgement was made as to which technique better demonstrated the aneurysm's relationship to surrounding vascular anatomy. CT angiography was found equivalent to DSA in 11 cases, better than DSA in three cases, and inferior to DSA in none. This was felt to be due to the three-dimensional nature of the display and the ability to view the aneurysm from any angle (Figure 2-7). Vascular relationships are also better seen on CTA because CT angiography opacifies the entire circle of Willis simultaneously (Figure 2-8). This latter feature can be particularly helpful when an aneursym is closely related to multiple segments of the circle of Willis, all of which rarely fill on a single catheter injection. This small series suggests that CT angiography may have a role in the preoperative diagnosis of intracranial aneurysms in patients with acute SAH.[31]

CT Angiography and Complications of Subarachnoid Hemorrhage

Rapid and accurate detection of aneurysms is not the only imaging concern in the patient with recent subarachnoid hemorrhage. The detection and management of vasospasm is of great importance. Onset of spasm typically occurs 4 to 11 days after hemorrhage in approximately 30 percent of patients. Vasospasm is responsible for about half of the deaths and disabilities in this subgroup.[32] Current therapy includes hypervolemic and pharmacologic therapy and its efficacy is well documented.[32] Recent advances in angioplasty techniques have led to improved outcome after such procedures,[33] and are generally

TABLE 2-4 Segments visualized by CTA vs. DSA

	CT Angiography	DSA
A1	29	30
A2	30	30
A Comm	14	14
M1	30	30
M2	30	30
P1	30	30
P2	30	30
P Comm	24	27

Comparison of vascular segments of the circle of Willis detected with CT angiography and DSA in a series of patients with acute subarachnoid hemorrhage.[31] Abbreviations: A1 = A1 segment of anterior cerebral artery (ACA), A2 = A2 segment of ACA, A Comm = anterior communicating artery, M1 = M1 segment of middle cerebral artery (MCA), M2 = M2 segment of (MCA), P1 = P1 segment of posterior cerebral artery (PCA), P2 = P2 segment of (PCA), P Comm = posterior communicating artery. Three posterior communicating arteries were not found with either technique.

reserved for patients who have not responded to conventional therapy. Current means of detection (aside from CT evidence of frank infarction) is limited to catheter angiography and, more recently, transcranial Doppler evaluation. The latter technique, while noninvasive, is dependent on flow velocity measurements rather than direct visualization of arterial anatomy. Doppler measurements are currently confined to the distal internal carotid, proximal middle and anterior circulations, and a limited evaluation of the posterior fossa. A complete examination requires transtemporal, bilateral transocular, and transoccipital views.[34] The middle cerebral artery is usually readily identified, but the anterior and posterior cerebral arteries can frequently be missed.[35] The technique is also limited in the presence or absence of vasospasm based solely on the basis of flow velocities and can lead to false negative results.[36] MR angiography will be restricted in the evaluation of these patients due to the presence of aneurysm clips and time constraints.

Preliminary work with CT angiography suggests that vasospasm can be seen with this technique. Several patients have been studied with both CT angiography and DSA at our

TABLE 2-5 Aneurysms detected with CTA vs. DSA

	CT Angiography	DSA
Aneurysms	14	14
Patients	11	11

Number of aneurysms detected with CT angiography and DSA in 15 consecutive patients with acute subarachnoid hemorrhage.[31] Four patients had no cause for hemorrhage found on either technique.

TABLE 2-6 Aneurysm location: CTA vs. DSA

	CT Angiography	DSA
A Comm	3	3
P Comm	6	6
MCA	2	2
PICA	1	1
PCA	1	1
Basilar tip	1	1

Comparison of aneurysm location between CT angiography and DSA in 15 consecutive patients with acute subarachnoid hemorrhage.[31]

institution, with good correlation. Findings of vasospasm were convincingly seen, even in the posterior fossa and in patients with aneurysm clips (see below). Aside from poor visualization of arterial segments seen previously, the axial source images can be particularly revealing, demonstrating not only the narrowed lumen but also the vessel wall (Figure 2-9). The latter may prove to be particularly important in the distinction between spasm and dissection (see Figure 2-5). Clearly, CT angiography has potential as a viable noninvasive imaging modality in these patients. Such a technique could prove useful for the detection of vasospasm as well as response to therapy. We have recently started to examine patients with suspected vasospasm with CT angiography in an attempt to correlate findings with DSA and transcranial Doppler. Once an aneurysm is identified and clipped, questions may arise as to the proper placement of the clip. The principle is to occlude the neck while leaving related vessels patent. The aneurysm is thereby isolated from the remainder of the circulation and risk of hemorrhage eliminated. One potential problem is to only partially clip the neck and allow continued filling of the aneurysm. Another is to inadvertently occlude vital vessels after improper placement. We have had the opportunity to use CT angiography in order to clarify such dilemmas. Remarkably, CT angiography is not severely degraded by the presence of nearby aneurysm clips.

TABLE 2-7 Aneurysm size: CTA vs. DSA

	CT Angiography	DSA
2–4 mm	10	10
5–7 mm	3	3
> 7 mm	1	1

Comparison of aneurysm size measurements between CT angiography and DSA in 15 consecutive patients with acute subarachnoid hemorrhage.[31]

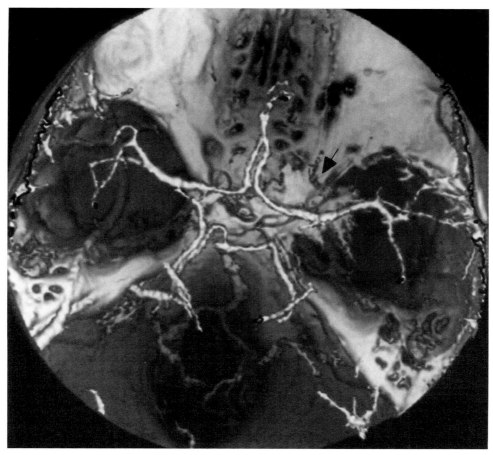

A

FIGURE 2-9A Vasospasm identified on CT angiography and DSA. This patient was initially studied for the evaluation of subarachnoid hemorrhage. (A) CT angiogram, shaded-surface display, viewed from above and behind showed no evidence of aneurysm. A starlike artifact (arrow) is seen arising from an old clip at the right posterior communicating artery.

I attribute this to the very thin collimation used (one mm) which seems to limit the severe beam-hardening artifacts seen in routine head studies. Depending on the size and orientation of the clip, a starshaped artifact in the immediate vicinity of the clip is seen in the x- and y-axes in the shaded-surface display. Often, quite a bit of detail of the clip itself can be seen. We have been able to demonstrate both residual aneurysm after clipping (Figure 2-10) as well as patency of vessels thought compromised by clip placement

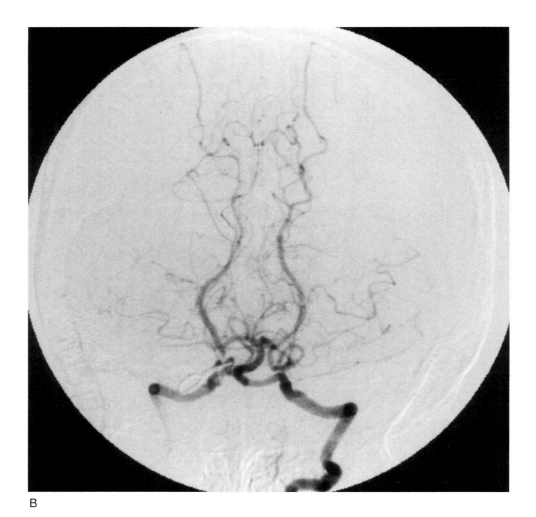

B

FIGURE 2-9B DSA, left vetebral artery injection, PA view was negative. No aneurysm was found with either technique. Ten days later, the patient clinically had vasospasm and was restudied with both techniques.

(Figure 2-11) despite this artifact. In the latter patient, transcranial Doppler was ineffective because of a large amount of postoperative air under the craniotomy flap. The expense and risk of catheter angiography was avoided in these two patients. Further work for advancement in this area could focus on further reduction of artifact and correlative studies with DSA.

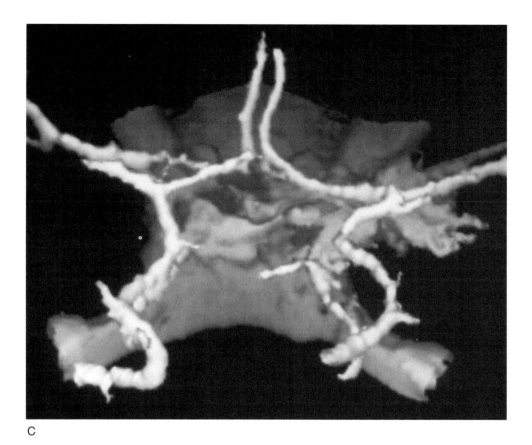

C

FIGURE 2-9C The CT angiogram, similar projection as (A), showed poor visualization of the vertebrobasilar system and the posterior cerebral arteries.

CT Angiography as an Aneurysm Screening Technique in the Absence of SAH

A frequent problem in clinical practice is screening for intracranial aneurysm. Often a patient will have signs or symptoms suggestive of the diagnosis without evidence of subarachnoid hemorrhage. In others there is a family history of the disease and the patient, though asymptomatic, is concerned that they may harbor an aneurysm as well. In these cases, the clinician is often unsure as to how to proceed. The prevalence of berry aneurysm in the general population is estimated at roughly one to two percent.[37] Should the patient be subjected to an expensive, invasive, and potentially morbid procedure (catheter angiography) to include or exclude the diagnosis, or should they simply be reassured? Most

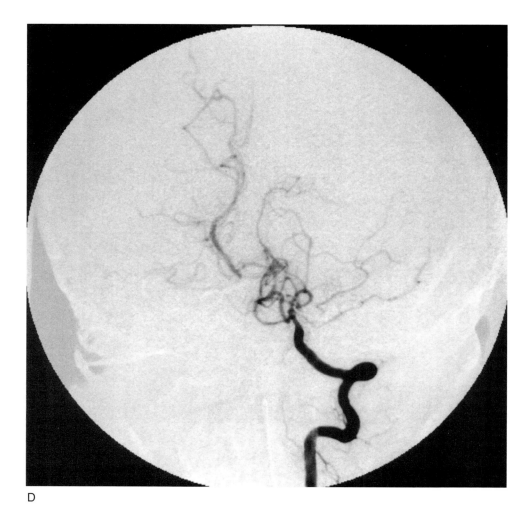

D

FIGURE 2-9D DSA vertebral artery injection, PA view shows severe vasospasm in a similar distribution.

clinicians will hesitate to order angiography on their patients due to real or imagined risks involved. Perhaps they should have routine CT scanning or MR imaging in the hopes that an aneurysm will be discovered. Does a negative conventional CT or MR study effectively exclude a small yet potentially fatal aneurysm? This is a critical question, as the mortality of a ruptured aneurysm is 50 to 60 percent while the corresponding figures for surgery to clip an unruptured aneurysm is close to 0 percent.[38] This has particular relevance in

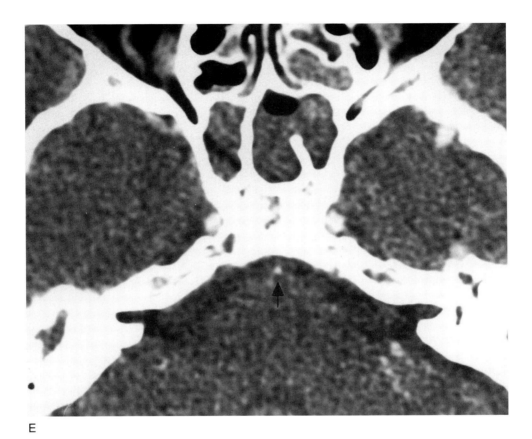

E

FIGURE 2-9E Axial source image used for the repeat CT angiogram showing the diminutive caliber of the vertebral artery secondary to spasm (arrow). The small size of these spastic vessels is below the resolution of the shaded-surface display model.

patients with conditions that have known associations with berry aneurysms such as adult polycystic kidney disease.[39] Given the presence of an aneurysm, the estimated rate of rupture is approximately one to two percent per aneurysm per year, and may be higher.[32] Until the advent of MR angiography, there was little recourse. However, the screening potential of MR angiography for intracranial aneurysm has yet to be determined, and its use, while widespread, is somewhat controversial.[40]

We have been able to use CT angiography at our institution for this purpose with encouraging preliminary results. This came about in part by necessity as MR angiography was not until recently available to us. We have detected two aneurysms in a series of seven such patients (unpublished data). All had DSA correlation soon after CT angiography with no false positive or false negative results. An example of a patient scanned for a strong

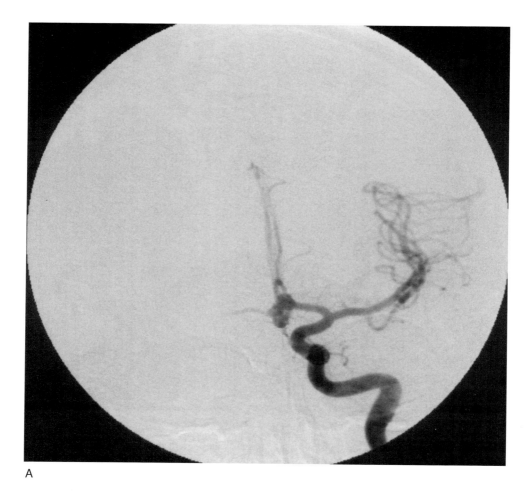

A

FIGURE 2-10A Residual aneurysm seen with CT angiography after clipping. This patient had a large bilobed anterior communicating artery aneurysm diagnosed by DSA (A) which the referring surgeon had difficulty clipping.

family history of aneurysm rupture is shown in Figure 2-12. While asymptomatic, this patient's mother was diagnosed with a ruptured aneurysm one month before. Multiple other family members had died from intracranial hemorrhage. Another patient had recent onset severe headaches with negative plain CT scan and lumbar puncture and was found to have a posterior communicating artery aneurysm. Both aneurysms were clipped in these patients and did well. In an additional case, CT angiography was able to convincingly demonstrate a suspected posterior fossa aneurysm as vertebro-basilar dolichoectasia (Figure 2-13), and

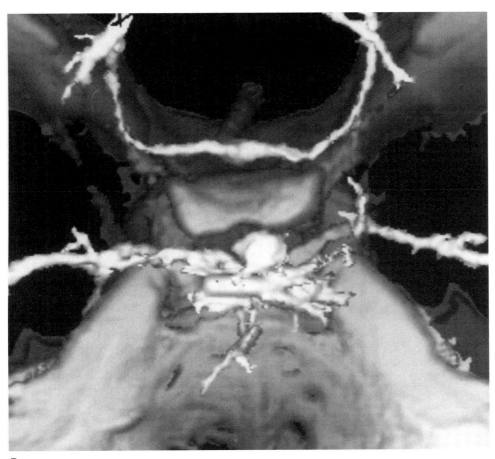

B

FIGURE 2-10B CT angiogram, shaded-surface display, viewed from above and in front shows the jaws of the aneurysm clip and the residual aneurysm sac just posteriorly. Note the minimal artifact from the clip on the model.

catheter angiography was avoided. This limited experience suggests that CT angiography may have a role in screening patients for intracranial aneurysm. Further work is needed to examine if CT angiography can replace MR angiography for screening purposes.

Other Intracranial Applications

Besides aneurysm detection and complications of subarachnoid hemorrhage, potential exists for CT angiography to reliably identify intracranial occlusive disease. An unfortunate

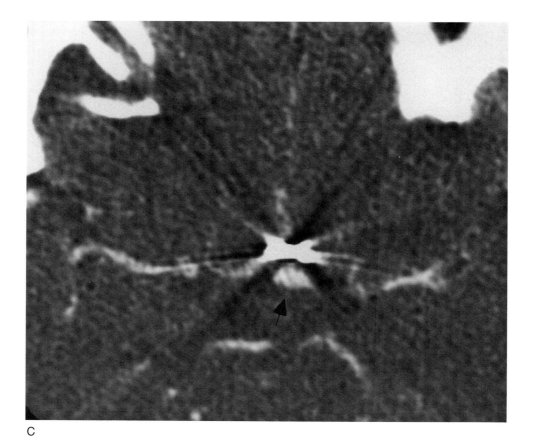

C

FIGURE 2-10C The axial source image confirms residual aneurysm (arrow). Repeat catheter angiography was avoided in this case.

anecdote in our experience is shown in Figure 2-14, a case of basilar tip thrombosis. This case underscores the risks of catheter angiography which conceivably could have been avoided. All necessary preoperative information was thought to have been given by the CT angiogram. The fatal complication was the result of conventional angiography that was used to confirm the diagnosis.

Aside from acute thrombosis, we have seen several patients in which the diagnosis of intracranial stenotic disease was made with CT angiography and confirmed with DSA. The sensitivity and specificity of such findings is not known. Further work is needed to see what role, if any, CT angiography has to play in these patients. It is doubtful that in its present form CT angiography will be able to reliably differentiate atherosclerotic disease from vasculitis, for example. However, CT angiography does seem to be able to

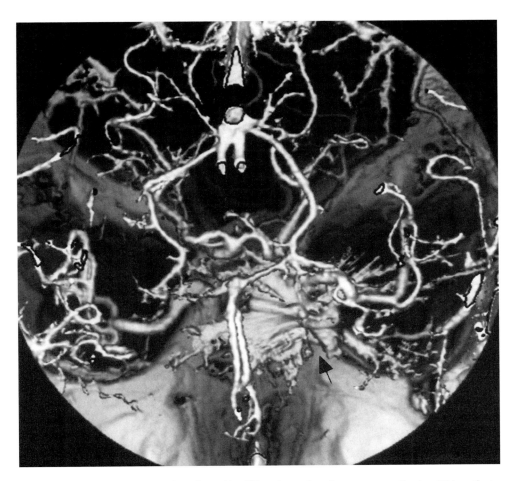

FIGURE 2-11 Patency of vessel confirmed by CT angiography after aneurysm clipping. This patient was studied after clipping of a left supraclinoid internal carotid artery aneurysm. The patient awoke from surgery aphasic and it was unclear whether postoperative edema or compromise of the middle cerebral artery (MCA) was the cause of the deficit. The CT angiogram in a shaded-surface display seen from in front and above shows some starlike artifact from the aneurysm clip (arrow). The MCA branches distal to the clip fill well; this study was interpreted as normal. Followup CT scans showed no evidence of infarction and the deficit reversed in two days. Catheter angiography was avoided in this case.

distinguish contour and occlusive abnormalities of the intracranial circulation with some fidelity (Figure 2-15).

Additional abnormalities that have been studied with CT angiography include several types of vascular malformations of the brain. One patient studied for acute subarachnoid hemorrhage was incidentally noted to have a venous angioma of the frontal lobe (Figure 2-16).

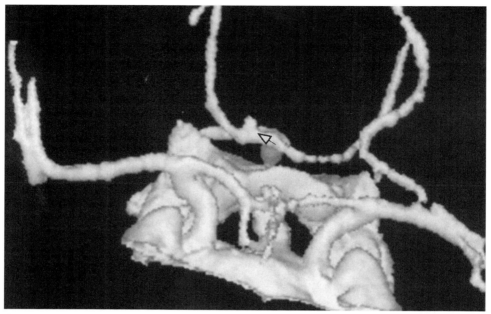

A

FIGURE 2-12A Postive screening examination for aneurysm with CT angiography with DSA correlation. This patient was studied for a strong family history of aneurysm rupture and was asymptomatic. (A) CT angiogram, shaded-surface display, viewed from above and in front demonstrates a small aneurysm arising from the P1 segment of the posterior cerebral artery on the right side (arrow).

This was diagnosed by CT angiography and confirmed with DSA. We also have studied arteriovenous malformations (Figure 2-17), and a dural AVM (Figure 2-18). In these cases, scanning the entire head is advantageous in order to identify all feeding vessels and draining veins. It was therefore necessary to appropriately modify the protocol (Table 2-8). In the latter case, the patient was studied for a large posterior fossa bleed. The CT angiogram was able to identify the venous aneurysm responsible.

Advantages, Pitfalls, and Limitations of CT Angiography of the Intracranial Circulation

The potential advantages of further refinement and use of CT angiography of the intracranial circulation are many. First and foremost is the speed of the technique. At the present time, a three-dimensional model of the circle of Willis can reliably be generated approximately five minutes after the initiation of scanning. This could have enormous impact on the management of acutely ill patients, such as those with subarachnoid hemorrhage.

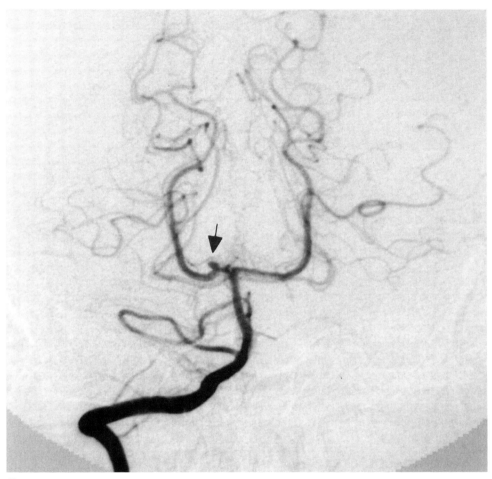

B

FIGURE 2-12B DSA, right vertebral artery injection, PA view, confirms the aneurysm (arrow). No other aneurysms were detected with either technique. The aneurysm was successfully clipped and the patient did well.

Instead of transferring the patient to the angiography suite, arranging technical support, and performing a lengthy and possibly morbid procedure, these patients can remain in the CT scanner and potentially have all the information necessary for operation in a very short period of time. MR angiography scan times do not yet approach this speed.[41] Technical advances will certainly make examination times even shorter (such as by increasing the pitch of the scans), and software refinements will also improve model generation time and

TABLE 2-8 Protocol for whole head CT angiography

Scan Mode	Helical
Gantry Angulation	None
Scan Parameters	120 kV, 280 mA, 1 sec
Field of view	20 cm
Pitch	1:1
Collimation	3 mm
Number of axial images	60 (may be less)
Area of interest	Foramen magnum to vertex
Patient instructions	Quiet breathing, no swallowing
Contrast	Nonionic, 300 mgI/mL
Amount	100 mL
Route	Intravenous via antecubital vein
Rate	2 mL/sec
Scan delay	20 sec
Reconstruction Algorithm	Standard
Images Used For Rendering	Overlapping—1 mm spacing
Threshold for 3-D Rendering	100 Hounsfield units
3-D Display Modes	Shaded-surface, MIP

fidelity. Preliminary work is limited but promising in terms of sensitivity and specificity. Much work needs to be done, particularly in the optimization of contrast delivery.

A great advatage that CT angiography has is the three-dimensional nature of the display. The radiologist can actively examine specific areas of interest on the model from any viewpoint, without exposing the patient to mulitple injections of contrast. This is done on a computer monitor in near real-time. The model can be modified in any way the examiner sees fit in order to analyze and display the findings to their best advantage. My neurosurgeon colleagues are very enthusiastic about the development of CT angiography at our institution. Aside from convenience and safety advantages for their patients, the models generated have been considered useful in operative planning.

The inclusion of venous anatomy, dicussed as a disadvantage above, can be an advantage in planning an operative approach. The surgeon can be provided with an image that will mimick the operative field if properly oriented, rather than inferring this information from the catheter angiogram. CT angiograms have also been considered a useful tool for resident teaching.

Another major step forward that CT angiography in this area could provide is a reasonable alternative to the expense and invasiveness of conventional angiography. Few clinicians would subject their patients to the risks and expense of catheter angiography if an infused CT scan of the head could provide the same diagnosis as reliably.

There can be pitfalls in the interpretation of these studies. Many of these are related to the proximity of the circle of Willis to the bony and venous anatomy of the skull base. I

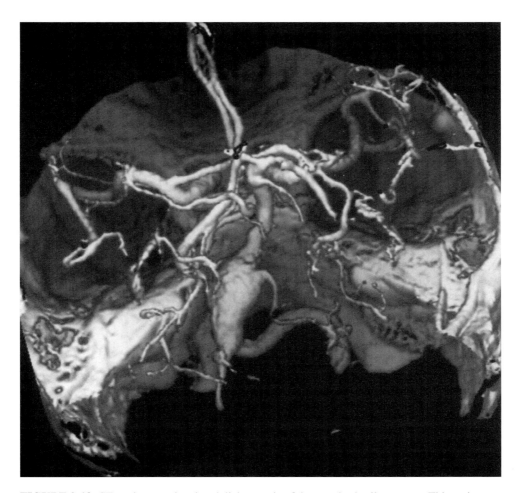

FIGURE 2-13 CT angiogram showing dolichoectasia of the vertebrobasilar system. This patient had a plain CT for the evaluation of what clinically was a brainstem transient ischemic attack. A posterior fossa aneurysm was suspected which prompted evaluation with CT angiography. On the basis of this study, the patient was thought not to represent an operative candidate. Catheter angiography was avoided in this case.

have seen quite large aneurysms difficult to appreciate on the shaded-surface display images which were immediately obvious on DSA. For example, a very common location of aneurysm rupture is from the posterior communicating artery. Because of its proximity to the cavernous sinus, it may be difficult to confidently detect on the shaded-surface display. This is because the aneurysm and the sinus will simultaneously be opacified with

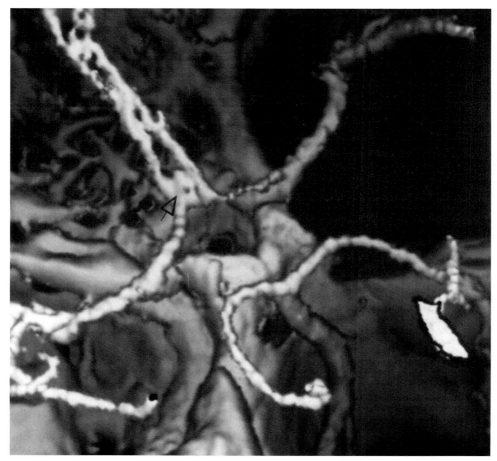

A

FIGURE 2-14A CT angiographic documentation of basilar tip thrombosis, a complication of catheter angiography. This patient presented with acute subarachnoid hemorrhage. (A) The CT angiogram demonstrated a small anterior communicating artery aneurysm (arrow) seen on this shaded-surface display from above, behind, and to the patient's left. Note the configuration of the widely patent distal basilar and the posterior cerebral arteries.

contrast, and also will be adjacent to the sphenoid bone. We have also seen one large intracavernous sinus aneurysm which was difficult to see on the shaded-surface display as it was surrounded by opacified sinus blood. All of these structures will have Hounsfield values of over 100 and therefore be included in the model as similar appearing structures. The potential also exists to miss pathology of the intrapetrous carotid as it is also surrounded

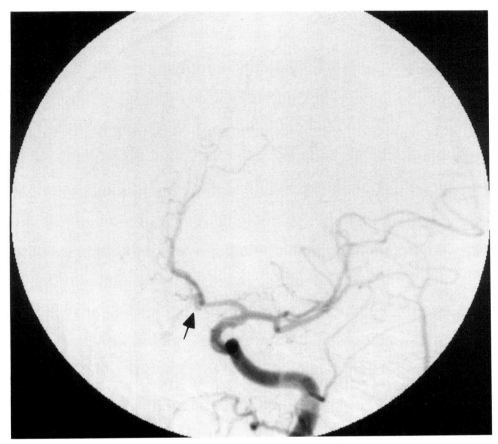

B

FIGURE 2-14B DSA, left internal carotid artery injection, oblique view, confirmed the aneurysm. A small left posterior inferior cerebellar artery aneurysm was also seen with both techniques (not shown). During vertebral catheterization, the patient suddenly became unresponsive and the catheter was immediately withdrawn.

by bone. In my experience, proper windowing of the source images will reliably differentiate bone from opacified lumen.

In an attempt to uncover pathology, a variable amount of anatomy will be lost by postprocessing such as electronic scalpel lines and threshold techniques. It is critical that a knowledgeable examiner decide on what information is to be discarded and what is to be kept for analysis. In this way, vital anatomy will not be missing for diagnosis. There is no substitute for the radiologist actively examining the model from many different

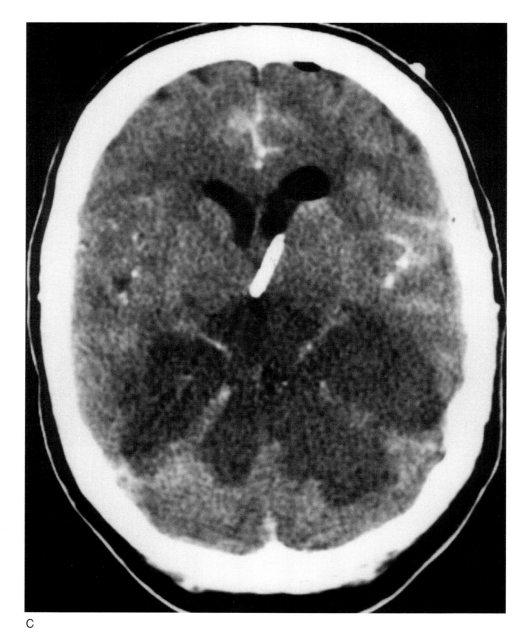

C

FIGURE 2-14C A CT scan the next day showed an infarct suggesting basilar tip thrombosis.

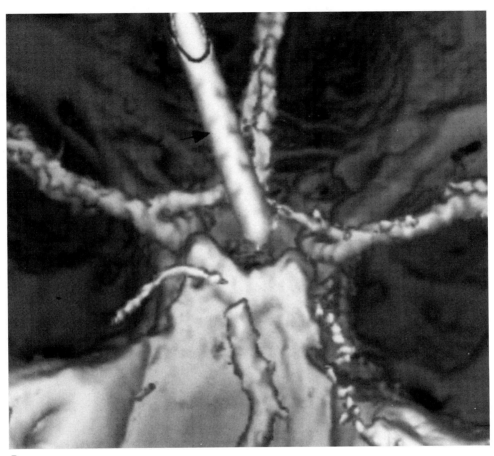

D

FIGURE 2-14D CT angiogram seen from above and behind done soon after. This showed abrupt termination of the basilar artery proximal to the tip, due to thrombus. Note also the appearance of the ventricular drain inserted in the interval (arrow). The patient died soon after.

perspectives in order to exclude or include an pathology such as an aneurysm. Often, only detailed review of the source images can provide a confident diagnosis, and this is done for every case. The importance of rigorous review of the axial source images cannot be overemphasized. It is easiest to examine each level in rapid succession at the workstation using the available interactive paging display. For these reasons, at our institution we do not rely on a routine filming protocol done by a nonradiologist as the sole source for images used for interpretation. As our position on the learning curve improves, this may become a reasonable option in the future.

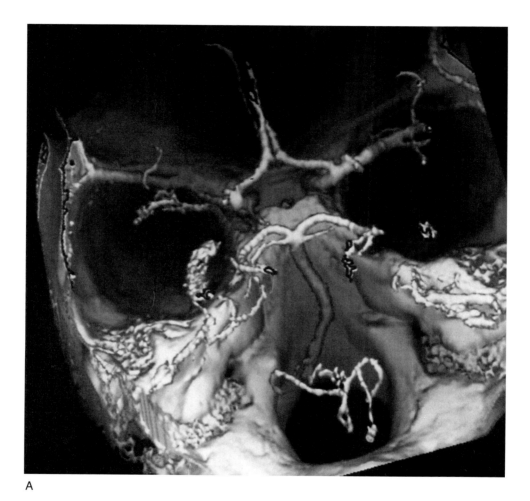

A

FIGURE 2-15A Intracranial occlusion diagnosed by CT angiography and DSA. This patient had a recent left middle cerebral artery (MCA) infarct diagnosed by plain CT scanning. (A) CT angiogram looking down from behind upon the left MCA region shows apparent discontinuity of the M1 segment of the MCA. There is also poor filling of the more distal branches in the Sylvian fissure when compared to the opposite side.

Another drawback is the inclusion of venous anatomy in the model. Even the rapid nature of the helical acquisition is not fast enough to exclude the venous phase, and at the present time there is little to be done about this. However, with time it is quite easy to identify major deep veins and either trim them away with postprocessing techniques, or simply "look around" them by manipulating the observer's viewpoint on the three-dimensional

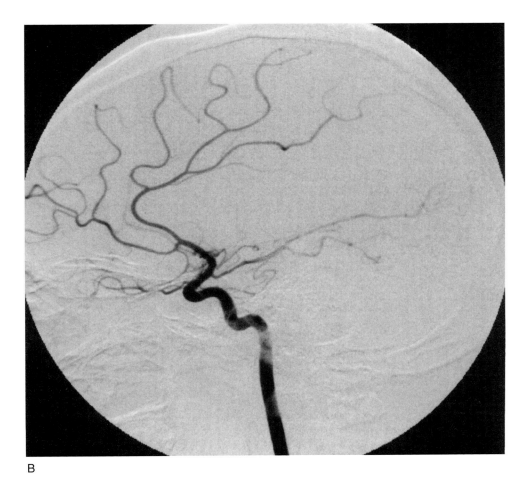

B

FIGURE 2-15B DSA, left internal carotid, lateral view, confirming the occlusion. There was delayed filling of Sylvian MCA vessels via collaterals from the arterior cerebral on the same side.

display. The basal veins of Rosenthal are usually the most prominent and problematic, as they follow a similar course through the perimesencephalic cistern as the posterior cerebral artery. Their size and proximity to the posterior cerebral artery will vary, but they should not be confused with a normal or abnormal artery (see Figure 2-19). Rarely, there can be prominent veins in the Sylvian fissure in close approximation to the middle cerebral artery bifurcation. This has simulated aneurysm in several cases, but was resolved by careful review of the source images. The more distal basal veins of Rosenthal, internal cerebral veins, and vein of Galen frequently will have to be removed for an unobstructed view of the posterior fossa.

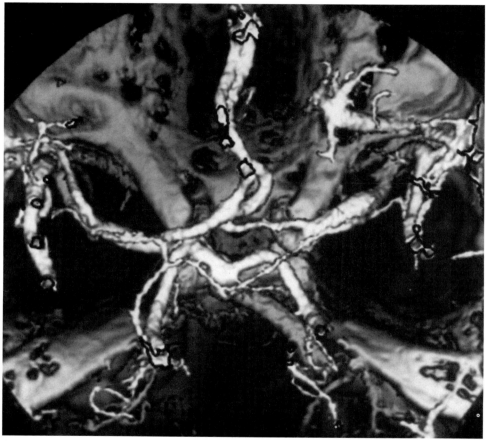

A

FIGURE 2-16A Venous angioma shown by CT angiography and DSA. This was an incidental finding on a patient with subarachnoid hemorrhage. (A) CT angiogram, shaded-surface display, viewed from above and behind showing a vascular structure in the frontal fossa on the right. The lesion has the characteristic "caput medusa" configuration of a venous angioma.

The posterior fossa veins themselves are infrequently visualized unless pathologically enlarged (see Figure 2-18).

Calcifications of any type will, by nature of their density, also be included in the volume of interest. The most frequent type that is encountered is the pineal, which can obscure the posterior fossa when looking from above. Choroid plexus calcifications are also often included, particularly those of the temporal horns (Figure 2-19A) and fourth ventricle. These are rarely confused with pathology. We have seen one case where physiologic calcification

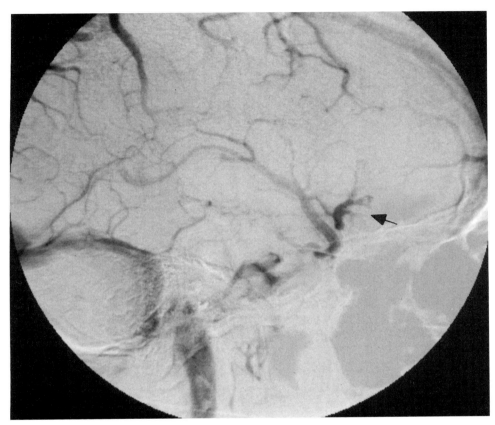

B

FIGURE 2-16B DSA, right internal carotid, lateral view, venous phase confirming the finding (arrow). No aneurysm was found with either technique, and this was not thought to represent the cause of bleeding as blood was confined low in the posterior fossa.

of the globus pallidus was superimposed upon the internal carotid bifurcation and simulated an aneurysm of this region (Figure 2-19B). Careful manipulation of the model and review of source images were able to show these structures as separate.

Physiologic enhancement will frequently be included as well and should not be confused with pathology. Normal enhancement of the choroid plexus of the temporal horns is often seen, as is the infundibulum and substance of the pituitary gland (Figure 2-19A). We have not had the opportunity to study patients with abnormal enhancment such as tumors.

A word of caution is in order regarding interpretation. From personal experience, model rendering is quite operator-dependent. I have found that three-dimensional models

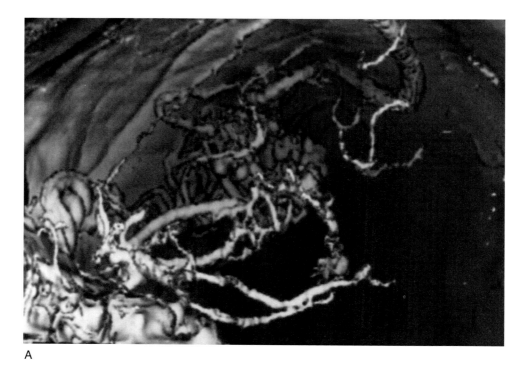

A

FIGURE 2-17A Arteriovenous malformation (AVM) of the right hemisphere shown by CT angiography and DSA. This was done with the whole head protocol outlined in Table 2-8. (A) CT angiogram, shaded-surface display, viewed from the patient's left. The right-sided structures have been electronically removed from the model for clarity. Enlarged middle cerebral artery branches, the nidus, and draining vein are well demonstrated.

may vary quite a bit in appearance depending on the radiologist who reconstructs and postprocesses the images. Similarly, interpretation will vary as well. In clinical situations like the detection of aneurysms with acute SAH, there will be little tolerance for poor sensitivity and specificity. In order to make this new technique a successful alternative to angiography, only experienced neuroradiologists with a thorough understanding of the anatomy, strengths, and pitfalls in this area should interpret these studies.

USE OF HELICAL SCANNING FOR ROUTINE HEAD STUDIES

Helical scanning techniques are seldom necessary for routine CT of the head. While the speed of helical CT is attractive in the setting of trauma, helical scanners can also be used nonhelically, and still result in a rapid examination. The GE HiSpeed will produce a nonhelical

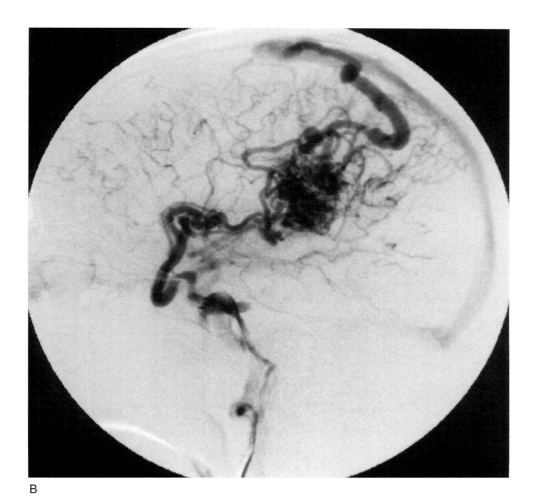

B

FIGURE 2-17B DSA, right internal carotid injection, lateral view, for correlation.

scan at a rate of one section every two sec. The entire examination may be completed in a minute or less.

Helical CT scanning of the head can cause artifacts that may simulate pathology. I have seen a case where axial images that were helically obtained showed evidence for acute subdural hematomas that were not present on conventional "step and shoot" scanning (Figure 2-20). This is due to partial voluming effects from z-axis translation as the patient moves through the gantry. The artifact is most pronounced at areas of great subject-to-background contrast difference, especially along cone-shaped or inclined surfaces (such as the

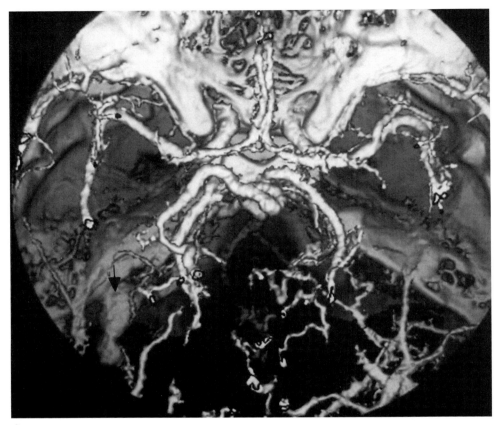

A

FIGURE 2-18A Dural arteriovenous malformation shown by CT angiography and DSA. This patient was evaluated for a large cerebellar hemorrhage on the left side. (A) CT angiogram, shaded-surface display, viewed from above and behind showing tortuous vessels in the posterior fossa, including a very large vessel related to the left petrous bone (arrow). This was interpreted as a probable venous aneurysm and the source of bleeding as this was adjacent to the hematoma.

skull-brain interface over the convexity). The result is a crescent-shaped band of increased density along the skull-brain interface that will simulate acute hemorrhage.[42]

An additional problem is the so-called "stairstep" artifact.[43] Recently described, this is also related to helical scanning of inclined surfaces such as the skull vault. This could lead to the false impression of a hypodense band at the periphery and simulate a chronic subdural hematoma or hygroma (Figure 2-21).

Partial volume averaging can be reduced by narrowing the collimation and pitch. Reducing collimation, reconstruction interval, and table feed speed can also reduce the

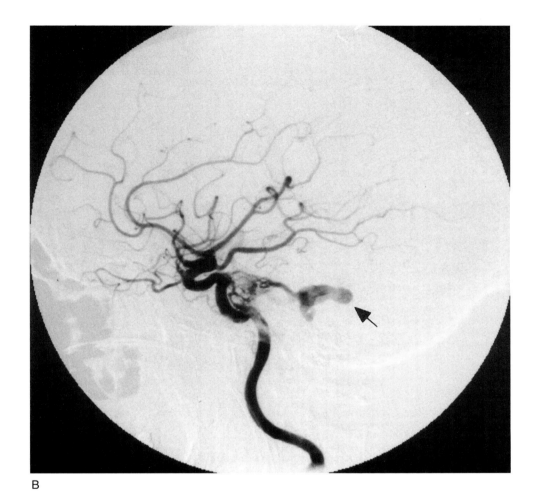

B

FIGURE 2-18B DSA, left internal carotid, lateral view, for correlation. The fistula was from the meningohypophyseal trunk to the superior petrosal sinus, and was not demonstrable on the CT angiogram. Multiple enlarged veins filled later on this injection that correlated well with the CT angiogram.

stairstep phenomenon. Newer interpolation techniques in the future may also eliminate the stairstep artifact as well.[43] False interpretation of a negative study for subdural hematoma could of course have disastrous consequences. Because of these problems, we do not use helical scanning for routine head examinations. Even where the speed of helical scanning would seem advantageous (such as trauma), it seems prudent to continue conventional

(Text continues on page 88)

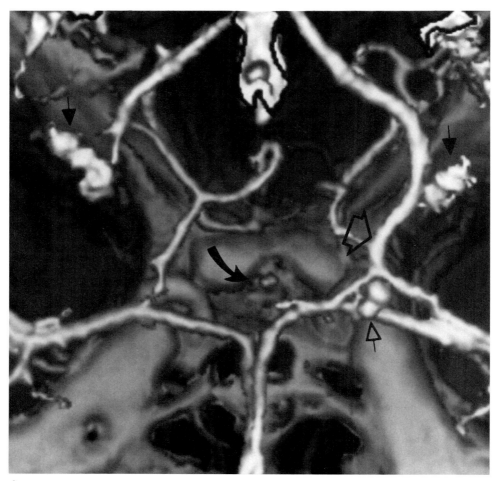

A

FIGURE 2-19A This patient's study contains pathology, as well as normal and variant anatomy that could simulate disease on CT angiography. Patient was studied for acute subarachnoid hemorrhage. (A) Because normal enhancement and calcifications will often be above the density threshold, they will very often be included as incidental findings. The shaded-surface display is seen from in front and above. Bilateral choroid plexus enhancement/calcifications are seen (closed arrows). Physiologic calcification of the globus pallidus on the patient's left can simulate an aneurysm of the internal carotid bifurcation on this one view (open arrow). The P1 segment on the left is atretic. Normal enhancement of the infundibulum and substance of the pituitary gland (curved arrow). The prominent basal vein of Rosenthal on the patient's left obscures the posterior communicator (open arrowhead).

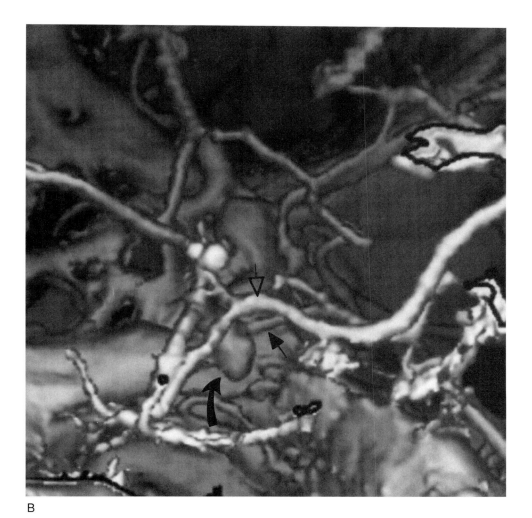

B

FIGURE 2-19B Same patient, viewed from the patient's left and from slightly above. This view allows separation of the posterior communicator (closed arrow) from the basal vein (open arrow). Also note the posterior communicating artery aneurysm (curved arrow). This is not an obvious finding as it blends with the opacified cavernous sinus and the bone of the skull base due to the nature of this display (see text).

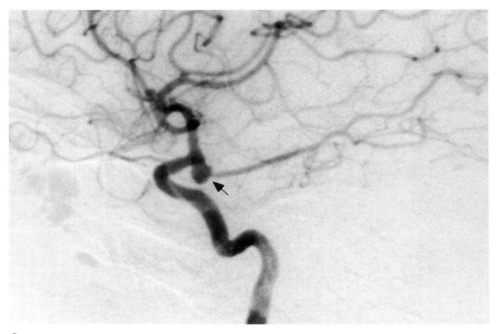

C

FIGURE 2-19C Left internal carotid artery injection DSA, lateral view, confirming the aneurysm seen in Figure 2-19B (arrow).

scanning until this problem is completely eliminated. Since these artifacts have little effect inside the substance of the brain itself, one can expect little interference with intracranial CT angiography.

HELICAL CT AND 3-D RENDERING OF THE FACIAL BONES

Three-dimensional display of CT scan data has been used for over a decade in assisting the surgeon to formulate the surgical approach to craniofacial disorders.[44–47] Using conventional CT, images were acquired with thin collimation and overlap specifically for 3-D rendering. This approach entailed significant radiation dose to the tissues in the region of overlapping acquisition. Given that many patients with craniofacial disorders are children, and need repeated exams, the radiation dose concerned many neuroradiologists. Helical CT offers the opportunity to retrospectively create overlapping sections, with no more radiation exposure than a nonoverlapping conventional CT scan.

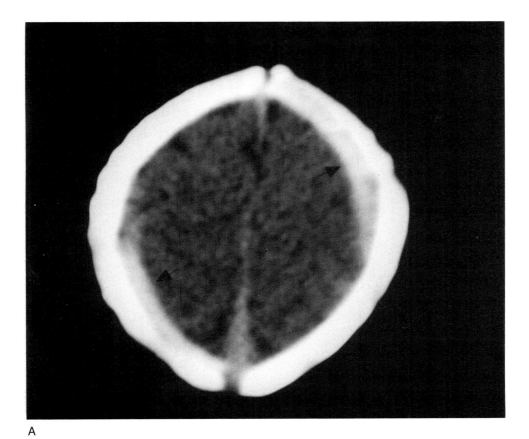

A

FIGURE 2-20A Helical CT artifact simulating bilateral acute subdural hematomas. The scan done helically (A) shows the artifacts (arrows).

There are a wide variety of congenital and post-traumatic craniofacial abnormalities for which 3-D models are useful. Plastic surgeons and neurosurgeons find that 3-D views give them a better appreciation of how the underlying anatomy contributes to the patient's external appearance. This information is not easily obtained from the axial sections. The models will also give an overview of relative intracranial volume and skull shape. This appears to be better assessed on 3-D than 2-D views.[47] Each patient is different, and we find it beneficial to discuss the case with the surgical team before rendering the model, so that important anatomic features are not omitted.

Our protocol for acquiring the helical scan is the same as that for whole head CT angiography (Table 2-8) except that contrast is not given, and five mm collimation is usually

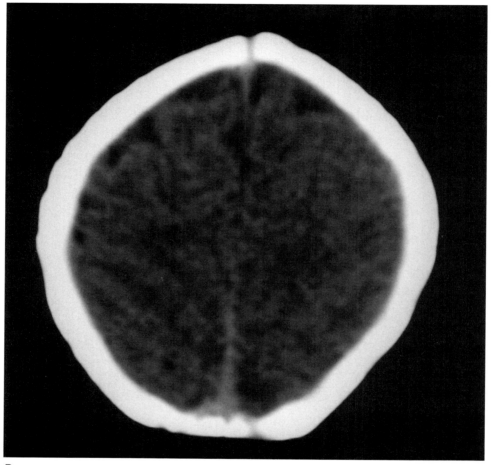

B

FIGURE 2-20B A conventional scan done immediately after confirms that the study is negative. This artifact is due to partial voluming effects secondary to z-axis translation during scanning *(Case courtesy of Dr. Keith White).*

sufficient for creation of photogenic models. The scans are reconstructed with two mm spacing and downloaded to the 3-D workstation. It is important to include the entire skull, especially if the intracranial volume or skull shape is in question. The threshold will initially be set low (70 H or less) so that a model which includes the soft-tissues will be rendered first. The threshold will then be raised to 200 to 300 H to display the underlying bony architecture (Figure 2-22). In patients with encephalocele, it is useful to create a low-threshold model which includes the brain and cerebrospinal fluid spaces, before rendering

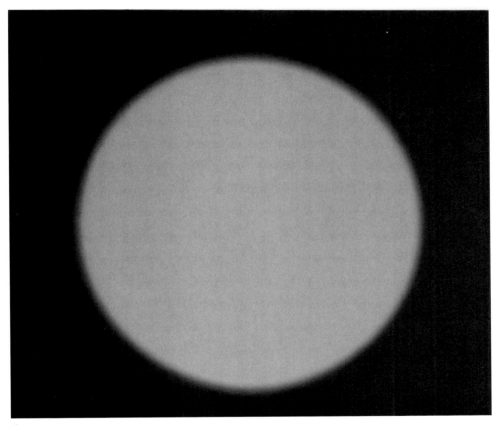

A

FIGURE 2-21A Demonstration of the stairstep artifact. A water-filled phantom with a spherical, inclined surface like the skull vault was scanned with conventional CT as well as helical CT with different pitches. (A) Conventional scan, 10 mm collimation.

the bony structures. On the low-threshold display, it is easy to electronically remove a "wedge" of tissue to show the relationship of the underlying brain to the bony defect in these patients.

Each institution should establish its own protocol for filming craniofacial 3-D studies. This will usually entail filming soft-tissue and bony threshold models in a variety of AP, lateral, and oblique views. We seldom archive images on videotape, but this may be helpful if the three-dimensional anatomy is difficult to visualize on static views. "Rocking" the model from side to side or recording movement of the model via an interactive track ball can really convey a greater sense of depth than filmed images. Occasionally ray-sum or MIP views are useful in postoperative patients. These views allow visualization of

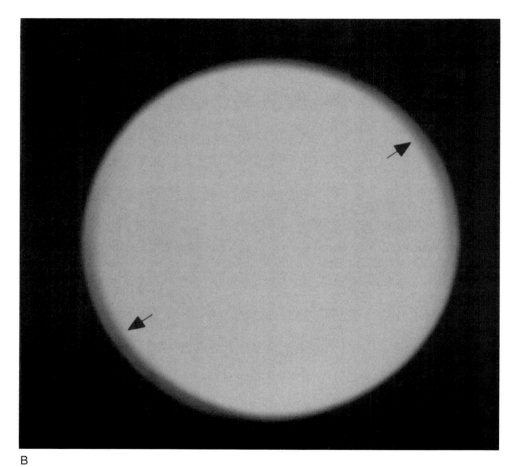

B

FIGURE 2-21B Helical scan, pitch 1:1, same collimation as A. Note the apparent discontinuity of the periphery, and the appearance of faint hypodense crescents (arrows).

metallic plates and other hardware, which could not otherwise be distinguished from bone on a surface model display.

HELICAL CT AND 3-D RENDERING OF THE LARYNX

Conventional CT scanning has generally replaced laryngography in the evaluation of laryngeal lesions. This has mainly been because of its ability to evaluate in the transaxial plain the

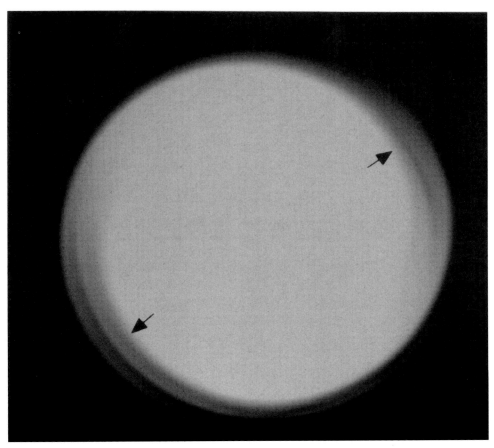

C

FIGURE 2-21C The pitch has been increased to 2:1, aggravating the artifact (arrows). These artifacts could simulate subdural hematomas.

deep spaces of the larynx. One limitation in assessing these radiographic studies is the ability to convey the information presented on the transaxial image to the surgeon whose approach is generally in a coronal plane. An advantage of an examination such as the laryngogram is that it allows visualization of the larynx with a single image in the coronal, conventional surgical plane. This provides a readily understandable assessment of the vertical extent of the lesion which is important in terms of tumor resectability.

(Text continues on page 96)

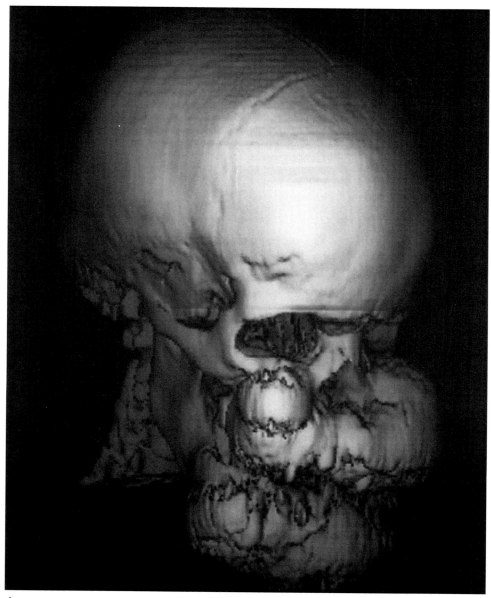

A

FIGURE 2-22A Three-dimensional rendering of child with cherubism. Oblique shaded-surface displays (A and B) demonstrate bony enlargement of the mandible and maxilla. The changes were due to fibrous dysplasia.

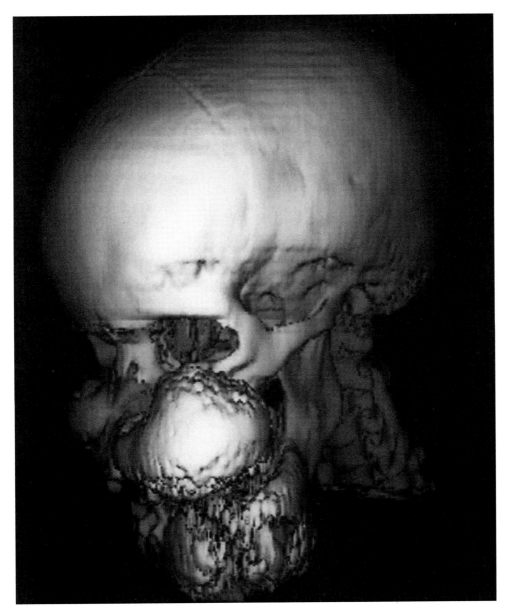

B

FIGURE 2-22B *(continued)*

Although currently 3-D imaging has been primarily used to evaluate vascular structures, we have adapted this technique to produce what we term "airway casts," which actually mimic the appearance of laryngogram (Figure 2-23). In addition to being noninvasive, these images can be rotated continuously along any axis of the airway to optimally assess pathology. Scans are acquired in the helical mode using a 1:1 pitch and either three or five mm collimation. If five mm continuous images are performed, the raw data should be saved and reconstructed at overlapping three mm intervals, the equivalent of a 60 percent overlap. These data sets are sent by local network to a workstation to generate the 3-D models.

In contrast to vascular models, these 3-D dimensional surface models are thresholded to include all structures that have CT attenuation between -1000 and -500 H. The result is a surface-shaded model in which all air-containing structures appear white while the soft tissues are removed. Disarticulation tools are used to separate the surface model from the air-skin interface along the outside of the patient. The creation of these models usually takes less than ten minutes to perform. We have found these images are complementary to the standard CT examination and most helpful to the head and neck surgeon in evaluating the larynx and upper airway, especially in the case of staging laryngeal carcinoma. At the present time, tumors can only be identified by their mass effect on the airway. New software developments suggest that we will be able to superimpose the actual tumor onto these models to provide an improved frame of reference and further enhance the utility of these models.

HELICAL CT OF THE SPINE

Applications of helical CT to the spine have been limited. In the lumbar spine, high techniques (up to 800 mAs) are often necessary for good image quality. For this reason, helical imaging presently provides little advantage. That is, the present tube-cooling requirements of our scanner do not allow a continuous acquisition along the entire z-axis (L3–S1) at this technique without multiple pauses. The time savings using helical instead of conventional "step and shoot" axial images are currently negligible in the lumbar spine, due to the pauses required. While helical acquisitions of good quality can be done, because of these problems we do not routinely use helical scanning in this region. Exceptions occur when high-quality three-dimensional models or multiplanar reconstructions are thought necessary.

Some preliminary work in the cervical spine has been done, however. Helical acquisitions show promise in this region due to the speed of scanning, as well as the high-fidelity multiplanar reconstructions. Nuñez et al.[48] studied the cervical spine in 800 patients with polytrauma. A summary of their protocol is given in Table 2-9. These studies were compared to the plain film findings in order to examine lesion detectability and influence on the patient's hospital course. Helical CT detected more than twice the number of fractures than did the plain films (Figure 2-24). The additional time of the patient in the scan room

(Text continues on page 99)

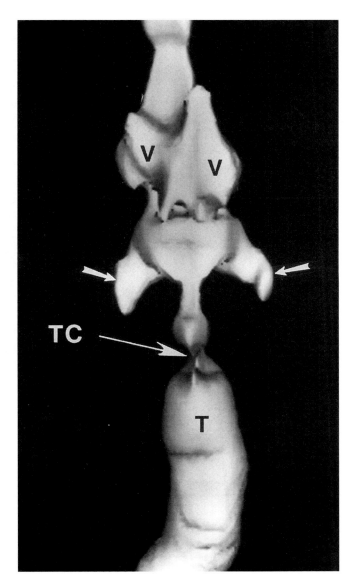

FIGURE 2-23 Three-dimensional model of the upper airway. By setting appropriate thresholds, a 3-D model can be developed that isolates the air-filled structures of the airway. The appearance is quite similar to a laryngogram, but noninvasively performed with helical CT. (arrows = pyriform sinuses, V = valleculae, T= trachea, TC = true cords).

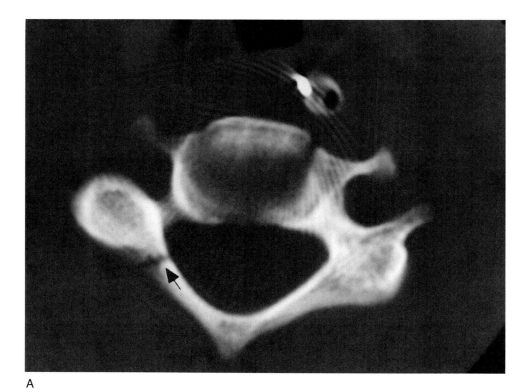

A

FIGURE 2-24A Screening examinations of the cervical spine in patients with polytrauma. The following are examples of fractures detected with the helical protocol in Table 2-9. These fractures were not visible on plain films. (A) Axial helical image showing a laminar fracture of C3 (arrow).

TABLE 2-9 Protocol for helical CT screening examination for cervical spine trauma[48]

Scan Mode	Helical
Gantry Angulation	None
Technique[a]	120 kV, 170 mA, 1 sec[a]
Field of view	13 cm
Pitch	1:1
Collimation	5 mm
Number of axial images	32 (average)
Area of interest	C1–C7
Patient instructions	Quiet breathing, no swallowing
Contrast	None

[a]Higher mA may be needed to adequately visualize C7

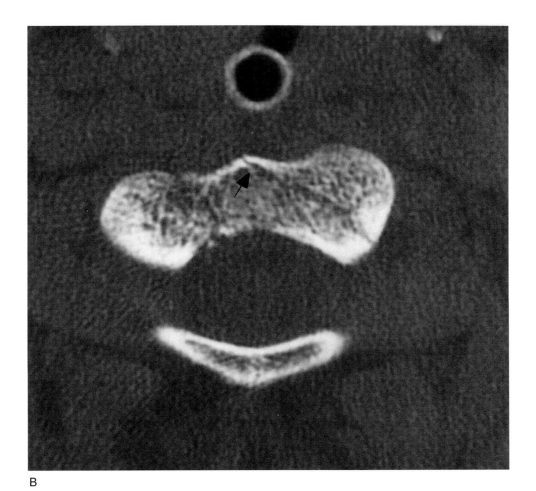

B

FIGURE 2-24B Minimally displaced fracture of C2 in another patient.

as a result of this additional imaging was on average eight minutes. The rapid exclusion or detection of fractures reduced patient time in the trauma resuscitation area by two hours. They conclude that routine screening of polytrauma patients with helical CT is more time-effective than the combination of plain radiographs followed by limited conventional CT at areas of suspected abnormalities.[48] They encourage helical CT scanning routinely in this subset of patients at high risk for cervical fracture. Further work could concentrate on whether such screening examinations would prove time and/or cost effective in different groups of patients or elsewhere in the spine.

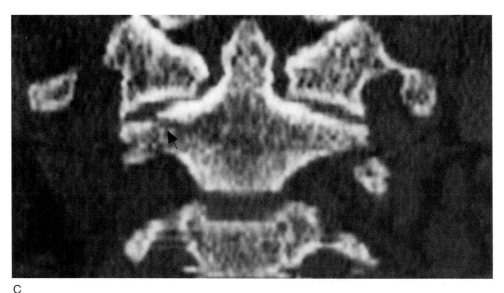

C

FIGURE 2-24C The coronal reconstruction also demonstrates this fracture in the same patient (arrow). *(Cases courtesy of Diego Nuñez, Jr.)*

CONCLUSION

Helical CT scanning of the head, neck, and spine is a modality in its infancy. Initial results in a variety of clinical situations are promising. There are many applications in which helical CT may play a significant role. Major advances over conventional CT include increased scan speed, superior three-dimensional and multiplanar reformatting, and CT angiography. Routine helical imaging of the head should be done with caution, if at all, because of the artifacts peculiar to this technique. These artifacts could simulate acute or chronic hematomas. Present experience in the spine is limited.

CT angiography shows great promise for noninvasive vascular imaging of the head and neck. Recent work in the evaluation of carotid stenosis is encouraging. CT angiography has potential for quickly and reliably imaging the intracranial circulation for aneurysm detection, vasospasm, screening examinations, clip placements, occlusive disease, and vascular malformations. In the latter case, CT angiography may play a role in stereotaxis and radiosurgery, perhaps taking the place of more invasive means currently employed.[49] Refinements of system hardware will allow more z-axis coverage, with similar or improved resolution. Software advances will improve speed of reconstruction and the fidelity of three-dimensonal models. Further work will undoubtedly clarify the indications, strengths, and limitations of this exciting new modality.

REFERENCES

1. Villafana T. Technologic advances in computed tomography. *Curr Opin Radiol* 1991; **3**:275–283
2. Polacin A, Kalender WA, Marchal G. Evaluation of section sensitivity profiles and image noise in spiral CT. *Radiology* 1992; **185**:29–35.
3. Rubin GD, Dake MD, Napel SA, McDonnell CH, Jeffrey RB Jr. Three-dimensional spiral CT angiography of the abdomen: initial clinical experience. *Radiology* 1993; **186**:147–152.
4. Dillon EH, van Leeuwen MS, Fernandez MA, Mali WP. Spiral CT angiography. *AJR* 1993; **160**:1273–1278.
5. Marks MP, Napel S, Jordan JE, Enzmann DR. Diagnosis of carotid artery disease: preliminary experience with maximum-intensity-projection spiral CT angiography. *AJR* 1993; **160**:1267–1271.
6. Napel S, Marks MP, Rubin GD, Dake MD, McDonnell CH, Song SM, Enzmann DR, Jeffrey RB Jr. CT angiography with spiral CT and maximum intensity projection. *Radiology* 1992; **185**:607–610.
7. Schwartz RB, Jones KM, Chernoff DM, Mukherji SK, Khorasani R, Tice HM, Kikinis R, Hooton SM, Stieg PE, Polak JF. Common carotid artery bifurcation: evaluation with spiral CT. Work in progress. *Radiology* 1992; **185**:513–519.
8. Castillo M. Diagnosis of disease of the common carotid artery bifurcation: CT angiography vs. catheter angiography. *AJR* 1993; **161**:395–398.
9. Galanski M, Prokop M, Chavan A, Schaefer CM, Jandeleit K, Nischelsky JE. Renal artery stenosis: spiral CT angiography. *Radiology* 1993; **189**:185–192.
10. Dillon EH, van Leeuwen MS, Fernandez MA, Eikelboom BC, Mali WP. CT angiography: application to the evaluation of carotid artery stenosis. *Radiology* 1993; **189**:211–219.
11. Riles TS, Posner MP, Cohen WS, Pinto R, Imparato AM, Baumann FG. The totally occluded carotid artery: preliminary observations using rapid sequential computerized tomographic scanning. *Arch Surg* 1982; **117**:1185–1188.
12. Heinz ER, Pizer SM, Fuchs H, Fram EK, Burger P, Drayer BP, Osborne DR. Examination of the extracranial caroid bifurcation by thin-section dynamic CT: direct visualization of intimal atheroma in man (part 1). *AJNR* 1984; **5**:355–359.
13. Heinz ER, Fuchs H, Osborne D, Drayer BP, Yeates A, Fuchs H, Pizer SM. Examination of the extracranial carotid bifurcation by thin-section dynamic CT: direct visualization of intimal atheroma in man (part 2). *AJNR* 1984; **5**:361–366.
14. Heiken JP, Brink JA, McClennan BL, Sagel SS, Forman HP, DiCroce J. Dynamic contrast-enhanced CT of the liver: comparison of contrast medium injection rates and uniphasic and biphasic injection protocols. *Radiology* 1993; **187**:327–331.
15. North American Symptomatic Carotid Endarterectomy Collaborators. Beneficial effect of carotid endarterectomy in symptomatic patients with high grade carotid stenosis. *N Eng J Med* 1991; **325**:445–453.
16. Masaryk TJ, Obuchowski NA. Noninvasive carotid imaging: caveat emptor. *Radiology* 1993; **186**:325–331.
17. Dobranowski J, Woods DM. Prostglandins: role in vascular radiology. In Taveras JM, Ferrucci, ed. *Radiology: Diagnosis—Imaging—-Intervention*. Philedelphia: JB Lippincott, 1991; (2)**140**:12.
18. Polak JF, Kalina P, Donalson MC, O'Leary DH, Whittemore AD, Mannick JA. Carotid endarterectomy: preoperative evaluation of candidates with combined doppler sonography and MR angiography. *Radiology* 1993; **186**:333–338.
19. Huston J, Lewis BD, Wiebers DO, Meyer FB, Riederer SJ, Weaver AL. Carotid artery: prospective blinded comparison of two-dimensional time-of-flight MR angiography with conventional angiography and duplex ultrasound. *Radiology* 1993; **186**:339–344.
20. McCormack J, Peyster RG, Brodner RA, Cooper VR. CT visualization of ruptured berry aneurysm within hematoma: the flip-flop sign. *J Comput Assist Tomogr* 1986; **10**:28–31.

21. LeRoux PD, Dailey AT, Newell DW, Grady MS, Winn HR. Emergent aneurysm clipping without angiography in the moribund patient with intracerebral hemorrhage: the use of infused computed tomography scans. *Neurosurgery* 1993; **33**:189–197.
22. Zouaoui A, Metzger J, Villanueva A, Feldman L, Arzimanoglou A, Kikhya F, Pertuiset B. Aneurysms of the circle of Willis. Comparison between computed tomography and angiography. *Acta Radiol Suppl* (Stochh) 1986; **369**:131-132.
23. Harbaugh RE, Schlusselberg DS, Jeffery R, Hatden S, Cromwell LD, Pluta D. Three-dimensional computerized tomography in the diagnosis of cerebrovascular disease. *J Neurosurg* 1992; **76**:408–414.
24. Aoki S, Sasaki Y, Machida T, Ohkubo T, Minami M, Sasaki Y. Cerebral aneurysms: detection and delineation using 3-D CT angiography. *AJNR* 1992; **13**:1115–1120.
25. Osborne A. *Introduction to cerebral angiography*. Philadelphia: Harper and Rowe, 1980; p. 146.
26. Wolpert SM, Caplan LR. Current role of cerebral angiography in the diagnosis of cerebrovascular disease. *Am J Radiol* 1992; **159**:191–197.
27. van Gijn J, van Dongen KJ. Computed tomography in the diagnosis of subarachnoid haemorrhage and ruptured aneurysm. *Clin Neurol Neurosurg* 1980; **82**:11-24.
28. Rinkel GJE, Wijdicks EFM, Vermeulen M, Ramos LMP, Tanghe HLJ, Hasan D, Meiners LC, van Gijn J. Nonaneurysmal perimesencephalic subarachnoid hemorrhage: CT and MR patterns that differ from aneurysmal rupture. *AJNR* 1991; **12**:829–834.
29. Kivel M, (ed.). FDA stresses need for caution during MR scanning of patients with aneurysm clips. In: *Medical Devices Bulletin* (1993) Volume XI, No. 3:1–2. Center for Devices and Radiological Health, United States Food and Drug Administration.
30. Klucznik RP, Carrier DA, Pyka R, Haid RW. Placement of a ferromagnetic intracerebral aneurysm clip in a magnetic field with a fatal outcome. *Radiology* 1993; **187**:855–856.
31. Vieco PT, Gross CE, Shuman WP. *Acute subarachnoid hemorrhage: detection of aneurysms of the circle of Willis with CT angiography and DSA*. Paper presented at the American Roentgen Ray Society 1994 Annual Meeting, New Orleans, LA.
32. Piepgras DG. Clinical decision making in intracranial aneurysms and aneurysmal subarachnoid hemorrhage—science and art. *Clin Neurosurg* 1992; **39**:68–75.
33. Higashida RT, Halbach VV, Cahan LD, et al. Transluminal angioplasty for treatment of intracranial arterial vasospasm. *J Neurosurg* 1989; **71**:648–653.
34. Fontaine S, Lafortune M, Lebrun LH, Couillard P. Le Doppler transcranien. Can Assoc Radiol J 1991; 42:389-96
35. Tsuchiya T, Yasaka M, Yamaguchi T, Kimura K, Omae T. Imaging of the basal cerebral arteries and measurement of blood velocity in adults by using transcranial real-time color flow Doppler sonography. *AJNR* 1991; **12**:497-502
36. Klingelhofer JD, Sander D, Holzgraefe M, Bischoff C, Conrad B. Cerebral vasospasm evaluated by transcranial Doppler ultrasonography at different intracranial pressures. *J Neurosurg* 1991; **75**:752–8.
37. Popovic EA, Siu K. Ruptured intracranial aneurysms: a 12 month prospective study. *Med J Aust* 1989; **150**:492, 496–497, 550–551.
38. Rosenorn J, Eskesen V, MadsenF, Schmidt K. Importance of cerebral pan-angiography for detection of multiple aneurysms with aneurysmal subarachnoid haemorrhage. *Acta Neurol Scand* 1993; **87**:215–218.
39. Stehbens WE. Etiology of intracranial berry aneurysms. *J Neurosurg* 1989; **70**:823–831.
40. Heinz ER. Aneurysms and MR angiography. *AJNR* 1993; **14**:974–977.
41. Ross JS, Masaryk TJ, Modic MT, Ruggieri PM, Haacke EM, Selman WR. Intracranial aneurysms: evaluation with MR angiography. *AJNR* 1990; **11**:449–456.
42. HiSpeed Advantage User's Guide, Rev. 0, Milwaukee, 1993, 2–69.
43. Wang G, Vannier MW. Stair-step artifacts in three-dimensional helical CT: an experimental study. *Radiology* 1994; **191**:79–83.

44. Hemmy C, Zonneveld FW, Lobregt S, Fukuta K. A decade of clinical three-dimensional imaging: a review. Part I. Historical development. *Invest Radiol* 1994; **29:**489–496
45. Vannier MW, Marsh JL, Warren JO. Three-dimensional CT reconstruction images for craniofacial surgical planning and evaluation. *Radiology* 1984; **150:**179–184
46. Herman GT, Liu HK. Display of three-dimensional information in computed tomography. *J Comput Assist Tomogr* 1977; **1:**155–160
47. Vannier MW, Hildeboldt CF, Marsh JL, et al. Craniosynostosis: diagnostic value of three-dimensional CT reconstruction. *Radiology* 1989; **173:**669–673
48. Nuñez DB, Ahmad AA, Coin CG, Becerra JL, Lentz KA, Quencer RM. *Cervical spine injury in multiple trauma victims: value of spiral CT as screening modality.* Paper presented at the American Society of Neuroradiology 1994 Annual Meeting, Nashville, TN.
49. Lunsford LD, Kondziolka D, Bissonette DJ, Maitz AH, Flickinger JC. Stereotactic radiosurgery of brain vascular malformations. *Neurosurg Clin N Am* 1992; **3:**79–98.

Chapter 3

Thorax

Philip Costello

INTRODUCTION

Spiral CT was first introduced into clinical practice in 1989 with the thorax as the first region studied in detail.[1,2] It has subsequently been embraced as the preferred means of performing chest CT. Potential limitations in tube current (milliAmperes) do not pose as great a problem in the thorax as in the abdomen, where there is far greater attenuation of the x-ray beam. In our center, virtually all CT scans of the chest are performed using spiral methodology.

ADVANTAGES AND DISADVANTAGES OF SPIRAL CT

Spiral CT allows for complete examination of a continuous anatomical region during one suspended respiration. With conventional CT, repeated consecutive breath-holds provide sections which may be at different levels of inspiration leading to the omission of small lesions. Scanning during one breath-hold increases the likelihood that focal lesions within the lungs are neither missed nor scanned twice. It also provides more accurate z-axis (cephalo-caudad) dimensions of focal lesions. In addition, since a true volume of data is acquired, retrospective overlapping reconstruction can be performed through the data volume at any point. Morphological and densitometric analysis of pulmonary nodules can, therefore, be made without the effects of partial volume averaging. Multiplanar and three-dimensional reformatting of the thorax is markedly improved compared to conventional CT due both to enhanced z-axis resolution inherent to spiral CT and to lack of motion.

The speed of spiral CT examination is an important factor for several reasons. Patient examination times are approximately 50 percent less than for conventional CT. This is particularly important for intensive care unit or critically ill or injured patients. Additionally, patients who find it uncomfortable to lie on the CT table can be examined in a minimum amount of time. Studies can be performed during maximal vessel enhancement with a small bolus of contrast material with image quality equivalent to conventional CT.[3] Vascular anomalies, aneurysms, tumors and pulmonary emboli are optimally demonstrated utilizing spiral CT. The radiation dose is similar to conventional CT but the need for repeat sections through lesions is eliminated due to the ability to reconstruct overlapping sections. This can be done retrospectively, even after the patient has left the CT suite.

The disadvantages of spiral CT relate to both the limitation in x-ray tube power required for continuous scanning and the interpolation process. As heat builds up during a spiral acquisition, the duration of exposure and tube current may be limited. X-ray tubes with increased power capacity should eliminate this problem in the future. Power limitations are far less of a disadvantage in the thorax than in the abdomen. Spiral CT results in a slight reduction in longitudinal resolution compared to conventional CT. This is due to broadening of the slice sensitivity profile by the reconstruction algorithm, and results in a minor degree of volume averaging (see chapter 1). For practical purposes, however, this minor degree of beam broadening does not adversely affect the image quality and diagnostic capabilities of spiral CT.

Because spiral scans are rapidly performed with high levels of circulating contrast material, there may be incomplete mixing of opacified and unopacified blood. This type of flow artifact, although infrequent, may occur in the superior vena cava. The inhomogeneity due to mixing should not be mistaken for venous thrombus. The most common location for these flow artifacts are where the contralateral (unopacified) inominate vein joins the superior vena cava, and at the level of the azygos arch.

INDICATIONS AND RECOMMENDED SCANNING TECHNIQUES

Spiral CT is routinely utilized at our institution on all patients undergoing thoracic imaging. A variety of protocols are used depending upon the specific clinical problem (Table 3-1). Our protocols are based on The Siemens Somatom scanner. Other scanners may offer higher milliAmperes, but this is usually not needed in the thorax. If higher milliAmperes is used, the kiloVolt peak can be reduced to 120. All studies are performed after careful patient explanation of the need for breath holding during spiral exposure. Patients are hyperventilated by three deep inspirations and expirations prior to scanning. The majority of patients can cooperate for a 32-sec breath-hold.

Most routine survey studies are performed to assess lung metastases, suspicious pulmonary nodules, lymphoma staging, or for tumor follow-up. There is still some debate as to the need for routine use of intravenous contrast in the evaluation of metastatic disease. Recognition of vascular involvement by tumor and differentiation of lymphadenopathy from prominent hilar vessels is aided by the use of contrast. Many radiologists will not use intravenous contrast for the follow-up evaluation of known tumors, where measurement of lesion size is all that is required.

For evaluation of the parenchyma images are reconstructed using a high resolution or bone algorithm. While we feel this optimizes resolution, some centers will use the standard algorithm for all their thoracic images. If a choice of interpolation algorithms is available, 180° linear or nonlinear interpolation should be used instead of 360° interpolation. The former will result in the thinnest effective slice thickness and the least partial volume averaging. In the initial staging of lung cancer, for mediastinal or hilar evaluation, intravenous contrast is infused at two ml/sec. Mediastinal images are reconstructed using a standard algorithm. A similar protocol to that for the mediastinum is used in the examination of patients with a clinical suspicion of aortic dissection.[4]

When a detailed analysis of the airways is required for tumors, strictures, or in patients with hemoptysis or suspected bronchiectasis, two consecutive spirals with five mm collimation and five mm/sec table increments are required.[5] Thin interval reconstructions at one to two mm facilitate the generation of elegant reformations (coronal or minimum intensity projection images).

Patients evaluated for interstitial lung disease have a screening spiral CT at eight mm increments followed by selected one mm collimation non-spiral high resolution CT (HRCT) sections. Characterization of a pulmonary nodule is performed with two mm collimation and a table incrementation of two mm/sec; allowing for accurate densitometric measurements. Increased pitch should not be used for attenuation measurement of nodules.

The role of spiral CT as a screen for pulmonary embolism is undergoing prospective evaluation but appears to be most useful in the detection of central emboli to the level of the third or fourth order vessels. Five mm collimation, five mm incrementation, and reconstructions at three mm provide a detailed analysis of the pulmonary vasculature. At our institution, 80 to 100 ml of contrast is infused at two and one-half ml/sec and scanning is started after a 15- to 20-second delay. Although scanning this early can cause streak artifacts to emanate from contrast within the superior vena cava, small pulmonary vessel opacification requires a dense contrast bolus. Some centers will use lower, while others will use higher injection rates.

CT angiography of the aorta provides angiographic-like images of the thoracic aorta in patients with known vascular pathology; e.g., anomalies, aneurysms, dissections, coarctations. The optimal technique is not yet decided, and will be discussed further in chapter 6. In many centers a test bolus is done prior to the CT angiogram. This serves to optimize the study by timing contrast delivery to the aorta since it is otherwise impossible to predict a time delay based on heart rate, age, or cardiovascular status. The typical delay between initiation of the contrast injection and scanning ranges from 12 to 24 sec when an injection rate of four ml/sec is used. The total volume is 120 ml. Other groups use a slower two and one-half to three ml/sec injection rate, a longer 30 to 40 sec delay before scanning, and find the test bolus unnecessary. Both of these techniques should be evaluated in the context of your practice to see which works best for you.

TABLE 3-1 Protocols for Thoracic Spiral CT

	A. Thoracic survey	B. Thoracic aortic dissection	C. Detailed thoracic evaluation for hemoptysis, bronchiectasis, etc.	D. Chest evaluation for interstitial lung disease
Scan Parameters	kVp: 137[a] mAs: 180	kVp: 120 mAs: 210	kVp: 137[a] mAs: 180	kVp: 137[a] mAs: 180
Slice Thickness	8 mm	8 mm	5 mm	8 mm (see comments)
Table Speed Incrementation	8–10 mm/sec	8–10 mm/sec	5 mm/sex	8–10 mm/sec (see comments)
Spiral Exposure	32 sec	32 sec	32 sec (2 overlapping spirals for full thoracic coverage)	32 sec
Reconstruction Interval	8 mm—supplemented by 4 mm for questionable findings	8 mm & 4 mm increments through pathology to improve multiplanar images	5 mm increments (1–2 mm through areas of pathology)	8 mm
Reconstruction Algorithm	a. High resolution algorithm for lung detail b. Standard algorithm used for mediastinal or hilar anatomy/pathology	Standard	High resolution	High resolution
Superior Extent	Superior margins of clavicles above lung apices	Lung apices	Lung apices	Lung apices
Inferior Extent	Posterior costophrenic sulci	At least to diaphragm, continue caudally if dissection extends into abdominal aorta	Posterior costophrenic sulci	Posterior costophrenic sulci
IV Contrast	Concentration: HOCM 282 mg iodine/ml (60% solution) or LOCM 300–320 mg iodine/ml	Concentration: LOCM 300–320 mg iodine/ml or HOCM 282 mg iodine/ml (60% solution)	None	None
Rate	2 ml sec	2 ml/sec		
Scan Delay	20 sec	20 sec		
Total Volume	80–100 ml	100 ml		
Comments	Include adrenals in patients with known bronchogenic carcinoma for initial staging or followup. IV contrast not necessary when simply following patients with pulmonary nodule(s) or for metastatic disease assessment	A few initial noncontrast scans of thoracic aorta may be obtained to look for displaced intimal calcification, but generally not needed. Supplemented by oblique, sagittal, and coronal reconstructions (need 4 mm interval reconstructions).	Coronal reconstructions through the airways require 1 mm or 2 mm interval reconstructions. Used for tracheal tumors, strictures, bronchial wall dehiscence, post-lung transplantation.	After spiral survey study, nonspiral thin scans using 1 mm collimation and the high spatial resolution reconstruction algorithm should be performed at each of these levels: aortic arch, q 3 cm down to mid portion of rt. hemidiaphragm. Targeted reconstruction of selected lung regions (small field of view) occas. improves detail

TABLE 3-1 Protocols for Thoracic Spiral CT (*continued*)

	E. Characterization of a Pulmonary Nodule	F. Pulmonary Embolus	G. CT Angiography of Thoracic Aorta	H. Multiplanar 3-D Imaging
Scan Parameters	kVp: 120[a] mAs: 150–250	kVp: 120 mAs: 210	kVp: 120[a] mAs: 210	kVp: 120[a] mAs: 150–250
Slice Thickness	2 mm	5 mm	3 mm	2–5 mm
Table Speed Incrementation	2 mm/sec	5 mm/sec	6 mm/sec	2–8 mm/sec
Spiral Exposure	Single spiral scan: scan duration > (lesion diameter/table incrementation) +2 tube rotation periods	32 sec	32 sec	Single spiral scan: scan duration > (lesion diameter/table incrementation) +2 tube rotation periods.
Reconstruction Interval	1–2 mm	3 mm	2 mm	1–2 mm
Reconstruction Algorithm	Standard	Standard	Standard	
Superior Extent	Superior to site of lesion	2 cm above top of aortic arch	2 cm above top of aortic arch	Superior to volume interest
Inferior Extent	Inferior to site of lesion	14 cm below aortic arch	16 cm below aortic arch	Inferior to volume interest
IV Contrast	None, unless a vascular malformation is suspected. Then, image dynamically at level where lesion is best seen following rapid bolus injection of contrast material.	Concentration: LOCM 300–320 mg iodine/ml or HOCM 282 mg iodine/ml (60% solution)		Concentration: LOCM 300–320 mg iodine/ml or HOCM 282 mg iodine/ml (60% solution)
Rate		2.5–3 ml/sec	4 ml/sec	2 ml/sec
Scan Delay		15 sec	see comments	20 sec
Total Volume		80–100 ml	120 ml	100 ml
Comments			An initial test bolus provides time delay for delivery of contrast (20 ml injected at 4 ml/sec). Single level scans at aortic arch during test infusion provides individualized time delay by ROI density analysis of aorta.	Oral Contrast: None, except when intrathoracic bowel herniation is suspected.

HOCM = High osmolarity contrast media
LOCM = Low osmolarity contrast media
[a]120 kVp may be used on devices that offer higher mA capability for extended helical scanning.

The CT angiogram is performed with a 32-sec spiral exposure, three mm collimation, and three to six mm/sec incrementation after the appropriate time delay. A pitch ratio of 1.5:1 or less results in minimal volume averaging. Pitch ratios in excess of 2:1 may result in failure to detect a subtle intimal flap, especially on 3-D rendered images. The raw data is stored and images are reconstructed at two mm increments. Image editing removes unwanted bones or soft-tissues and postprocessing of the images provides either maximum intensity projection images (MIP) or shaded-surface displays (SSD). SSD relies on a thresholding technique in which CT attenuation data is lost but SSD displays are useful in demonstrating tortuous anatomy. MIP displays provide angiographic-like depiction in which the density differences between calcium, contrast, and thrombus can be appreciated. Some workstations offer ray-sum projection views which depict the additive pixel values analogous to a conventional x-ray. These are more translucent than SSD or MIP views, and can be helpful in studying tortuous, redundant vessels and seeing "through" calcification. In most patients these studies can replace catheter angiography prior to surgery.

SPIRAL CT OF THE PULMONARY PARENCHYMA

Paranjpe and Bergin performed phantom, whole lung, and human subject examinations in order to optimize spiral CT techniques for lung parenchyma imaging.[6] Collimations of one, three, five, and eight mm were used together with pitch of one and two. Display kernels were varied and scans were assessed for each technique for edge sharpness, contrast resolution, vessel visibility, and noise. For line bars parallel to the z-axis, a spatial resolution of 7.7 lines per centimeter was obtained with all collimation thickness for both spiral and conventional CT. The z-axis resolution decreased more with spiral CT than conventional CT with increasing collimation. Optimal visualization of structures in the lung parenchyma was obtained with three mm collimation and an ultrahigh display kernel so that spiral CT scans with narrow collimation and ultrahigh display kernel provides the best image resolution. Table speed with pitch of up to two did not seem to affect the image quality of scans in human subjects. Since they found no differences with a faster table speed at a pitch of two, a greater range of coverage can be obtained.

CT scans of the lungs obtained using spiral and conventional modes at five and eight mm collimation showed no differences in resolution but at a lower collimation (one or three mm) curved structures such as walls of bullae and fissures become less distinct. Although scans obtained at one and three mm collimation provide the best image resolution and are most suitable for a detailed analysis of focal pulmonary abnormalities, a practical approach for chest coverage suggests that five or eight mm collimation is appropriate for screening examinations. When a detailed study of the lung parenchyma is needed, one or three mm collimation with two or six mm/sec table feeds may be utilized. Currently we utilize either five or eight mm collimation scans (Figure 3-1) to screen the lung parenchyma and one mm thick HRCT nonspiral sections for a detailed structural analysis.

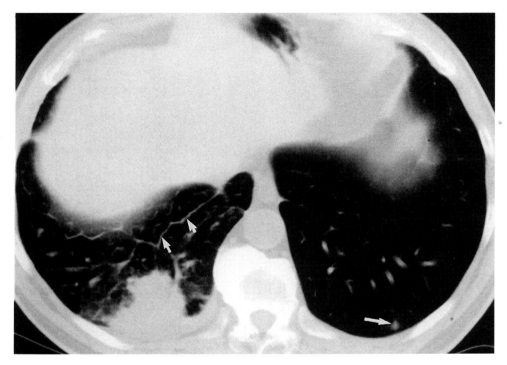

FIGURE 3-1 Lung Carcinoma with Lymphangitic and Hematogenous Metastases. Thickened interlobular septae (arrows) in the right lower lobe seen with slice collimation of eight mm and eight mm/sec table incrementation. In the left lower lobe periphery there is a five mm nodular density with a vessel leading into it representing a hematogenous metastasis (arrow) not seen on conventional CT at eight mm intervals.

Pulmonary Nodule Assessment

Assessment of focal lung disease by conventional CT is a commonly requested examination in an attempt to distinguish between benign granuloma and primary bronchogenic carcinoma. In some series, neoplasms represent only 40 to 60 percent of all resected pulmonary nodules.[7,8] Spiral CT can assist both in the detection and characterization of pulmonary nodules.[9] Absence of respiratory misregistration and the use of coronal or sagittal imaging facilitates identification of the intrapulmonary location of nodules. Volume scanning with multiplanar reconstructions can differentiate a true from a pseudo-nodule (Figure 3-2).

The most convincing radiographic evidence sign that a lung nodule is benign is the absence of growth over at least two years. However, if comparative studies are not available,

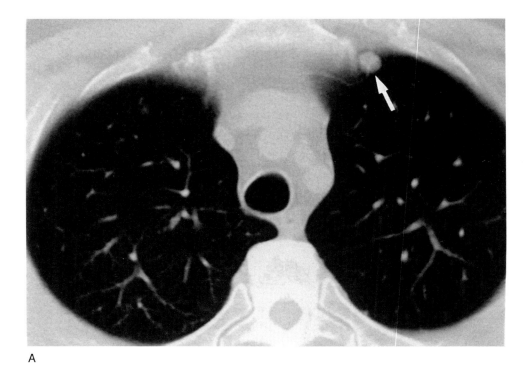

A

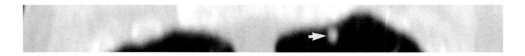

B

FIGURE 3-2 Pulmonary Metastasis. A. Transverse section at the level of the manubrium shows a one cm density (arrow) adjacent to the left first costochondral junction. B. Coronal reconstruction shows the one cm nodule lies in the lung parenchyma and represents a pulmonary metastasis from a renal cell carcinoma (arrow).

the next best finding for benignancy is the presence of diffuse, central, or laminated and concentric calcification within the lesion. Spiral CT sections with slice collimation less than half the thickness of the suspected pulmonary nodule provide accurate data for densitometric measurements (Figures 3-3, 3-4). Thin section spiral CT provides data which can be reconstructed retrospectively through the exact center of detected pulmonary

(Text continues on page 115)

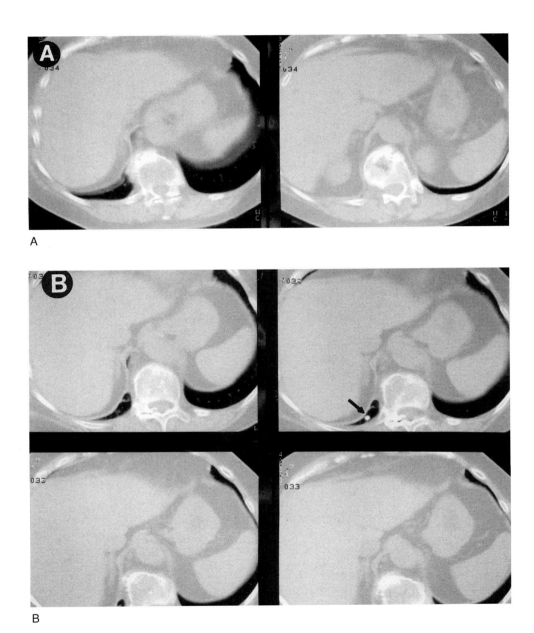

FIGURE 3-3 Peripheral Lung Nodule. A. Conventional eight mm thick CT sections at eight mm increments through the right lower lobe failed to show a lung nodule. B. Spiral CT of same patient with 8mm collimation and eight mm/sec table feed. Four millimeter incremental reconstructions show a calcified granuloma (arrow) in the right lower lobe.

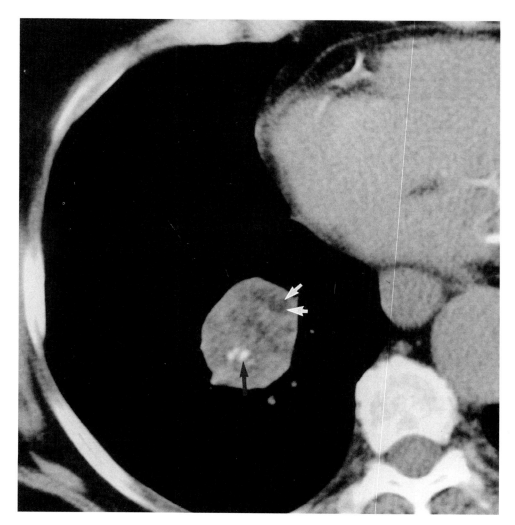

FIGURE 3-4 Pulmonary Hamartoma. Spiral CT section through a right lung mass contains fat (double arrows) and calcification (single arrow). Spiral acquisition obtained with four mm collimation and four mm/sec table feed with two mm incremental reconstructions provides accurate densitometric measurements.

nodules eliminating partial volume effects.[10] Consequently, reliable measurements of nodule density by thin incremental section analysis is possible. CT densitometry is most useful in nodules less than two cm in dimension with smooth or slightly lobulated borders. The finding of calcific deposits in at least 10 to 20 percent of the volume of the nodule, located near its center, is the most reliable indicators of benignancy. However, calcification in a solitary nodule is not a specific sign of benignancy, since a carcinoma can develop near a preexisting calcified scar or granuloma.[11,12] Although diffuse calcification can occur within a carcinoma, most cancers exhibit punctate or peripheral scattered calcifications and occupy only a small proportion of the lesion. Spiculated lesions greater than one and one-half cm in dimension should be considered suspicious for malignancy even if gross calcifications are present. For lesions greater than three cm in dimension, CT is not recommended unless there is a clinical suggestion of benign disease.[13]

Metastatic Disease

Examination of the thorax in patients with known extrathoracic malignancies is one of the most common indications for thoracic CT. Tumors which frequently produce metastases to the lung include: choriocarcinoma, renal cell carcinoma, testicular tumors, melanoma, bone and soft-tissue sarcomas.[14] In the majority of patients, 60 percent of lesions lie in an immediate pleural or subpleural location with 25 percent additional lesions in the outer one-third of the lung. Two-thirds of metastatic lesions occur in the lower lobes.[15] In a patient with a normal chest radiograph or an apparent solitary pulmonary nodule, the identification of multiple lesions on thoracic CT is critical in planning appropriate therapy. Should multiple pulmonary nodules be detected by CT, systemic chemotherapy may be given rather than major local tumor resection.

Conventional CT depicts more pulmonary nodules of a smaller size and at an earlier time than linear tomography.[16–28] Conventional CT is, however, associated with false negative examinations due to partial volume averaging, respiratory motion artifacts and variations in the depth of respiration between sections.[20,23–27] Variable respiratory cycles are probably the most common cause of missing pulmonary nodules at CT. The greatest degrees of pulmonary excursion occur in the vertical axis near the diaphragm and lesions as large as two cm in dimension can escape detection with conventional CT.[26] The peripheral lung also undergoes transverse excursion and can result in missed lesions since this is a predominant location for metastases.[28]

Several studies have assessed the utility of spiral CT in the detection and analysis of pulmonary nodules.[9,29,30] Twenty patients with suspected nodules less than one cm in dimension on plain radiographs were examined by both conventional and spiral CT.[9] Four nodules were detected by spiral CT with reconstructions at four mm increments that were not seen with conventional CT (Figure 3-5). The average size of the additional nodules was four and one-half mm and three were located in the periphery of the lower lobes.

Spiral CT was compared to incremental CT in a group of 39 patients by Remy-Jardin et al.[30] There were 23 patients with extrathoracic malignancies assessed for the presence of

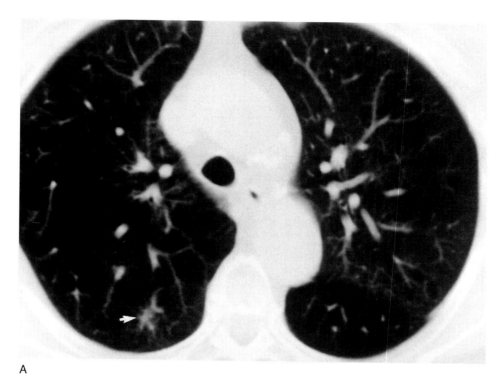

A

FIGURE 3-5A Adenocarcinoma. A. Contiguous eight mm thick conventional axial CT sections at eight mm intervals shows a "scar" (arrow) where a nodule was suspected on chest radiographs.

pulmonary metastases, seven patients with Osler-Weber-Rendu syndrome, and nine patients with solitary or multiple nodules detected with routine chest radiography. Conventional CT was performed with one-sec scan times and contiguous 10 mm thick sections; the spiral CT protocol consisted of 10 mm/sec table feed and reconstructions at 10 mm increments. A 24-sec spiral exposure enabled assessment of the entire lung in 21 patients and a second short exposure was obtained to screen the entire lung in 18 patients. Without knowledge of clinical data or chest radiographic findings, the presence of pulmonary nodules were assessed independently by two observers for each group of CT studies. The nodules were scored as either positive or negative for pulmonary nodules and their segmental location and central or peripheral distribution were recorded. The size of the nodules were stratified into small nodules less than five mm in dimension, median sized (5 to 10 mm) and large nodules greater than 10 mm in dimension. In addition, the edge characteristics and the presence of calcification was assessed.

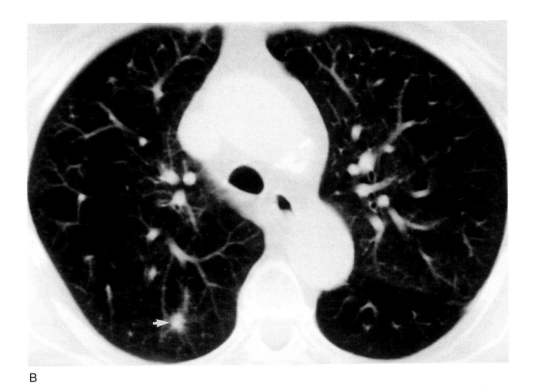

B

FIGURE 3-5B A spiral CT acquired the same day with eight mm collimation and eight mm/sec table feed was reconstructed at four mm increments. There is an eight mm nodule (arrow) with irregular margins representing a surgically proven adenocarcinoma of the lung.

The results of these authors merit detailed discussion. Four hundred ninety-seven nodules were detected by conventional CT, whereas spiral CT detected 42 percent more, a total of 705 nodules. The mean number of nodules detected per patient was 18 ± 4.5 with spiral CT and 12.5 ± 3.2 on conventional CT. Spiral CT detected two patients with two pulmonary nodules, each in whom conventional CT was normal. Of five patients thought on conventional CT to have single nodules, three had additional nodules seen on spiral CT. Of 29 patients with multiple nodules by both studies, a greater number of nodules were detected on spiral CT. There were more nodules less than five mm in dimension per patient demonstrated on spiral CT versus conventional CT, 12.7 ± 3.7 versus 8.4 ± 2.3 (p is less than .05). In addition, more nodules five to 10 mm in dimension were also demonstrated $2.9 \pm .09$ versus 2.4 ± 0.8 (p is less than 0.5). Respiratory motion artifacts were observed in four patients (10 percent) studied by conventional CT requiring repeat CT sections at the levels of respiratory motion, whereas none occurred with spiral CT.

This study conclusively showed that spiral CT demonstrates a greater number of pulmonary nodules than conventional CT. Most importantly, in patients whose chest x-rays were felt to be either normal or demonstrate a solitary pulmonary nodule, the detection of multiple pulmonary nodules influenced treatment. The inherent volume acquisition of spiral CT enables anatomically contiguous scanning of the thorax during a single suspended respiration enabling lesions to be detected at any point within the scanned volume. Only a modest degree of patient cooperation is required to breath-hold for 24 or even 32 sec, enabling a thoracic survey to be performed very rapidly. Careful attention to breathing instructions facilitates an optimal study and patients are hyperventilated prior to spiral CT exposure. Cardiac motion artifacts, which may prevent detection of small nodules, are also reduced by spiral CT, possibly as a result of the image reconstruction process which involves both spatial and temporal interpolation.

The increased sensitivity of spiral CT leads to the discovery of many incidental benign focal pulmonary abnormalities. Even with conventional CT, which is more effective than conventional linear tomography for nodules in the three to six mm range, 60 percent of the nodules detected proved to be granulomas or pleural-based lymph nodes at resection.[16] In Schaner's series, one-third of the nodules discovered by CT could not be found at thoracic surgery. Detection of small pulmonary nodules in the oncological patient raises a diagnostic and therapeutic dilemma. Metastatic lesions are similar morphologically to benign lesions and most metastases less than two cm in dimension have a smooth, rounded contour. Occasionally a connection between the metastatic nodule and adjacent branch of the pulmonary artery can be shown when vessels are horizontal to the scanned plane.[31,32] Prior microangiographic studies have shown a connection between pulmonary arteries and metastatic nodules seen on CT. Another sign occasionally seen with metastatic nodules is a zone of hypodensity distal to the metastatic nodule, possibly representing hypoperfusion beyond the vessel occluded by the metastasis.

Unfortunately, in many instances it is not possible to be certain of the nature of nodules discovered at spiral CT. The lesions may be too small for percutaneous needle biopsy and to resolve this difficulty, sequential CT examinations are used to assess tumor growth rate. We recommend repeat thoracic CT examinations for many incidentally discovered nodules at three- to six-month intervals to monitor growth rate.

Arteriovenous Malformations

Arteriovenous malformations may be either congenital or traumatic. The most common variant is a single artery and vein, although multiple arteries and veins may be present. In 33 percent of patients, arteriovenous malformations may be multiple and 40 to 60 percent are associated with hereditary hemorrhagic telangiectasia (HHT). Spiral CT with three-dimensional reconstructions generated from overlapping sections combined with transverse section analysis is as sensitive as angiography in detecting and displaying the vascular connections of arteriovenous malformations (Figure 3-6).[33,34] The procedure can be

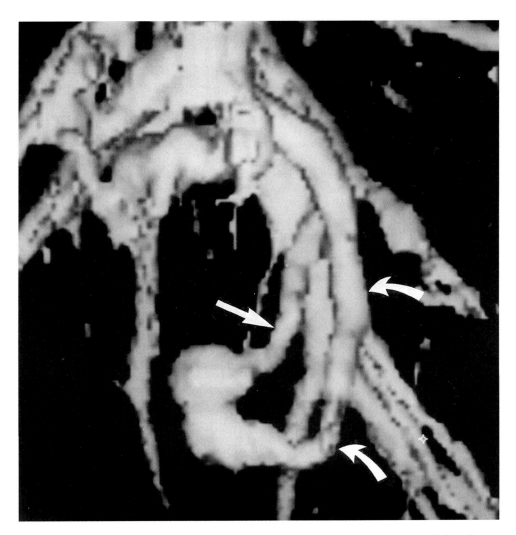

FIGURE 3-6 Pulmonary Arteriovenous Malformation. Fifty-eight year-old female with hereditary hemorrhagic telangiectasia and pulmonary arteriovenous malformations. Three-dimensional shaded surface reconstruction from spiral CT (five mm thickness/five mm increments). There is a simple arteriovenous malformation in the right lower lobe. The feeding artery (arrow) and draining vein (curved arrows) are clearly identified without contrast enhancement.

performed without intravenous contrast both pre- and postembolotherapy in these patients and could be used to screen families with HHT.

Bronchogenic Carcinoma Assessment

CT is used to assess mediastinal nodes in patients with bronchogenic carcinoma and is the imaging method of choice. Spiral CT provides a more accurate evaluation of hilar and mediastinal nodes due both to the consistent vascular opacification and to thin section analysis of the hilum (Figure 3-7). Despite a wide range of sensitivity and specificity in staging mediastinal nodal metastases, important information can be obtained. Identification and anatomic localization of enlarged nodes aides in the selection of the appropriate invasive procedure for surgical staging. Either mediastinoscopy, Wang needle biopsy, or percutaneous needle biopsy may be chosen.

Conventional CT is limited in its ability to detect parietal pleural and chest wall invasion with a sensitivity of 38 to 78 percent and specificity of 40 to 59 percent.[35,36] Peripheral tumors greater than three cm in dimension or tumors of any size associated with visceral pleural invasion are classified as T2 lesions, whereas lesions with direct extension into the parietal pleural or chest wall are classified as T3. Forty-two patients underwent conventional two-dimensional CT and three dimensional reconstructions through peripheral lung carcinomas for the assessment of pleural invasion.[37] The use of 3-D imaging allowed the detection of visceral pleural invasion not apparent on 2-D CT images (Figure 3-8). Evidence of visceral pleural invasion was identified with 3-D CT in 92 percent of patients compared to only 17 percent of patients with the use of 2-D CT imaging. Although the sensitivity of pleural puckering was high, its specificity was still only 76 percent, and could be seen not only with tumor invasion but with fibrotic changes in the pleura. This preliminary work suggests that spiral CT may help determine the presence of pleural invasion in patients with peripheral bronchogenic carcinoma. Tumors undergoing radiation or chemotherapy are followed more precisely by spiral CT than conventional CT because it provides accurate bidirectional and volumetric measurements.

SPIRAL CT OF THE MEDIASTINAL AND THORACIC VESSELS

Suspected Mediastinal Mass

Conventional CT is accepted as the premier technique for the diagnosis and differentiation of mediastinal pathology. Masses can be anatomically localized by CT and a specific diagnosis of certain conditions can often be made based upon attenuation characteristics. For example, fatty and cystic lesions of the mediastinum can be differentiated from lymphadenopathy and solid masses. Because of the shortened acquisition time of spiral CT, it is possible to obtain optimal enhancement of the mediastinal vascular structures. Contrast material is necessary in the assessment of mediastinal masses for a number of reasons.

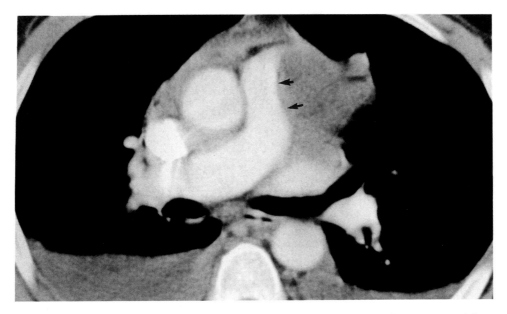

FIGURE 3-7 Small Cell Carcinoma. Spiral CT scan during an 80 ml bolus of contrast material shows a mass compressing the main pulmonary artery (arrows); diagnosed on biopsy as small cell carcinoma of the lung.

Firstly, masses arising adjacent to the aorta and pulmonary arteries can be distinguished from vascular anomalies and aneurysms (Figure 3-9); secondly, tumors may compress or invade mediastinal vessels. Thirdly, the blood supply of enhancing mediastinal masses such as Castleman's disease is well delineated with high levels of contrast and can further be assessed by the application of multiplanar imaging (Figure 3-10).

Thoracic spiral CT examinations are performed with significant reduction in the volume of intravenous contrast material compared to conventional CT. As little as 60 ml of 60 percent contrast can be used to assess the mediastinum.[3] Since nonionic contrast agents cost 10 to 15 times as much as ionic contrast, the ability to perform studies of the thorax with reduced contrast volumes enables significant cost savings.

Mediastinal Vascular Anomalies

Most mediastinal vascular anomalies are frequently detected on CT scans as an incidental finding; it is important to distinguish these abnormalities from lymphadenopathy or other masses. In other individuals, the plain radiographs may be abnormal, prompting a CT

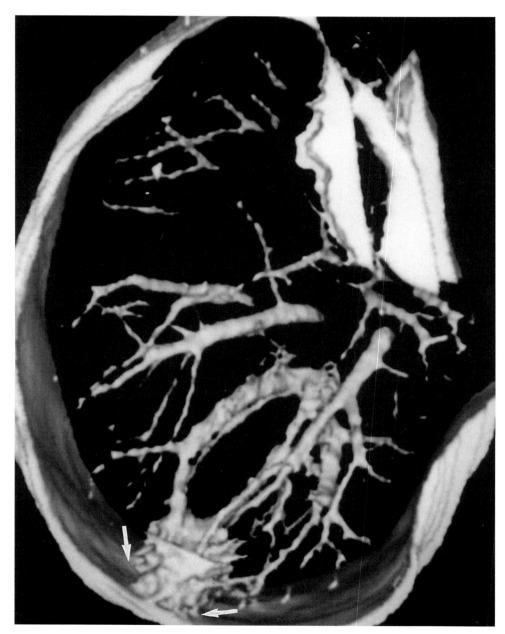

FIGURE 3-8 Carcinoma with Pleural Invasion. Seventy year-old male with a peripheral right lower lobe adenocarcinoma with pleural invasion. Shaded surface 3-D display reveals puckering (arrows) of the pleura indicative of pleural invasion not apparent on 2-D transverse sections.

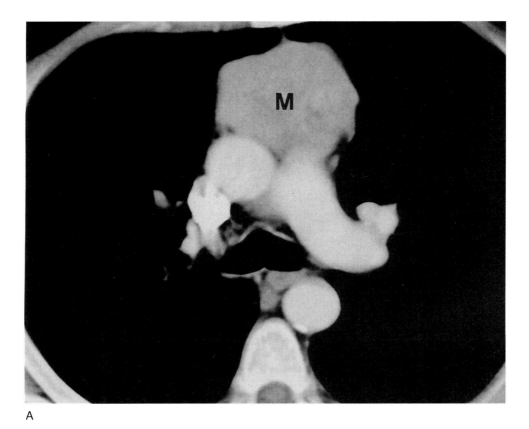

A

FIGURE 3-9A Thymoma. A. Transverse CT through a moderately vascular anterior mediastinal mass (M).

examination. An aberrant right subclavian artery arising from the normal left aortic arch causes posterior indentation upon the trachea. In many instances, it is dilated at its origin but may become aneurysmal throughout its entire course causing striking radiographic abnormalities (Figure 3-11 and see Figure 6-10). Pseudocoarctation is an unusual anomaly, which can simulate a mediastinal mass on chest radiographs and is often mistaken for true coarctation. The ascending aorta is normal but the aortic arch is very high and kinks at the level of the ligamentum arteriosum. Spiral CT with shaded-surface display and maximum intensity projection imaging provide angiographic-like images which confirm the diagnosis of these abnormalities replacing angiography (Figure 3-12). An artifact seen only in the ascending aorta can simulate the appearance of an aortic dissection and should be recognized by those interpreting spiral CT studies.[38] This artifact is thought to result from a combination of z-axis blurring and aortic motion and can be minimized by decreasing the pitch.

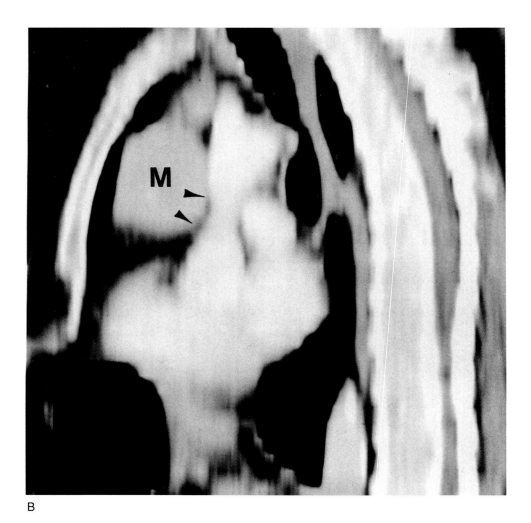

B

FIGURE 3-9B Oblique coronal reconstruction shows the mass (M) as separate from but indenting the ascending aorta (arrowheads).

Aortic Aneurysms

CT is a well-established technique for the diagnosis of aneurysm and in characterizing aneurysm size and extent. The amount of intraluminal thrombus and degree of involvement of major vessels can be precisely delineated by spiral CT. Measurements of aneurysms can be difficult on axial sections, particularly when the aorta is tortuous and

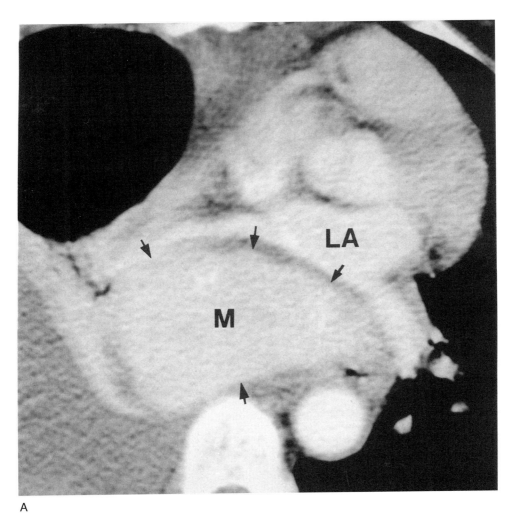

A

FIGURE 3-10A Castleman's Disease. A. Contrast-enhanced spiral CT shows a mediastinal mass (M, arrows) posterior to the left atrium (LA). The mass exhibits dense contrast enhancement. Biopsy-proven Castleman's disease.

coursing through the transverse CT plane obliquely.[39] Multiplanar reconstructions and the angiographic-like renderings of spiral CT provide valuable information in these cases prior to surgery.[4]

(Text continues on page 129)

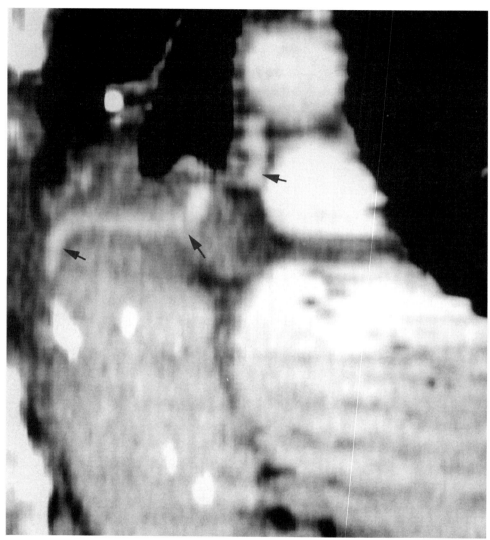

B

FIGURE 3-20B Curved coronal reconstruction through the mediastinum reveals a hypertrophied bronchial artery (arrows) supplying the vascular mediastinal mass.

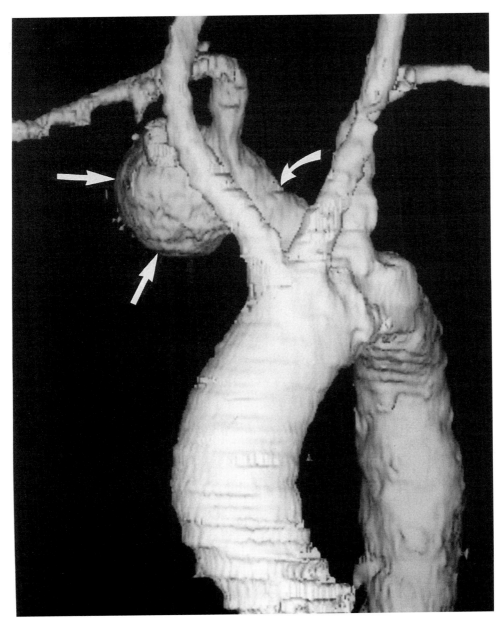

FIGURE 3-11 Aberrant Right Subclavian Artery Aneurysm. Three-dimensional shaded-surface display of the aorta reveals an aneurysm (arrows) of an aberrant right subclavian artery (curved arrow)

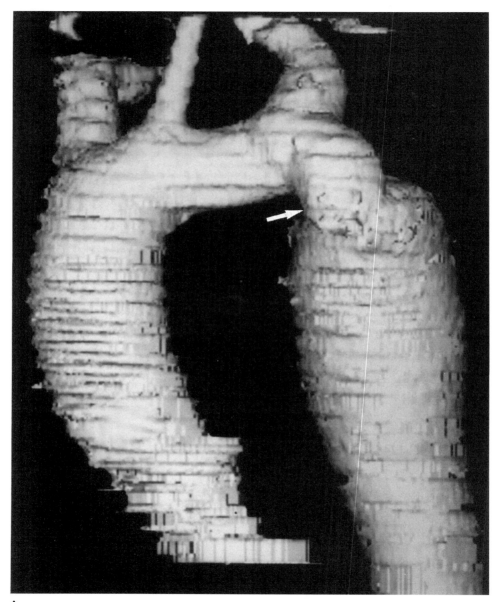

A

FIGURE 3-12A Pseudocoarctation of the Aorta (64-year-old female). A. 3-D shaded surface display reveals a very tortuous, kinked aorta at the level of the ligamentum arteriosum (arrow). The left subclavian artery and descending aorta are dilated.

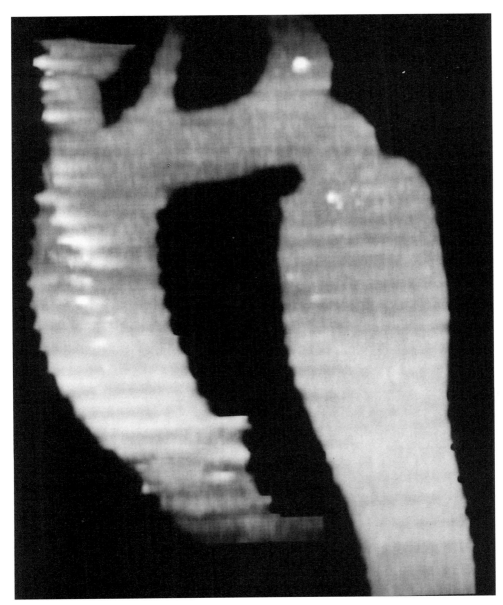

FIGURE 3-12B Maximum intensity projection image clearly demonstrates the pseudocoarctation and dilated descending aorta.

Aortic Dissection

The prompt diagnosis of acute aortic dissection is essential for successful therapy and with the appropriate institution of medical or surgical therapy, survival can be improved. The prognosis and treatment of aortic dissection depends upon the anatomical site of origin. Type A aortic dissections involving the ascending aorta usually undergo immediate surgery because of the high risk of the hematoma extending proximally into the pericardium or aortic valve, or occlusion of the coronary arteries and brachiocephalic vessels. Uncomplicated, Type B dissections involving the descending aorta are usually treated successfully with medical therapy by reducing peak systolic pressure. Current surgical treatment of Type A dissections involves insertion of a graft and resection of the proximal portion of the aorta; the coronary arteries may be reimplanted and aortic valve reconstructed as necessary. The sensitivity and specificity of CT and MR imaging are similar to that of aortography in the diagnosis of aortic dissection.[40–43] Identification of the intimal flap, delayed opacification of the false lumen and opacification of the compressed true lumen can be distinguished on CT. Identification of the intimal flap requires optimal aortic opacification and was not always shown consistently in studies using older CT equipment.[41] Angiography does not always show conclusive evidence of an aortic dissection since the separated intima may not be imaged tangentially, or the false lumen may fail to opacify at the time of the examination. It may be very difficult to precisely delineate the location and extent of the intimal tear constituting the entry site at angiography. CT similarly does not depict the site of an intimal tear, nor does it allow assessment of the aortic valve or coronary arteries.

The major advantages of spiral CT relate to a lack of arterial catheterization and examination speed which allows for rapid diagnosis or exclusion of dissecting aneurysm. Since the entire thorax can be examined rapidly in a single contrast bolus, high quality multiplanar imaging of the aorta and its branches is possible (Figure 3-13). Three-dimensional rendering may also be helpful in depicting the relationship between the intimal flap and the left subclavian artery (see Figure 6-9). CT is accomplished more rapidly then MR imaging and is easier to perform in many patients who may be clinically unstable, requiring close monitoring. Patients may be followed by either CT or MR since they are at risk to redissection or extension of the dissection.

Coronary Artery Bypass Grafts

Spiral CT is a useful technique in the assessment of patency of coronary artery bypass grafts. It can establish graft patency with a sensitivity of 85.7 percent and 100 percent specificity compared to angiography. The three-dimensional reconstruction capabilities can clarify complex tortuous graft anatomy and enhance clinician acceptance of the technique.[44]

Penetrating Atherosclerotic Ulcer

This condition occurring in the descending thoracic aorta can be confused clinically with aortic dissection.[45–47] Most patients are hypertensive and require distinction from a Type B dissection since surgical treatment may be implemented if the intramural hematoma

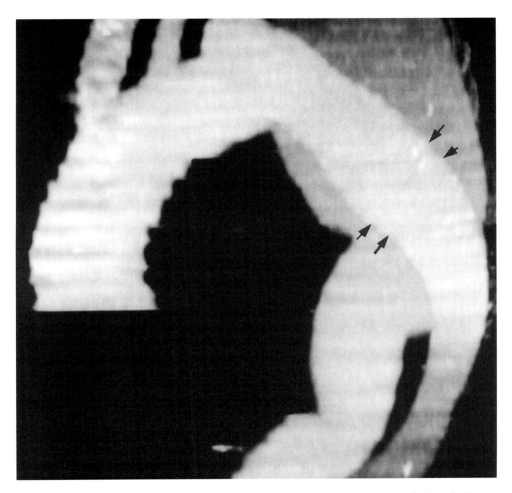

FIGURE 3-13 Type B Dissecting Aortic Aneurysm. Maximum intensity projection display of a Type B descending aorta dissection; the true lumen (arrows) is denser and smaller than the false lumen.

extends or a pseudoaneurysm develops at the site of ulceration. Aortic ulcers are easily seen on spiral CT because of optimized vessel enhancement (Figure 3-14).

Pulmonary Thromboembolic Disease

Pulmonary emboli are found in up to 60 percent of routine autopsies[48] with an estimated incidence of 630,000 cases per year in the United States.[49] The condition can be fatal in up to 30 percent of untreated cases and although anticoagulant therapy can reduce the

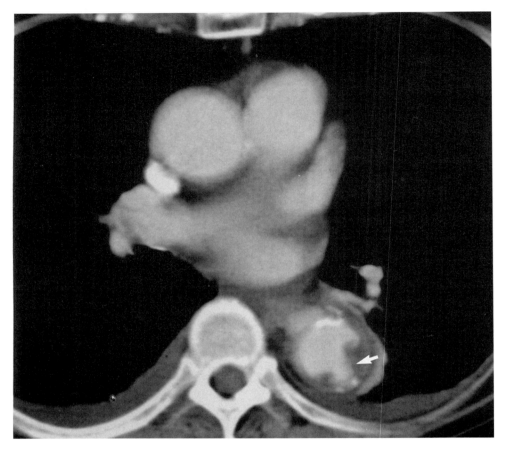

FIGURE 3-14 Aortic Ulcer. CT scan of a 73-year-old woman with atherosclerotic aorta, mural thrombus with ulceration (arrow), calcified aortic wall, adjacent pulmonary atelectasis, and fluid in left pleura.

mortality rate to 8 percent,[50,51] treatment is not without risks. Complications can occur in as many as 15 percent of patients.[52] Because of the variable symptoms and nonspecific radiographic appearance of pulmonary embolism, the condition is often undiagnosed, and an accurate noninvasive screening technique is desirable. Noninvasive imaging procedures that have been used to date include: ventilation perfusion scanning (V/Q),[53–60] MR imaging[56–59] and conventional computed tomography (CT).[60–67]

At most institutions, V/Q scanning is the primary screening test for patients with suspected pulmonary embolism (PE). A comprehensive prospective evaluation of V/Q scanning is included in the PIOPED study.[53] In patients with high probability V/Q scans

(13 percent of patients), positive angiography was obtained in 88 percent. However, patients with normal or near-normal V/Q scans, 14 percent had positive angiography (9 percent of patients). Low-probability V/Q scans with positive angiography (16 percent of patients) and intermediate probability scans with positive angiograms in 33 percent of patients constituted 73 percent of cases. The lack of specificity of the V/Q scan in such a high percentage of patients makes additional studies necessary. In some patients, impedance plethysmography or Doppler ultrasonography of the lower extremities may establish a diagnosis of deep venous thrombosis, a common source of emboli. Pulmonary angiography has long been considered the gold standard for defining the presence of emboli in segmental or larger pulmonary arteries. Even with angiography, however, there is considerable interobserver variability in the diagnosis of embolic disease in peripheral branches.[68] Angiography is associated with a small but measurable morbidity (4 percent) and mortality rate (0.2 percent) and in certain situations may be contraindicated.[69–71]

Conventional CT has been used over the past decade with anecdotal reports of its use in the diagnosis of pulmonary emboli.[60–67] Conventional CT scanners are limited by scan times of one to two sec and interscan delays of six to eight sec so that pulmonary vascular opacification is not always optimal throughout the entire examination. Many believe that spiral CT may ultimately become the screening exam of choice for the detection of clinically significant pulmonary emboli.

The potential of spiral CT for the detection of central thromboembolic disease has been shown in patients with acute and chronic pulmonary emboli.[72,73] In a prospective study of acute pulmonary embolism in 42 patients, a high degree of accuracy for spiral CT was reported when compared to conventional angiography.[72] The pulmonary vascular bed was examined using five mm thick collimation and a five mm/sec table feed with three mm incremental reconstructions and a scan volume of 12 cm (24 sec exposure). Studies were commenced at the level of the aortic arch with intravenous injection of contrast through an 18 gauge catheter in an antecubital vein and a five-sec delay to scanning. A 12 to 30 percent iodine concentration and volumes of up to 90 to 120 ml were infused at five to seven ml/sec. Both selective pulmonary angiography and spiral CT were analyzed independently of each other. All but seven of the 42 patients were able to sustain breath-holding for 24 sec and vascular opacification was considered excellent or good in 98 percent of patients. The mediastinal windows used for pulmonary emboli detection were not impaired by minor respiratory motion. Central pulmonary emboli were excluded by spiral CT and confirmed normal at angiography in 23 patients. In 19 patients, spiral CT showed changes consistent with pulmonary thromboembolism and pulmonary angiography substantiated the diagnosis in 18 of 19 patients. There was one false positive spiral CT study in a patient with asymmetrical pulmonary vascular opacification due to increased pulmonary arterial resistance.

Using selective pulmonary angiography as the diagnostic standard, there were no false negative studies on spiral CT with a sensitivity of 100 percent and specificity of 96 percent. A total of 112 thromboemboli were depicted on spiral CT and pulmonary angiography in 18 patients. The emboli were in the main (8), lobar (28), and segmental (76) pulmonary artery branches. CT signs were partial filling defects (37 percent), complete filling defects (45 percent), "railway-track" sign (five percent) and mural defects (13 percent) (Figure 3-15). Direct evidence of intraluminal filling defects was seen in 58 pulmonary arteries on spiral CT, whereas, angiography showed only indirect signs such as regional perfusion defects[45] or abrupt cutoffs.[13] Several intersegmental lymph nodes were initially misinterpreted as representing thrombi but on review correctly interpreted as representing lymph nodes. The amount of adherent thrombotic material was underestimated by angiography and additionally the multiplanar reconstruction capabilities of spiral CT were useful in predicting the length and course of adherent thrombotic material. All pulmonary emboli diagnosed on spiral CT were present in the second to fourth division pulmonary arterial branches. The advantages of spiral CT relate to its rapid scan time, volumetric data acquisition, and optimal degree of vascular enhancement.

Electron beam CT (EBT) with images obtained in 100 msec has been used to demonstrate emboli in both in vitro and in vivo studies.[74-76] Breath-holding is not necessary with electron beam CT and similar to spiral CT, as a result of the rapid examination time, the pulmonary arteries can be optimally enhanced with a small volume of intravenous contrast material. In a group of 86 patients suspected of having pulmonary embolism, thrombotic material was demonstrated in 39 patients.[76] Of 25 patients with angiographic or pathologic proof, there were 19 positive CT scans, four proved negative scans, one false negative and one false positive scan. There was agreement between the CT findings and angiography in 85 percent of patients studied by both modalities (231 anatomic zones). Of the 18 zones judged positive on angiography alone, nine showed angiographic evidence of chronic thromboembolic disease in segmental vessels. Seven additional zones were seen at angiography to involve acute emboli in segmental vessels in the upper or middle lobes not detected by CT. There were 17 zones scored positive by CT alone and 10 showed clear evidence of thrombotic material in the central pulmonary vasculature not found on angiography; most of these were in patients with chronic thromboembolic disease.

Both spiral CT and electron beam CT suffer several limitations in the detection of emboli; horizontal vessels in the right middle lobe and lingular may be poorly visualized because of volume averaging. For spiral CT, this can be minimized by using pitch ratios as close as 1:1 as possible. The peripheral portions of the upper and lower lobes may be inadequately scanned by both techniques possibly related to insufficient time delays between contrast initiation and scan performance. In order to correctly utilize spiral CT, a precise knowledge of the broncho-vascular system is essential and scans should be scrutinized for the presence of intersegmental lymph nodes which may cause false positive studies. The use of multiplanar reconstructions in coronal, sagittal and oblique planes may help differentiate intraluminal thrombi from extrinsic lesions such as nodes. CT fails to depict discrete stenoses and webs in segmental vessels seen with chronic PE. Central pulmonary emboli are, however, often better shown on CT than angiography because the emboli are seen frequently en face. Thrombi that are chronic and adherent to the arterial wall are more susceptible to be overlooked at angiography (Figure 3-16). Vertically oriented vessels containing emboli are readily demonstrated on CT as filling defects surrounded by contrast material or as zones of transition from enhanced to nonenhanced vessel.

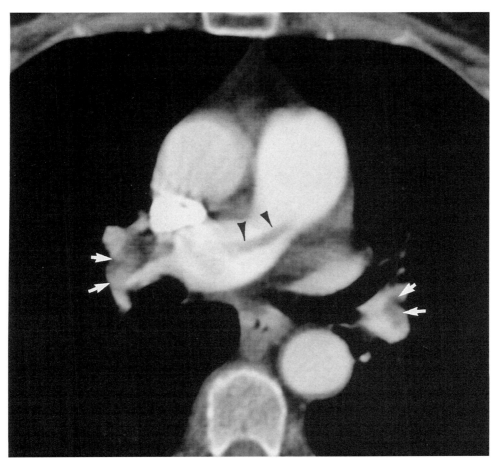

A

FIGURE 3-15A Acute Pulmonary Embolus. A. Spiral CT scan through the main pulmonary artery reveals bilateral pulmonary emboli (arrows) with a linear thrombus in the right pulmonary artery (arrowheads).

Although spiral CT is a powerful tool for the detection of emboli in the second to fourth division pulmonary arteries, it does not replace angiography in every instance. Spiral CT is a relatively fast, noninvasive way to detect acute emboli avoiding the cost and potential complications of pulmonary angiography. It is useful in monitoring patients with documented central emboli as the vascular bed recanalizes. Further prospective multi-institutional investigations will be necessary to determine if electron beam CT or spiral CT can be offered as an alternative to V/Q scanning as the primary noninvasive screening

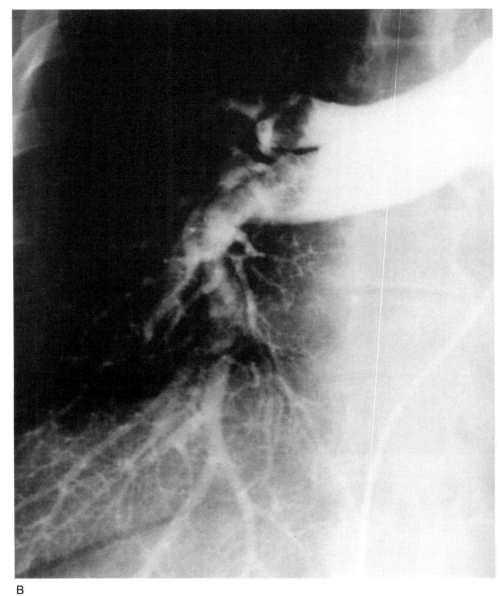

B

FIGURE 3-15B Selective right pulmonary angiogram confirms the lobar emboli. The linear thrombus in the right main pulmonary artery is not seen.

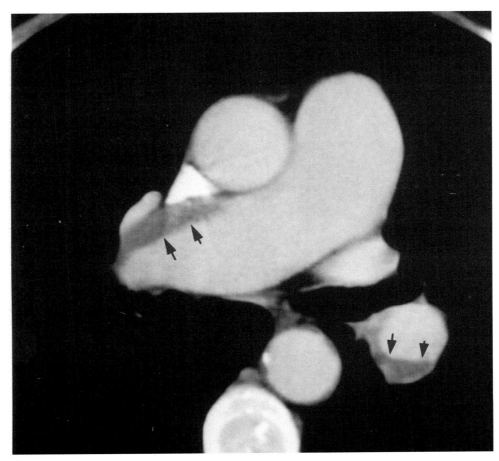

A

FIGURE 3-16A Chronic Pulmonary Emboli. Sixty-seven-year-old male with recent myocardial infarction and coronary angioplasty. A. Contrast enhanced thoracic CT study was performed to exclude a thymoma. Both pulmonary arteries are enlarged with chronic thrombi (arrows) in both right and left pulmonary arteries.

tool for acute thromboembolic disease. Reasonably small volumes of contrast material can be used and although it may not replace angiography entirely, it may obviate or alter the performance of angiography in some patients.

Both spiral CT and EBT are clearly useful in the diagnosis and assessment of chronic PE. This group of patients with secondary pulmonary hypertension may benefit from surgical thromboendarterectomy. Surgical candidates require demonstration of thrombi in the

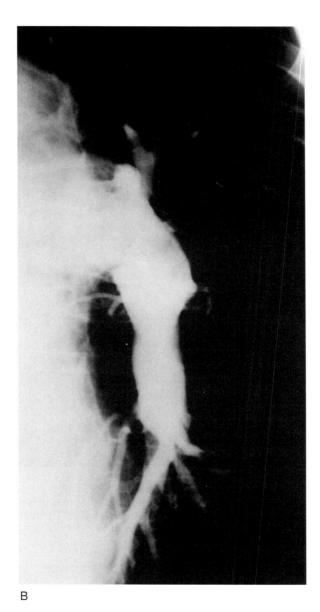

B

FIGURE 3-16B Selective left pulmonary angiogram fails to identify the mural embolus. The caliber change in the artery was felt not to be a specific finding for this entity.

main, lobar, or segmental pulmonary arteries. Organization of embolic material to the vessel wall with adherence, recanalization and retraction are responsible for the angiographic findings and shows as a crescentic filling defect on CT.[77] In the setting of chronic thromboembolic pulmonary hypertension, angiography may underestimate the amount of thrombus present.[78] For this reason, CT and angiography are complimentary to each other in assessing patients with severe pulmonary hypertension undergoing consideration for thromboendarterectomy.

SPIRAL CT OF THE DIAPHRAGM, CHEST WALL, AND AIRWAYS

Diaphragm

Conventional CT has difficulties in the assessment of lesions arising on or adjacent to the diaphragm. With spiral CT, the thorax and upper abdomen can be examined in a single breath, eliminating respiratory misregistration. From the data volume acquired through the diaphragm, overlapping sections can be retrospectively reconstructed generating high-quality multiplanar reformations. For optimal quality images, slice collimation from two to five mm and table increments from two to six mm/sec are used. Axial images are reconstructed from the spiral data set at one to two mm increments providing idealized multiplanar reconstructions. Using this technique, we have found spiral CT to be extremely useful in distinguishing and characterizing masses arising in the lung parenchyma, pleura, diaphragm, and subdiaphragmatic space (Figures 3-17, 3-18).[79]

Chest Wall Tumors

Lack of rib and sternal motion during spiral data acquisition makes it possible to generate high-quality 3-D images of tumors involving the chest wall (Figure 3-19). Osseous or cartilaginous tumors and inflammatory lesions can be outlined prior to reconstructive surgery. We use spiral CT to plan tangential radiotherapy fields in patients with breast carcinoma with the goal of reducing the dose delivered to the left coronary artery and left ventricle.[80] Spiral CT image data is transferred to a radiation therapy workstation where treatment fields are planned based on consistent CT data.

The Airways

It is essential that the airways be assessed with a detailed knowledge of normal anatomy and variants with careful attention to CT technique.[81-87] Slice collimation should be proportional to the airway being assessed and since lobar bronchi range between three and five mm in dimension, they are most reliably assessed by a slice thickness of less than five mm. Spiral CT facilitates airway assessment by its ability to reconstruct sections at any point within the data volume; additionally, high-quality multiplanar and three-dimensional images of the airways can be generated. Three-dimensional images of the airway have been correlated with bronchoscopy in a variety of central airway lesions.[88]

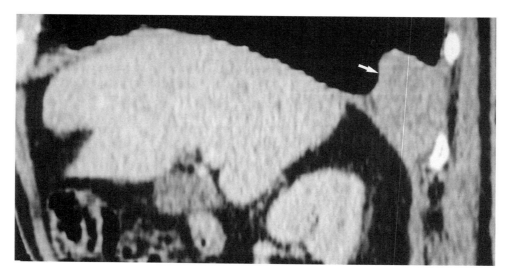

FIGURE 3-17 Metastasis to Pleura. Sagittal reconstruction through the right diaphragm shows a mass in the pleural space (arrow). Biopsy confirmed this mass to be a metastasis from a clinically occult renal cell carcinoma.

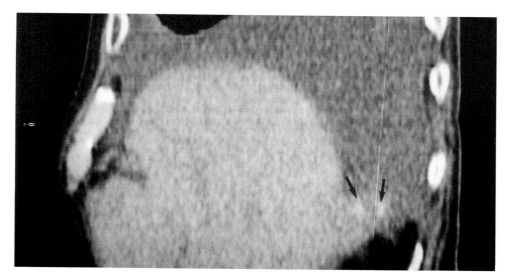

FIGURE 3-18 Gallstones Perforating the Diaphragm. Sagittal reconstruction through the mid portion of the right diaphragm in a 90-year-old male with an empyema. At laparoscopic cholecystectomy, gallstones were lost intraperitoneally and are seen perforating the diaphragm (arrows) posterior to the liver causing an empyema.

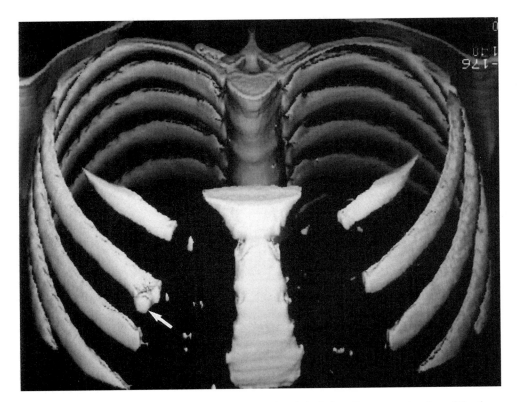

FIGURE 3-19 Rib Osteochondroma. Three-dimensional shaded-surface reconstruction of the thorax in a 16-year-old female with an osteochondroma projecting from the right fourth rib (arrow). Excellent detail of the ribs and sternum without motion artifacts.

CT is established for the diagnosis of both neoplastic and inflammatory lesions involving the airways.[89-93] Bronchiectasis is readily diagnosed by CT and is usually established by recognition of the characteristic signs including the presence of signet rings. Mucoid impaction is clearly demonstrated by spiral CT, particularly on multiplanar reconstructions (Figure 3-20).

Prior to resection of tracheal tumors, spiral CT is extremely valuable. Tumors of the central airways can be assessed for longitudinal and transverse extent by spiral CT, greatly assisting surgical planning (Figure 3-21). Following lobectomy or pneumonectomy, the anastomosis can be assessed for tumor recurrence, stricture, or dehiscence (Figures 3-22, 3-23).

CT is accurate in identifying central airway pathology but it is not precise in the determination of whether a lesion is primarily endobronchial, submucosal, or extrinsic. CT is very useful in delineating the extent of peribronchial abnormalities and has proved to be

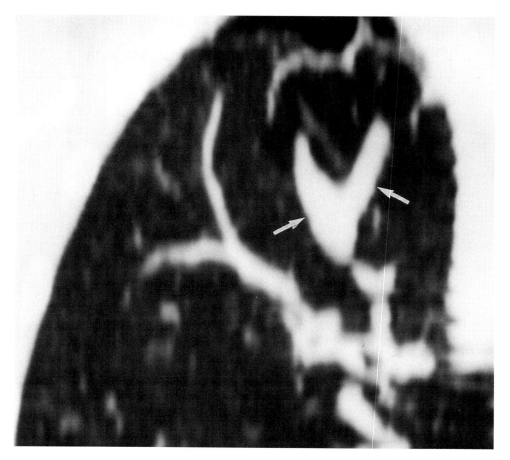

FIGURE 3-20 Mucoid Impaction. An oblique reconstruction through the apical segmental bronchus in this 42-year-old asthmatic confirms the diagnosis of mucoid impaction shown as a branching tubular structure (arrows).

most valuable in the assessment of disease extent in patients with known or suspected lung cancer.

Patients with hemoptysis and a nonlocalizing chest radiograph require thin section CT examinations of the airways.[94–96] Several studies have demonstrated a clinical role for demonstrating abnormalities on CT as a cause of hemoptysis. A variety of techniques have been proposed consisting of one to two mm sections at eight to ten mm from the thoracic inlet to the carina followed by five mm contiguous sections to the level of the inferior

(Text continues on page 145)

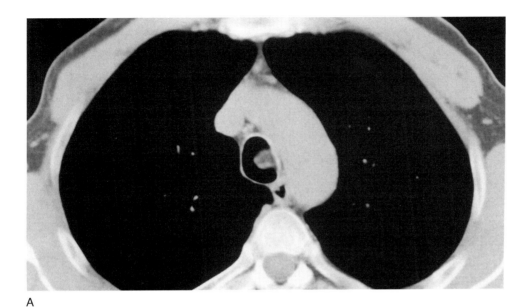

A

FIGURE 3-21A Tracheal Hamartoma. A 59-year-old male with a rounded density projecting into the tracheal lumen on a lateral chest radiograph. A. Transverse CT section shows a mass within the trachea containing fat.

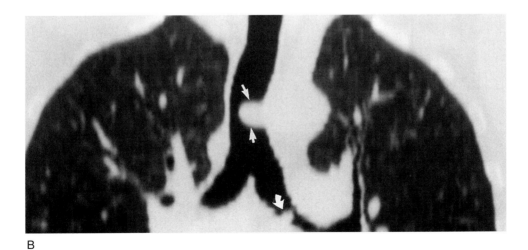

B

FIGURE 3-21B Coronal reconstruction through the trachea generated from spiral CT data reveals two endoluminal masses (arrows). Their length and location are precisely defined prior to surgery. The larger proximal lesion is a tracheal hamartoma (double arrows) and the second lesion in the left main bronchus a granulomatous web (curved arrow).

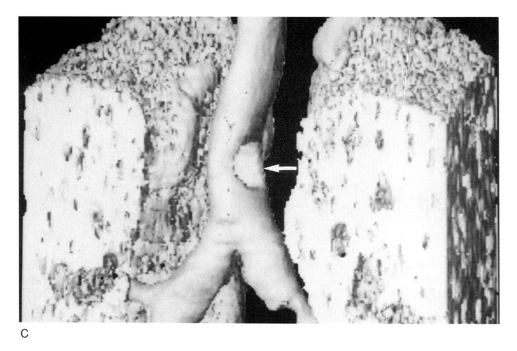

FIGURE 3-21C A surface-shaded 3-D image generated using reconstructions at one mm increments shows the mass projecting into the tracheal lumen (arrow).

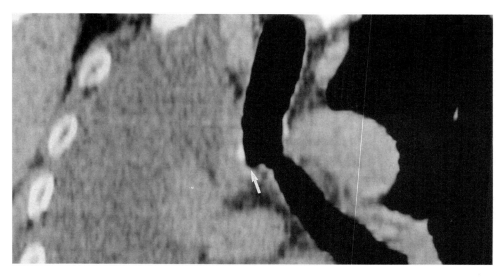

FIGURE 3-22 Postpneumonectomy Appearance. A 58-year-old male, status postpneumonectomy, who was studied because of persistent cough. A coronal reconstruction through the trachea confirms the resection site to be intact (arrow). Note the smooth contours caused by the lack of respiratory misregistration and the use of one mm reconstruction intervals.

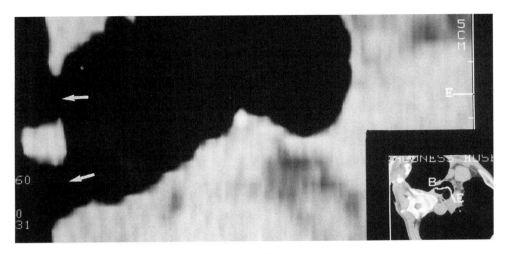

FIGURE 3-23 Bronchopleural Fistula. A 56-year-old male, status post right pneumonectomy for adenocarcinoma. He presents six months after surgery and radiation therapy with a large air collection in the right pleural space indicative of a bronchopleural fistula. Curved coronal reconstruction through the carina and right mainstem bronchus confirms two communications into the pleural space (arrows). This coronal reconstruction assisted surgical planning.

pulmonary veins. Our spiral CT technique uses five mm collimation and five mm incrementation with reconstructions at three mm intervals beginning at the bifurcation of the right upper lobe bronchus and ending at the level of the inferior pulmonary veins.

Transbronchial biopsy procedures are facilitated by the use of spiral CT which acts as a road map (Figure 3-24) or in assessing patients with central tumors to predict those who will benefit from photodynamic therapy by delineating tumor extent (Figure 3-25).[97] "Virtual bronchoscopy" is a computer simulation technique for viewing spiral CT data from the perspective of a bronchoscopist.[98] It can provide a road map prior to bronchoscopy and assist in planning transbronchial biopsy as both endobronchial and peribronchial structures can be displayed at the same level by rendering the airway walls transparent. Advances in computer technology will reduce the postprocessing time, and new methods for effective image segmentation of soft tissues are being developed.

Spiral CT with multiplanar and minimum intensity projection reconstructions has proven to be extremely valuable following lung transplantation.[99,100] Complications at sites of tracheobronchial anastomoses are common after lung transplantation. Small peribronchial air collections indicating dehiscence may be detected on overlapping axial spiral CT sections even when conventional CT is normal. Larger areas of dehiscence requiring stenting to prevent delayed stricture formation are best shown on minimum intensity projection images (Figure 3-26). The length and width of bronchial stenoses and the location of stents (Figure 3-27) are best shown on multiplanar reconstructions along the axis of a bronchus.

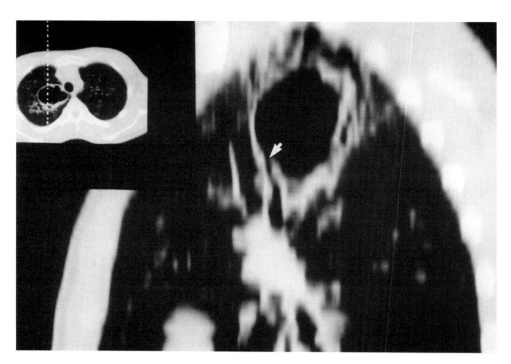

FIGURE 3-24 Lung Abscess. Sagittal reconstruction through a cavitary lesion in the right lung confirms the apical segmental bronchus communicates with it directly (arrow) facilitating transbronchial sampling.

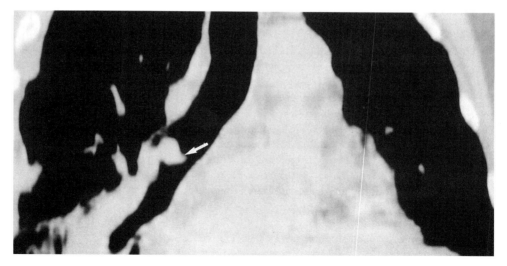

FIGURE 3-25 Endobronchial Metastasis. Oblique coronal reconstruction from spiral CT scan shows an endobronchial metastasis (arrow) from a renal cell carcinoma. Images used during laser resection.

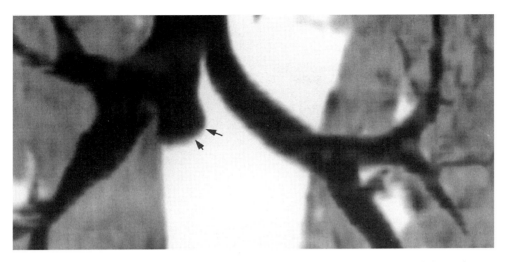

FIGURE 3-26 Bronchial wall dehiscence following lung transplantation. Coronal minimum intensity projection image through the carina after lung transplantation shows a large diverticulum (arrows) projecting from the inferior wall of the right mainstem bronchus requiring stent placement. *(Courtesy of Dr. C. M. Schaefer, Hanover, Germany.)*

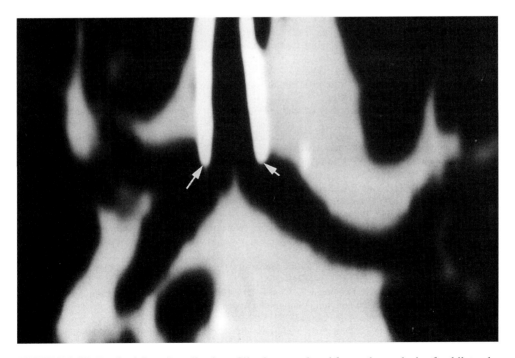

FIGURE 3-27 Tracheal Stent Localization. Silastic stent placed for tracheomalacia after bilateral lung transplantation. The stent is too low in position almost touching the carina (arrows). *(Courtesy of Dr. C. M. Schaefer, Hanover, Germany.)*

CONCLUSION

Spiral CT of the thorax has resulted in major refinements in our ability to detect and stage pulmonary neoplasms. The vascular applications of spiral CT have fueled a resurgence of interest in CT, but further investigation remains needed to determine if this breakthrough technology can replace existing methods of evaluation.

REFERENCES

1. Yock P, Soucek M, et al. Lung: spiral volumetric CT with single-breath-hold technique. *Radiology* 1990; **176:**864–867.
2. Kalender WA, Seissler W, et al. Spiral volumetric CT with single-breath-hold technique, continuous transport, and continuous scanner rotation. *Radiology* 1990; **76:**181–183.
3. Costello, Dupuy DE, Ecker CP, et al. Spiral CT of the thorax with reduced volume of contrast material: a comparative study. *Radiology* 1992; **183:**663–665.
4. Costello P, Ecker CP, Tello R, et al. Assessment of the thoracic aorta by spiral CT. *AJR* 1992; **158:**1127–1130.
5. Costello P, Kruskal J, Dupuy D, et al. Evaluation of the tracheobronchial tree with spiral CT (abstr). *Radiology* 1992; **185:**355.
6. Paranjpe DV, Bergin CJ. Spiral CT of the lungs. *AJR* 1994; **162:**561–567.
7. Steele JD. The solitary pulmonary nodule: report of a cooperative study of resected asymptomatic solitary pulmonary nodules in males. *J Thorac Cardiovasc Surg* 1963; **46:**21–39.
8. Toomes H, Delphendah A, Milne HG, et al. The coin lesion of the lung. A review of 955 resected coin lesions. *Cancer* 1983; **51:**534–537.
9. Costello P, Anderson W, Blume D. Pulmonary nodule: evaluation with spiral volumetric CT. *Radiology* 1991; **179:**875–876.
10. Cann CE. Quantitative accuracy of spiral versus discrete volume CT scanning (abstr). *Radiology* 1992; **85**(P):126–127.
11. Zerhouni EA, Stitik FP, Siegelman SS, Naidich DP, et al. CT of the pulmonary nodule: a comparative study. *Radiology* 1986; **160:**319–327.
12. Siegelman SS, Khouri NF, Leo FP, Fishman EK, et al. Solitary pulmonary nodules: CT assessment. *Radiology* 1986; **160:**307–312.
13. Naidich DP, Zerhouni EA, Siegelman SS. Focal lung disease, in Naidich DP, Zerhouni EA, Siegelman SS (eds) *Computed Tomography and Magnetic Resonance of the Thorax,* 2nd ed. Raven Press, New York, NY **1991:**303–340.
14. Gilbert HA, Kagan AR. Metastases: incidence, detection and evaluation without histologic confirmation, in Weiss L (ed) *Fundamental Aspects of Metastasis.* Amsterdam: North-Holland Publishing 1976.
15. Scholten ET, Kreel L. Distribution of lung metastases in the axial plane: a radiological-pathological study. *Radiol Clin* (Basel) 1977; **46:**248–265.
16. Schaner EG, Chang AE, Doppman JL, Conkle DM, Flye MW, Rosenberg SA. Comparison of computed and conventional whole lung tomography in detecting pulmonary nodules: a prospective radiologic–pathologic study. *AJR* 1978; **131:**51–54.
17. Peuchot M, Libshitz H. Pulmonary metastatic disease: radiologic-surgical correlation. *Radiology* 1987; **164:**719–722.
18. Sagel SS, Stanley RJ, Evans RG. Early clinical experience with motionless whole body computed tomography. *Radiology* 1976; **119:**321–330.
19. Muhm JR, Brown LR, Crowe JK. Detection of pulmonary nodules by computed tomography. *AJR* 1977; **128:**267–270.

20. Lund G, Heilo A. Computed tomography of pulmonary metastases. *Acta Radiol* 1982; **23**:617–620.
21. Gross BH, Glazer GM, Bookstein FL. Multiple pulmonary nodules detected by computed tomography: diagnostic implications. *J Comput Assist Tomogr* 1985; **9**:880–885.
22. Pass HI, Dwyer A, Makuch R, Roth JA. Detection of pulmonary metastases in patients with osteogenic and soft-tissue sarcomas: the superiority of CT scans compared with conventional linear tomograms using dynamic analysis. *J Clin Oncol* 1985; **3**:1261–1265.
23. Robertson PL, Boldt DW, DeCampo JF. Paediatric pulmonary nodules: a comparison of computed tomography, thoracotomy findings and histology. *Clin Radiol* 1988; **39**:607–610.
24. Chang AE, Schaner EG, Conkle DM, Flye MW, et al. Evaluation of computed tomography in the detection of pulmonary metastases: a prospective study. *Cancer* 1979; **43**:913–916.
25. Vanel D, Henry-Amar M, Lumbroso J, et al. Pulmonary evaluation of patients with osteosarcoma: roles of standard radiography, tomography, CT, scintigraphy and tomoscintigraphy. *AJR* 1984; **143**:519–523.
26. Krudy AG, Doppman JL, Herdt JR. Failure to detect a 1.5 centimeter lung nodule by chest computed tomography. *J Comput Assist Tomogr* 1982; **6**:1178–1180.
27. Cohen M, Grosfeld J, Baehner R, Weetman R. Lung CT for detection of metastases: solid tissue neoplasms in children. *AJR* 1982; **139**:895–898.
28. Gurney JW. Cross-sectional physiology of the lung. *Radiology* 1991; **178**:1–10.
29. Heywang-Koebrunner SH, Lommatzsch B, Fink U, Mayr B. Comparison of spiral and conventional CT in the detection of pulmonary nodules (abstr). *Radiology* 1992; **185**:131.
30. Remy-Jardin M, Remy J, Giraud F, Marquette CH. Pulmonary nodules. Detection with thick-section spiral CT versus conventional CT. *Radiology* 1993; **187**:513–520.
31. Meziane MA, Hruban RH, Zerhouni EA, Wheeler PS, Khouri NF, et al. High resolution CT of the lung parenchyma with pathologic correlation. *Radiographics* 1988; **8**(1):27–54.
32. Milne ENC, Zerhouni EA. Blood supply of pulmonary metastases. *J Thorac Imag* 1987; **2**(4):15–23.
33. Remy J, Remy-Jardin M, Giraud F, Wattinne L. Angioarchitecture of pulmonary arteriovenous malformations: clinical utility of three-dimensional helical CT. *Radiology* 1994; **191**:657–664.
34. White RI, Pollak JS, Pulmonary arteriovenous malformations: Diagnosis with three-dimensional helical CT— a breakthrough without contrast media. *Radiology* 1994; **191**:613–614.
35. Glazer HS, Duncan Mayer J, Aronberg DJ, Moran JF, et al. Pleural and chest wall invasion in bronchogenic carcinoma: CT evaluation. *Radiology* 1985; **57**:191–194.
36. Pennes DR, Glazer GM, Wimbish KJ, Gross BH, et al. Chest wall invasion by lung cancer: limitations of chest CT. *AJR* 1985; **144**:507–511.
37. Kuriyama K, Tateishi R, Kumatani T, Kodama K, Doi O, et al. Pleural invasion by peripheral bronchogenic carcinoma: assessment with three-dimensional helical CT. *Radiology* 1994; **191**:365–369.
38. Rosniak VH, Olson MC, Demos TC. Aortic motion artifact simulating dissection on CT scans: elimination with reconstructive segmented images. *AJR* 1993; **161**:557–558.
39. Posniak HV, Olsen MC, Demos TC, et al. CT of thoracic aortic aneurysm. *Radiographics* 1990; **10**:839–855.
40. Thorsen MK, San Dretto MA, Lawson TL, et al. Dissecting aortic aneurysms: accuracy of computed tomographic diagnosis. *Radiology* 1983; **148**:773–777.
41. Vasile N, Mathieu D, Keita K, Lellouche D, et al. Computed tomography of thoracic aortic dissection: accuracy and pitfalls. *J Comput Assist Tomogr* 1986; **10**:211–215.
42. Nienaber CA, von Kodolitsch Y, Nicolas V, et al. The diagnosis of thoracic aortic dissection by noninvasive imaging procedures. *N Engl J Med* 1993; **328**:1–9.
43. Nienaber CA, Spielmann RP, von Kodolitach Y, et al. Diagnosis of thoracic aortic dissection: magnetic resonance imaging versus transesophageal echocardiography. *Circulation* 1992; **85**:434–447.
44. Tello R, Costello P, Ecker C, Hartnell G. Spiral CT evaluation of coronary artery bypass graft patency. *J Comput Tomogr* 1993; **17**(2):253–259.
45. Kazerooni EA, Bree RL, Williams DM. Penetrating atherosclerotic ulcers of the descending thoracic aorta: evaluation with CT and distinction from aortic dissection. *Radiology* 1992; **183**:759–765.

46. Welch TJ, Stanson AW, Sheedy PF II, et al. Radiologic evaluation of penetrating aortic atherosclerotic ulcer. *Radiographics* 1990; **10**:675–685.
47. Yucel EK, Steinberg FL, Egglin TK, et al. Penetrating aortic ulcers: diagnosis with MR imaging. *Radiology* 1990; **177**:779–781.
48. Freiman DG, Suyemoto J, Wessler S. Frequency of pulmonary thromboembolism in man. *N Engl J Med* 1965; **272**:1278–1280.
49. Dalen JE, Alpert JS. Natural history of pulmonary embolism. *Prog Cardiovasc Dis* 1975; **17**:259–270.
50. Hermann RE, Davis JH, Holden WD. Pulmonary embolism: a clinical and pathologic study with emphasis on the effect of prophylactic therapy with anticoagulants. *Am J Surg* 1961; **102**:19–28.
51. Morrell MT, Truelove SC, Barr A. Pulmonary embolism. *Br Med J* 1963; **2**:830–835.
52. Remy-Jardin M, Remy J, Wattinne L, Giraud F. Central pulmonary thromboembolism: diagnosis with spiral volumetric CT with the single-breath-hold technique—comparison with pulmonary angiography. *Radiology* 1992; **185**:381–387.
53. PIOPED investigators. Value of the ventilation/perfusion scan in acute pulmonary embolism. *JAMA* 1990; **263**:2753–2759.
54. Hull RD, Hirsch J, Carter CJ, et al. Diagnostic value of ventilation/perfusion lung scanning in patients with suspected pulmonary embolism. *Chest* 1985; **88**:819–827.
55. Hanson MW, Coleman RE. Pulmonary nuclear medicine evaluation of thromboembolic disease. *J Thorac Imaging* 1989; **4**:40–57.
56. Spies WG, Burnstein SP, Dillehay GL, Vogelzang RL, Spies SM. Ventilation-perfusion scintigraphy in suspected pulmonary embolism: Correlation with pulmonary angiography and refinement of criteria of interpretation. *Radiology* 1986; **159**:383–390.
57. White RD, Winkler ML, Higgins CB. MR imaging of pulmonary arterial hypertension and pulmonary emboli. *AJR* 1987; **149**:15–21.
58. Ovenfors CO, Batra P. Diagnosis of peripheral pulmonary emboli by MR imaging; an experimental study in dogs. *Magn Reson Imaging* 1988; **6**:487–491.
59. Shah HR, Buckner B, Purness GL, Walker CW. Computed tomography and magnetic resonance imaging in the diagnosis of pulmonary thromboembolic disease. *J Thorac Imaging* 1989; **4**:58–61.
60. Sinner NW. Computed tomographic patterns of pulmonary thromboembolism and infarction. *J Comput Assist Tomogr* 1978; **2**:395–399.
61. Godwin JD, Webb WR, Gamsu G, Ovenfors CO. Computed tomography of pulmonary embolism. *AJR* 1980; **135**:691–695.
62. Ovenfors CO, Godwin JD, Brito AC. Diagnosis of peripheral pulmonary emboli by computed tomography in the living dog. *Radiology* 1981; **141**:519–523.
63. Sinner WN. Computed tomography of pulmonary thromboembolism. *Eur J Radiol* 1982; **2**:8–13.
64. DiCarlo LA, Schiller NB, Herfkens RL, Brundage BH, Lipton MJ. Noninvasive detection of proximal pulmonary artery thrombosis by two-dimensional echocardiography and computed tomography. *Am Heart J* 1982; **104**:879–881.
65. Breatnah E, Stanley RJ. CT diagnosis of segmental pulmonary artery embolus. *J Comput Assist Tomogr* 1984; **8**:762–764.
66. Goodman LR, Gurney J. Computed tomography of pulmonary thromboembolism and infarction. *J Comput Assist Tomogr* 1988; **12**:533–559.
67. Kalebo P, Wallin J. Computed tomography in massive pulmonary embolism. *Acta Radiol* 1989; **30**:105–107.
68. Quinn MR, Lundell CJ, Klotz TA, et al. Reliability of selective pulmonary arteriography in the diagnosis of pulmonary embolism. *AJR* 1987; **149**:469–471.
69. Newman GE. Pulmonary angiography in pulmonary embolic disease. *J Thorac Imaging* 1989; **4**:28–39.
70. National Heart and Lung Institute. The Urokinase Pulmonary Embolism Trial: a national cooperative study. *Circulation* 1973; **47**(suppl 2):1–108.
71. Mills SR, Jackson DC, Older RA, Heaston DK, Moore AV. The incidence, etiologies, and avoidance of complications of pulmonary angiography in a large series. *Radiology* 1980; **136**:295–299.

72. Remy-Jardin M, Remy J, Wattinne L, Giraud F. Central pulmonary thromboembolism: diagnosis with spiral volumetric CT with the single breath-hold technique: comparison with pulmonary angiography. *Radiology* 1992; **185**:381–387.
73. Schwickert VH, Schweden F, Schild H, Duber C, Iversen S. Darstellung der chronisch rezidivierenden lungenembolie mit der spiral CT. *Fortschr Rontgenstr* 1993; **158**(4):308–313.
74. Geraghty JJ, Stanford W, Landas SK, Galvin JR. Ultrafast computed tomography in experimental pulmonary embolism. *Invest Radiol* 1992; **27**:60–63.
75. Rooholamini SA, Galvin JR, Stanford W. Ultrafast CT for detection of intracardiac and proximal pulmonary artery thromboembolism (abstr). *Radiology* 1989; **173**(P):481.
76. Teigen CL, Maus TP, Sheedy PF, Johnson CM, et al. Pulmonary embolism: diagnosis with electron beam, CT. *Radiology* 1993; **188**:839–845.
77. Auger WR, Fedullo PF, Moser KM, Buchbinder M, Peterson KL. Chronic major-vessel thromboembolic pulmonary artery obstruction: appearance at angiography. *Radiology* 1992; **182**:393–398.
78. Brown KT, Bach AM. Paucity of angiographic findings despite extensive organized thrombus in chronic thromboembolic pulmonary hypertension. *JVIR* 1992; **3**:99–102.
79. Brink J, Heiken JP, Semenkowich J, Teefey SA, et al. Abnormalities of the diaphragm and adjacent structures: findings on multiplanar spiral CT scans. *AJR* 1994; **163**:307–310.
80. Plunkett ME, Bornstein BA, Costello P, Kjewski PK, Harris JR. Use of spiral CT in the assessment of cardiac structures for planning 3-D volumetric radiation treatment of the breast (abstr). *Radiology* 1993; **189**:355.
81. Lee K, Im J-G, Bae WK, et al. CT anatomy of the lingular segmental bronchi. *J Comput Assist Tomogr* 1991; **15**:86–91.
82. Naidich DP, Terry PB, Stitik FP, Siegelman SS. Computed tomography of the bronchi: 1. Normal anatomy. *J Comput Assist Tomogr* 1980; **4**:746–753.
83. Naidich DP, Zinn WL, Ettenger NA, McCauley DI, Garray SM. Basilar segmental bronchi: thin-section CT evaluation. *Radiology* 1988; **169**:11–16.
84. Lee KS, Bae WK, Lee BH, Kim HY, Choi EW, Lee BH. Bronchovascular anatomy of the upper lobes: evaluation with thin-section CT. *Radiology* 1991; **181**:765–772.
85. Bhalla M, Noble ER, Shepard JAO, McLoud T. Normal position of trachea and anterior junction line on CT. *J Comput Assist Tomogr* 1993; **17**:714–718.
86 Morrison SC. Demonstration of tracheal bronchus by computed tomography. *Clin Radiol* 1988; **39**:208–209.
87. McGinness G, Naidich DP, Garay SM, Davis AL, Boyd AD. Accessory cardiac bronchus: CT features and clinical significance. *Radiology* 1993; **189**:563–566.
88. Murakami J, Murayama S, Tori Y, Masuda K. Three-dimensional images of tracheobronchial diseases obtained with helical CT (abstr). *Radiology* 1993; **189**(P):436.
89. Davis SD, Maldjian C, Perone RW, Yankelevitz DF, Knapp PH, Henschke CI. CT of the airways. *Clin Imag* 1990; **14**:280–300.
90. Gamsu G, Webb WR. Computed tomography of the trachea and mainstem bronchi. *Semin Roentgenol* 1983; **18**:51–60.
91. Henschke CI, Davis SD, Auh PR, Westcott J, Berkman YM, Kazam E. Detection of bronchial abnormalities: comparison of CT and bronchoscopy. *J Comput Assist Tomogr* 1987; **11**:432–435.
92. Naidich DP, Lee JJ, Garay SM, McCauley DI, Aranda CP, Boyd AD. Comparison of CT and fiberoptic bronchoscopy in the evaluation of bronchial disease. *AJR* 1987; **148**:1–7.
93. McGinness G, Naidich DP, McAuley DI. Bronchiectasis: CT evaluation (pictorial essay). *AJR* 1993; **160**:253–259.
94. Naidich DP, Funt S, Ettenger NA, Arranda C. Hemoptysis: CT-bronchoscopic correlations in 58 cases. *Radiology* 1990; **177**:357–362.
95. McGinness G, Beacher JR, Harkin TJ, Garay SM, Rom WN, Naidich DP. Hemoptysis: prospective high-resolution CT/bronchoscopic correlation. *Chest* 1994 (in press).

96. Millar A, Boothroyd A, Edwards D, Hetzel M. The role of computed tomography (CT) in the investigation of unexplained hemoptysis. *Respir Med* 1992; **86**:39–44.
97. Gelb AF, Aberle DR, Schein MJ, Naidich DP, Epstein JD. Computed tomography and bronchoscopy in chest radiographically occult main-stem neoplasm: diagnosis and Nd-YAG laser treatment in 8 patients. *West J Med* 1990; **153**:385–389.
98. Vining DJ, Padhani AR, Wood MS, Zerhouni EA, Fishman EK, Kuhlman JE. Virtual bronchoscopy: a new prospective for viewing the tracheobronchial tree (abstr). *Radiology* 1993; **189**(P):438.
99. Schaefer CM, Prokop M, Doehring W, et al. Spiral CT of the tracheobronchial system: optimized technique and clinical applications (abstr). *Radiology* 1991; **181**(P):274.
100. Schaefer CM, Prokop M, Charvan A, Schafers J, Zink C, Galanski M. Spiral CT of anastomotic complications after lung transplantation (abstr). *Radiology* 1993; **189**(P):263.

Chapter 4

Abdomen and Pelvis

Robert K. Zeman / Paul M. Silverman

INTRODUCTION

As helical scanning techniques have been refined, so has our ability to detect abdominal and pelvic pathology. This chapter will focus on the helical scan methodology and clinical utility of helical CT in a wide range of abdominal disease processes. Several recurrent themes will be apparent; adapting contrast administration strategies to take advantage of the speed of helical CT, overlapping reconstruction, and 3-D rendering are all important for optimal use of this new technology.[1]

ADVANTAGES AND DISADVANTAGES OF HELICAL CT

For scanning the abdomen, helical CT has both advantages and disadvantages. The speed of helical CT is a major advantage. Using conventional "stop-and-go" scanners, it may require two to three minutes to scan the liver and even longer to scan the entire abdomen. During helical CT, it takes 20 to 30 sec to scan the liver depending on the collimation used. While speed results in improved throughput, it also results in improved recognition of abnormalities because the entire scan can be acquired while contrast levels are at or near their peak. The ability to detect tumors in the liver and pancreas requires that scanning be completed prior to significant contrast equilibration with the extracellular water. *Contrast equilibration is the enemy of diagnosis.* Scans acquired between one and two minutes after the start of the contrast injection will result in the greatest diagnostic accuracy. For the radiologist who performs abdominal CT, this is the "golden" minute. The principles of contrast dynamics are found in detail later in this chapter.

Another advantage of helical CT is its reduction of misregistration artifacts compared to conventional, nonhelical CT. During conventional CT scanning, the patient will exhale then inhale before each individual section or cluster of sections. While many patients are consistent in their degree of inspiration, many are not. This can result in uneven spacing of the sections, potential gaps in coverage, and even failure to detect small structures or abnormalities.[2] Because helical scans are acquired as a single, prolonged x-ray exposure during a single, prolonged breath-hold, misregistration is minimized. In 50 patients we evaluated by both helical and nonhelical CT, misregistration was present on only one helical scan, but on 12 nonhelical scans.[2] For patients who cannot hold their breath for a full 30 sec, breathing intervals can be added (Figure 4-1), but this does increase the risk of misregistration.

Because helical scanning results in a volumetric acquisition, scans may be reconstructed at any location and with any spacing over the length of the helix. This may be potentially of value in visualizing small structures such as vessels or small abnormalities by reducing partial volume averaging. The collimation (slice thickness) is prospectively

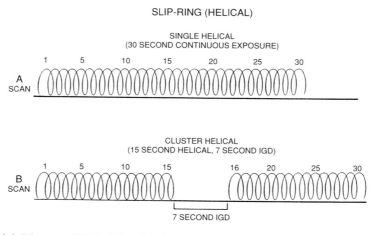

FIGURE 4-1 Diagram of Helical Scan Timing. A. Most helical scans are done as a single prolonged exposure of 30 or 32 sec. Because the exposure is made during a single breath-hold, there will be minimal misregistration artifact. B. In patients who cannot hold their breath for the full duration of the helical exposure, the helix may be briefly paused for a short breathing interval. We find that a minimum of seven sec is necessary for the patient to inhale and exhale. The patient should be instructed to take approximately the same depth of inspiration during this breathing interval as taken prior to the beginning of the helical scan. This will help minimize misregistration that might occur during the pause in exposure. Some vendors call the brief interval when scanning is paused the "intergroup delay" (IGD).

set prior to beginning the scan acquisition, but the spacing may be selected at any time, prior to or even after the scan has been completed. The raw data files must still be on-line (stored on a system disk or other magnetic hard disk) to allow reconstruction of images with varied spacing. Most vendors preserve the raw data for several hours after acquisition for this purpose.

If the selected reconstruction spacing is less than the collimation that was used, overlapping sections will result. We do not routinely view overlapping scans, but they are useful in selected cases. For example, when scanning the liver, we routinely use seven mm collimation and prospectively reconstruct the scans at seven mm intervals. The images which result have no overlap. They are filmed, interpreted and archived (on both film and optical disk). If an area of suspected abnormality associated with partial volume averaging is identified, a second set of scans will be reconstructed at three or four mm intervals. This increases the number of images in the set of scans by approximately 50 percent, compared to the set reconstructed without overlap. The additional sections lie "in-between" those of the initially reconstructed scans. As will be shown later in this chapter, these "in-between" scans often show structures and abnormalities not seen on sections reconstructed without overlap.

One of the most exciting advantages of helical CT is the ability to render high-quality three-dimensional models using graphics workstations. In the abdomen this has been most useful in the evaluation of the vascular system, especially for detection of renal artery stenosis, tumor encasement of major vessels, and extent of abdominal aortic aneurysms.

The key to high-quality 3-D rendering is use of overlapping source images. Prior to helical CT this could only be accomplished by acquiring overlapping scans as individual sections. This entailed a substantially increased radiation exposure to the patient. In helical CT the radiation dose is not increased, because the overlapping sections are created by interpolation and shifting the center of the reconstructed slice, not additional x-ray exposure. Within the computational limits of the workstation, increasing overlap reduces aliasing (jagged edges and a stairstep appearance to the model). Use of thin collimation and at least 40 percent overlap results in photogenic and accurate models for diagnostic interpretation and surgical planning. The techniques and clinical applications of 3-D will be discussed in this chapter and partially in chapter 6.

There are two disadvantages associated with helical CT. The first is a minor disadvantage which is no longer of clinical significance due to refinements in reconstruction algorithms. As discussed in chapter 1, the section sensitivity profile (i.e., effective slice thickness) for scans reconstructed from helical data is slightly greater than that for nonhelically acquired scans. In theory this could produce blurring and partial volume averaging artifacts. Using the older 360° linear interpolation algorithm, the section sensitivity profile for spiral CT was up to 30 percent greater than the nominal slice thickness. In other words, a five mm nominal slice thickness would have an effective slice thickness of six and a half mm. Most vendors now use newer reconstruction algorithms such as 180° linear interpolation. With this algorithm, broadening of the slice thickness is minimal, except when scanning with increased pitch. When blinded observers compared 1:1 pitch helical scans reconstructed with 180° linear interpolation to nonhelical scans in 50 patients, there was no significant difference in image quality, nor could they distinguish which scans were helical versus nonhelical (Figure 4-2). Thus, the increased effective slice thickness seen during helical or spiral CT is not clinically significant when using 1:1 pitch.

The second disadvantage of helical CT is of greater significance. Because of heat accumulation during the x-ray exposure, there are limitations in tube current and the length of exposure. The latter is important because it directly translates into limitations of coverage in the z-direction (from head to foot). While many vendors have extended the length of

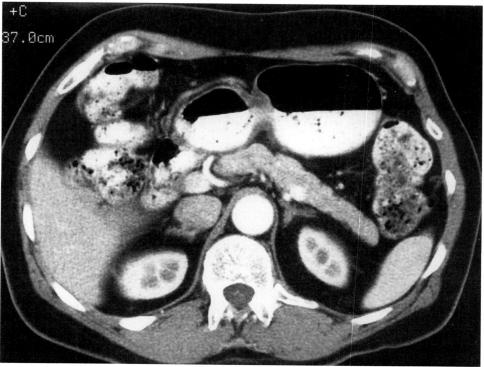

A

FIGURE 4-2A Image Quality of Helical Versus Nonhelical Scans. A. Because helical scans were initially felt to have a slightly wider beam profile, concerns were expressed that image quality might not be as good as that for conventional scans. To the contrary, we have found no difference in helical versus nonhelical image quality in routine clinical practice. This seven mm collimation scan shows excellent vascular opacification. There is no evidence of blurring of small structures such as the adrenal glands or pancreas.

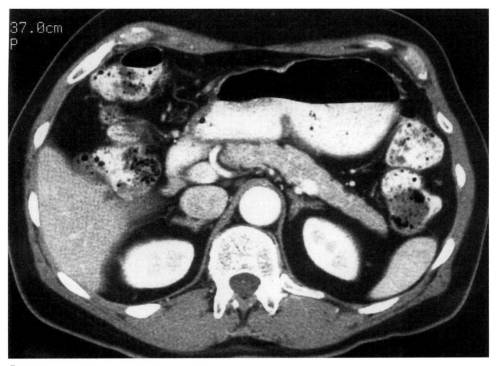

B

FIGURE 4-2B Nonhelical scan in the same patient shows comparable image quality. This scan was performed later than the section in 2A. This accounts for the slightly lower level of vascular contrast. Experienced radiologists could not differentiate the helical from nonhelical sections during blind review.

their helical scan up to 60 sec or more, usually only 32 sec or less may be performed at the maximum milliAmperage. Scanning beyond 32 sec may require lowering the milli-Amperage to potentially unacceptable levels.

As was stressed in chapter 1, there is an inherent relationship between the coverage, length of exposure, collimation, and pitch. During a 32-sec exposure using one cm collimation and table incrementation of one cm/sec, 32 cm of z-direction coverage will be achieved (32 sec × 1cm/sec = 32 cm). If five mm collimation is used, the coverage during an exposure of the same duration would decrease to 16 cm (32 sec × .5 cm/sec = 16 cm). This example illustrates how use of thin collimation during helical or spiral scanning can introduce coverage constraints. While increasing the pitch (by increasing the rate of table travel) can offset some of these constraints, it introduces other problems such as increased partial volume averaging. As we discuss our scanning techniques in the abdomen, some of these considerations will be presented in detail.

INDICATIONS AND RECOMMENDED SCANNING TECHNIQUES

Virtually all of our abdominal studies are performed helically. The only exception to this is when CT is used as guidance for abdominal interventional procedures. Although helical scanning allows rapid localization of the needle tip for intervention, this is also easily accomplished by conventional CT. We believe it is important to tailor the examination of the abdomen based on the clinical indication. The quality of the exam and its diagnostic accuracy ultimately depends on the scanning parameters which have been selected. In helical CT, the positioning of the helix, the collimation, the pitch ratio, exposure factors, and reconstruction parameters all affects exam quality.

There are six common clinical situations that we encounter in our practice and for which CT of the abdomen is requested. These are: (1) routine survey of the abdomen for nonspecific symptoms, symptoms suggestive of an inflammatory process or acute abdomen, and/or trauma; (2) metastatic survey of the abdomen, chest, and pelvis; (3) metastatic survey focused on the liver; (4) suspected pancreatic or biliary disease; (5) suspected renal mass; and (6) suspected vascular abnormality such as abdominal aortic aneurysm, aneurysm of other vessels, or renal artery stenosis. The exam techniques for the first two areas will be presented in tabular form (Tables 4-1, 4-2), and discussed in detail in this section. Technique tables for the other clinical indications (Tables 4-3–4-5) will be presented here but discussed later in this chapter. Evaluation of the vascular system will be presented in chapter 6 because of its relation to 3-D CT Angiography.

Routine Survey Exam

The routine survey exam encompasses a wide range of clinical indications, ranging from nonspecific symptoms to symptoms of an acute abdominal process or even trauma. In general we will conduct all abdominal studies as helical exams which begin at the diaphragm and end at the level of the iliac crest (Table 4-1). If the pelvis is to be studied, as we routinely do in trauma or the acute abdomen, we will usually perform the pelvic portion of the study nonhelically. Philosophically, we feel the speed of helical scanning is not necessary for scanning the pelvis, because contrast equilibration is not an issue. On the GE HiSpeed scanner, the delay between completion of the helical abdominal scan and the beginning of the nonhelical pelvic scans is negligible. We will usually allow a short 7 to 10 sec breathing interval after completion of the helix before beginning the pelvic portion of the study. Because the delay between helical and nonhelical scans is so short, the contrast level within the pelvic vessels is excellent (Figure 4-3). The bladder is usually partially opacified. If bladder opacification is not adequate, a few delayed, nonhelical sections may be taken one to two minutes after conclusion of all the other images.

For those devices which do not allow a second helix or nonhelical scans to rapidly be performed after helical scans, scanning of the pelvis is problematic. There are two alternatives. The pelvis can be scanned as part of the abdominal helix using increased pitch ratio or collimation, so that the coverage includes the pelvis. Partial volume averaging may be present on the resulting scans and the bladder will usually not be opacified adequately. The second

TABLE 4-1 Protocol for routine abdominal scan

Scan mode	Helical
Gantry angulation	None
Scan parameters	120 kVp, 280 mA[a], 1 sec
Length of helical exposure	30 sec
Field of view	30 to 40 cm
Pitch	1:1[b]
Collimation	7 mm[c]
Number of sections	30 (approximate)
Area of interest	From diaphragm to iliac crest[d]
Patient instructions	Breath-hold in midinspiration[e]
Contrast	Prefer nonionic 300 mgI/mL
Volume	140 mL
Administration route	Intravenous via antecubital vein
Rate	2–3 mL/sec
Scan delay	70 sec[f]
Reconstruction algorithm	Standard
Reconstruction spacing	Equal to collimation[g]

[a] Minimum suggested mA on GE HiSpeed. Adjust appropriately for other scanners. Lower mA may be used in thin patients. If five mm collimation is used, sections will look photopenic, if less than 280 mA
[b] Increased pitch will cause undesirable partial volume averaging when used in conjunction with collimation beyond five mm
[c] If cannot achieve adequate z-axis coverage, use eight mm or one cm collimation
[d] Use scanogram to localize starting location. May scan cephalad to caudad or vice versa. If combined exam to include thorax, start at bottom of liver and scan cephalad as described in text
[e] If patient cannot hold breath, split helix with seven sec pause after 15 to 20 sec
[f] Optimal for two mL/sec injection. Reduce to 45 to 55 sec for three mL/sec
[g] Overlapping reconstruction at three mm intervals in selected cases

alternative is more prevalent. After scanning the abdomen helically, either a delayed second helix or delayed nonhelical scans of the pelvis are performed. The length of the delay will depend on the interval needed to allow for tube cooling, and for the software to reset to allow additional scanning. This interval could be as long as several minutes on some devices. While the vascular level of contrast will drop during this "waiting" interval, this is only clinically significant in patients with confusing anatomy or in whom adenopathy is difficult to distinguish from pelvic vessels. All the vendors who have not yet eliminated these types of "waiting" intervals are diligently attempting to address this problem.

For our routine survey studies of the abdomen we administer 900 mL of dilute oral barium to opacify the gastrointestinal tract. Six-hundred mL is given 30 to 45 min prior to the exam and 300 ml is given at the time of the exam. If perforation is possible, as in the setting of trauma, water soluble oral contrast is used. Intravenous contrast material is absolutely essential for evaluation of the abdomen. We inject two mL/sec via a mechanical

TABLE 4-2 Protocol for chest, abdomen, pelvis survey

Scan mode	Helical, followed by cluster nonhelical
Gantry angulation	None
Scan parameters	120 kVp, 280 mA[a], 1 sec
Length of helical exposure	50 sec
Field of view	30 to 40 cm
Pitch	1:1[b]
Collimation	7 mm chest/abdomen, 10 mm pelvis[c]
Number of sections	50 helical, 15 nonhelical (approximate)
Area of interest	From lung apex to symphysis[d]
Patient instructions	Breath-hold in midinspiration[e]
Contrast	Prefer nonionic 300 mgI/mL
Volume	140 mL
Administration route	Intravenous via antecubital vein
Rate	2–3 mL/sec
Scan delay	70 sec[f]
Reconstruction algorithm	Standard
Reconstruction spacing	Equal to collimation[g]

[a]Minimum suggested mA for abdomen and pelvis on GE HiSpeed. Adjust appropriately for other scanners. Lower mA may be used in thin patients. If five mm collimation is used for abdomen, sections will look photopenic, if less than 280 mA. For chest 220 to 250 mA acceptable.
[b]Increased pitch will cause undesirable partial volume averaging when used in conjunction with collimation beyond five mm
[c]If cannot achieve adequate z-axis coverage, use one cm collimation for abdomen and chest. Alternative for chest is to mix collimation within helix: ten mm at the lung apex and base and five mm at hila
[d]Use scanogram to localize starting location. Scan cephalad. Start at bottom of liver and scan as described in text. After helical scans return to iliac crest and scan nonhelically to symphysis
[e]Split helix with seven sec pause after completing abdomen (20 to 25 sec). Scan thorax after breathing interval
[f]Optimal for two mL/sec injection. Reduce to 45 to 55 sec for three mL/sec
[g]Overlapping reconstruction at three mm intervals in selected cases

power injector (Medrad Inc, Pittsburgh, PA), for a total dose of 120 to 150 mL. We routinely use either 60 percent ionic contrast or 300 mgI/mL nonionic contrast. The latter often results in a better exam with less motion due to nausea. In spite of better-quality exams, the high cost of nonionic contrast has forced many centers to switch back to ionic contrast. The reader is cautioned against using markedly smaller volumes or lesser concentrations of contrast. These will result in less vascular and hepatic enhancement than the doses and concentrations recommended throughout this chapter. If a power injector with only a 100 ml capacity is used, either 320 or 350 mgI/mL concentration nonionic contrast should be used.

For the routine survey exam, noncontrast sections are not routinely performed. Following a localizing "scanogram," the start of the helix is programmed to begin at the

TABLE 4-3 Protocol for focused exam of liver

Scan mode	Helical[a]
Gantry angulation	None
Scan parameters	120 kVp, 280 mA[b], 1 sec
Length of helical exposure	30 sec (40–45 sec for dual-phase)
Field of view	30 to 40 cm
Pitch	1:1[c]
Collimation	7 mm[d]
Number of sections	30 (40 to 45 for dual-phase)
Area of interest	From diaphragm to iliac crest[e]
Patient instructions	Breath-hold in midinspiration[f]
Contrast	Prefer nonionic 300 mgI/mL
Volume	140 mL
Administration route	Intravenous via antecubital vein
Rate	2–3 mL/sec
Scan delay	70 sec (25–35 sec for dual-phase)[g]
Reconstruction algorithm	Standard
Reconstruction spacing	Equal to collimation[h]

[a]Add noncontrast, nonhelical scans if breast cancer or known hypervascular primary tumor with suspected metastases

[b]Minimum suggested mA on GE HiSpeed. Adjust appropriately for other scanners. Lower mA may be used in thin patients. If five mm collimation is used, sections will look photopenic, if less than 280 mA

[c]Increased pitch will cause undesirable partial volume averaging when used in conjunction with collimation beyond five mm

[d]Five to eight mm collimation is acceptable

[e]Use scanogram to localize starting location. May scan cephalad to caudad or vice versa. If combined exam to include thorax, start at bottom of liver and scan cephalad as described in text. The abdomen below the liver may be scanned nonhelically if necessary

[f]If patient cannot hold breath for single phase study, split helix with seven sec pause after 15 to 20 sec. If dual-phase study, allow breathing between first and second phase

[g]Optimal for two mL/sec injection. If dual-phase study, begin second phase at 70 sec. For three mL/sec, reduce injection delay to 45 to 55 sec for single phase study. If dual phase study, scan at 25 and 55 sec for respective phases

[h]Can be viewed on console. Film at spacing equal collimation

diaphragm and extend inferiorly to the iliac crest. We use seven mm collimation routinely, although eight mm collimation can also be used. A 30-second exposure and a pitch ratio of one will easily allow the entire abdomen to be scanned (30-sec × 7 mm/sec = 21.0 cm of coverage). If only a 24-second or less exposure is allowed, coverage of the abdomen is more difficult but can be accomplished by either increasing the collimation to one cm or increasing the pitch ratio to 1.5:1. Both of these strategies negate some of the benefit of helical scanning, but still can result in acceptable images.

The milliAmperage used will vary for different devices; on the GE HiSpeed with solid state detectors of 80 percent efficiency, we will usually use 300 to 320 mA. Approximately

TABLE 4-4 Protocol for focused exam of pancreas

Scan mode	Nonhelical without contrast to localize pancrease, followed by helical
Gantry angulation	None
Scan parameters	120 kVp, 280 mA[a], 1 sec
Length of helical exposure	30 sec (40–45 sec for dual-phase)[b]
Field of view	30 to 40 cm
Pitch	1:1[c]
Collimation	5 mm[d]
Number of sections	30 (40 to 45 for dual-phase)
Area of interest	From below uncinate to diaphragm[e]
Patient instructions	Breath-hold in midinspiration[f]
Contrast	Prefer nonionic 300 mgI/mL
Volume	140 mL
Administration route	Intravenous via antecubital vein
Rate	2–3 mL/sec
Scan delay	70 sec (30–40 sec for dual-phase)[g]
Reconstruction algorithm	Standard
Reconstruction spacing	2 mm intervals[h]

[a]Minimum suggested mA on GE HiSpeed. Adjust appropriately for other scanners. Lower mA may be used in thin patients. If less than five mm collimation is used, sections will look photopenic, if less than 280 mA

[b]For dual-phase, carry second helix up through liver. If necessary because of tube cooling, complete liver nonhelically

[c]Increased pitch will cause partial volume averaging

[d]Some centers use three mm collimation

[e]Use noncontrast sections to localize bottom of pancreas. Scan from caudad to cephalad

[f]If patient cannot hold breath for single phase study, split helix with seven sec pause after 15 to 20 sec. If dual-phase study, allow breathing between first and second phase

[g]Optimal for two mL/sec injection. If dual-phase study, begin second phase at 70 sec. For three mL/sec, reduce injection delay to 45 to 55 sec for single phase study. If dual phase study, scan at 25 and 55 sec for respective phases

[h]May be reviewed on console. Film images reconstructed with five mm spacing

280 mA is the minimum current that will produce high-quality scans in all patients. Lower milliAmperes (200 to 250mA) may be acceptable, but only in thin patients. If collimation less than seven mm is to be used for specific indications, the milliAmperes should be increased to 300 or higher to maintain adequate photon flux. One hundred twenty kVp should be used. Some vendors suggest using 130 kVp to increase exposure without having to use high milliAmperage. This approach produces less heating of the x-ray tube and has proven useful on those scanners with tubes possessing inadequate heat capacity. Unfortunately, there have been insufficient validation studies showing that the reduction in contrast resolution at 130 kVp is clinically acceptable.

TABLE 4-5 Protocol for focused exam of kidney "Rule Out Renal Mass"

Scan mode	Helical[a]
Gantry angulation	None
Scan parameters	120 kVp, 280 mA[b], 1 sec
Length of helical exposure	30 sec
Field of view	30 to 40 cm
Pitch	1:1[c]
Collimation	5 mm[d]
Number of sections	30 (approximate)
Area of interest	From upper to lower pole of kidneys[e]
Patient instructions	Breath-hold in midinspiration[f]
Contrast	Prefer nonionic 300 mgI/mL
Volume	100–120 mL
Administration route	Intravenous via antecubital vein
Rate	2 mL/sec
Scan delay	70 sec[g]
Reconstruction algorithm	Standard
Reconstruction spacing	2 mm and 5 mm intervals[h]

[a]Nonconstrast scans should be performed nonhelically prior to helical scans. Use comparable collimation. Delayed nonhelical sections should be done approximately two min after helix

[b]Minimum suggested mA on GE HiSpeed. Adjust appropriately for other scanners. Lower mA may be used in thin patients. If less than five mm collimation is used, sections will look photopenic, if less than 280 mA

[c]Increased pitch will cause undesirable partial volume averaging when used in conjunction with collimation beyond five mm

[d]If cannot achieve adequate z-axis coverage, use seven mm collimation. May need to do additional thinner sections for CT numbers

[e]Use noncontrast scans to localize starting location. May scan cephalad to caudad or vice versa. If combined exam to include thorax, start at bottom of kidney and scan cephalad. May require reducing mA or completing theorax nonhelically

[f]If patient cannot hold breath, split helix with seven sec pause after 15 to 20 sec

[g]Optimal for two mL/sec injection.Reduce to 45 to 55 sec for three mL/sec

[h]May be reviewed on console. Film images reconstructed with five mm spacing

For the routine survey study, the images will be reconstructed at an interval equal to the collimation, i.e., seven mm collimation scans will be reconstructed at seven mm intervals. It is this set of reconstructed scans that are used for interpretation and archiving in the patient's film jacket. At times overlapping scans may provide additional information. We choose to reconstruct overlapping sections as a second series of scans, but view them only when equivocal or confusing findings are present. On most systems, these images may be reconstructed by the computer "in background," and results in no penalty or slowdown in acquiring additional sections. If the overlapping scans are not useful, they may

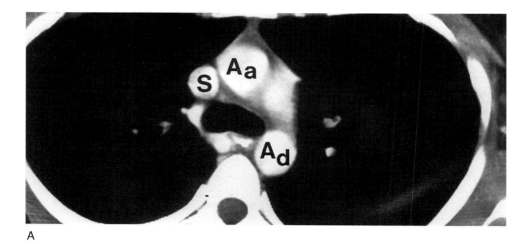

A

FIGURE 4-3A Excellent Vascular Opacification During a Combined Helical Examination of the Thorax, Abdomen, and Pelvis. A. Since the entire helical examination is rapidly performed, it is not uncommon to see excellent vascular opacification at all scan locations in a combined exam. This patient was studied using a 70-sec delay between the initiation of the contrast injection and scanning. The abdomen and thorax were scanned helically, followed by nonhelical sections through the pelvis. The ascending aorta (Aa) and descending aorta (Ad) are well opacified. The superior vena cava (S) is also clearly identified. Because this scan was obtained shortly after the conclusion of the contrast injection, the contrast within the superior vena cava is partially recirculated, and not giving rise to streak artifact.

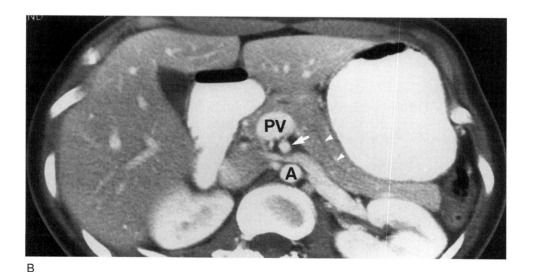

B

FIGURE 4-3B Uniform enhancement of the abdominal vessels is noted. The aorta (A), superior mesenteric artery (arrow), and portal vein (PV) are all well enhanced. By scanning with a 70-sec delay, the portal vein is near its peak enhancement. The normal sized pancreatic duct (arrowheads) is also identified.

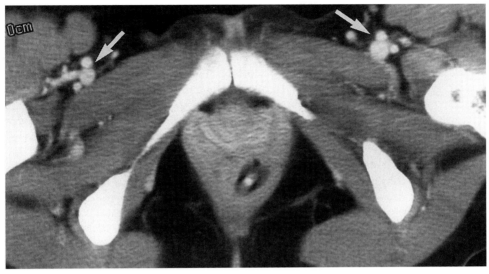

C

FIGURE 4-3C The pelvis was scanned with only a 10-sec delay after the conclusion of the helical sections through the abdomen and thorax. This means that only one to one and one-half minutes has elapsed from the end of the contrast injection before scanning the pelvis. The femoral arteries and veins (arrow) have high levels of contrast material. Enhancement of the vaginal and periurethral tissues is common when scanning with high levels of vascular contrast.

be electronically discarded. If reconstruction of overlapping scans does slowdown the acquisition of additional scans (this is true on some systems), overlapping sections should be reconstructed only in selected cases and at times when patients are not being scanned.

Metastatic Survey of the Chest, Abdomen, and Pelvis

Many of the principles for the complete evaluation of the oncologic patient are similar to those for the routine survey exam of the abdomen (Table 4-2). A full load of oral and intravenous contrast material is required. The scanning approach will vary depending upon the type of scanner used. In general the critical organ, with regard to contrast administration and scan timing, is the liver. Having enhancement of the vessels in the chest and pelvis is useful and simplifies interpretation of the scan. The precise timing in relation to the contrast injection, however, is not as important as for the liver, where scanning too early or late can mask significant disease.

Our goal is to scan the liver somewhere during the "golden minute," between one and two minutes following the start of the contrast injection. Scanning of the chest and pelvis must be done at times other than this crucial interval. While it may seem logical to scan through the chest prior to scanning the liver, on many devices this may not be the best approach for helical scanning, due to idiosyncrasies in x-ray tube cooling (see below).

We will use our full milliAmperage capability (300 to 320 mA on the GE HiSpeed) for the liver and scan helically from the bottom of the liver up to the diaphragm. The scan is started at 60 to 70 sec after beginning the contrast injection. It typically takes 20 to 25 sec, using seven mm collimation and 1:1 pitch, to scan the abdomen. If increased pitch or collimation is used, the exposure length will be reduced. We allow a short seven to ten sec breathing interval after the liver has been scanned, before continuing our scan up into the chest.

As scanning is continued into the chest we will reduce the milliAmperage to a lower level (usually 250 mA on the HiSpeed). Higher milliAmperage than this is not necessary in the chest where noise and quantum mottle are not a problem. The chest is studied during 20 to 30 sec of exposure with the scan continued to the level of the lung apices. If heat buildup prevents scanning the entire lung, we will either decrease our milliAmperage, increase the collimation, or scan the lung apices nonhelically after completion of the helix. We generally will not increase the pitch because of the real concern that pulmonary nodules may be obscured due to partial volume averaging.

Why not scan the chest first? In helical scanning, x-ray tubes cool faster when they are hotter. Using the higher milliAmperes setting first, for the abdomen, results in more efficient tube cooling. If the tube was "warmed up" by first scanning the chest, the tube cooling algorithm would try to protect the tube by limiting the jump in milliAmperes needed to scan the abdomen. This would compromise the quality of the abdominal study either because of increased noise or reduced coverage.

Once we have scanned the abdomen and chest, what about the pelvis? The entire chest and abdomen have been scanned in approximately 60 sec. Since scanning was begun about one minute into the contrast injection, there should still be very high levels of contrast in the pelvic vessels. When we scan the pelvis we do so nonhelically as cluster scans (three scans every seven sec followed by a short breathing interval).[3] We begin at the iliac crest and scan inferiorly to the bottom of the symphysis. Regardless if seven or 10 mm collimation is used, the entire pelvis can be scanned in about one minute. If the bladder is not adequately opacified, a few nonhelical delayed scans can be obtained.

Using this approach, the entire chest, abdomen, and pelvis are completed within three to four minutes of starting the contrast injection. Evaluation of the abdomen is optimized while vascular opacification is generally excellent in all areas scanned (Figure 4-3). Scanners that must introduce lengthy tube cooling or software delays between helices or helical and nonhelical scans may not allow use of this approach at the present time. Should that be the case on your scanner, it may be necessary to split the contrast injection or settle for suboptimal vascular opacification in the pelvis. CT vendors now increasingly understand that these delays are unacceptable and must be eliminated if helical CT is to be used effectively.

INTERPRETATION OF THE NORMAL STUDY, VARIANTS, AND PITFALLS

The major abdominal imaging and CT textbooks nicely address normal abdominal anatomy.[4-7] Specific anatomic features for the liver, pancreatobiliary system, and kidney will be discussed in those specific sections later in this chapter.

There are unique anatomic and physiologic features to be kept in mind when interpreting helical scans. Helical CT is very fast. Its easy to "beat" the intravenous contrast material to the abdomen if meticulous technique is not exercised. While there may be a role for early (20 to 40 sec) scanning of the liver (see below), the hepatic veins and even the portal venous branches may not be opacified prior to 60 to 70 sec. It is easy to confuse unopacified vessels with focal hepatic masses or even dilated biliary ducts (Figure 4-4). Even when using 60- to 70-sec contrast injection delays, poor mixing of contrast may be identified within major veins, such as the inferior vena cava (Figure 4-5) and superior mesenteric vein (Figure 4-6). For the inferior vena cava, mixing artifact may mimic clot especially at the level of the renal veins. Unopacified blood from the lower abdomen and

(Text continues on page 170)

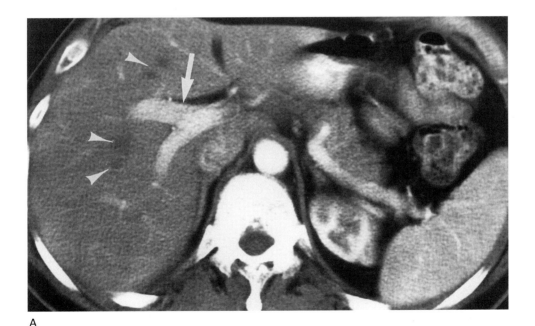

A

FIGURE 4-4A Unopacified Vessels Mimicking Space-Occupying Lesions in the Liver. A. CT scan 50 sec after contrast administration demonstrates dense opacification of the aorta and main portal vein (arrow). Multiple low attenuation areas in the liver could represent unopacified portal vein branches, hepatic veins, or small metastases (arrowheads).

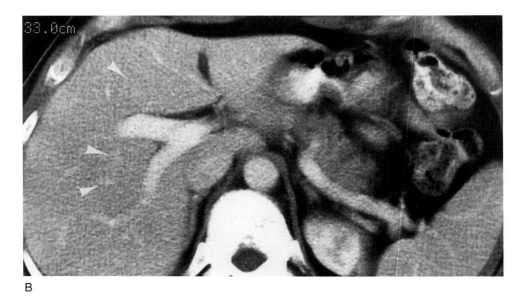

FIGURE 4-4B Scan at 75 sec demonstrates that these areas are opacified with contrast indicating that they simply represent vessels that were unopacified on the earlier scan (arrowheads).

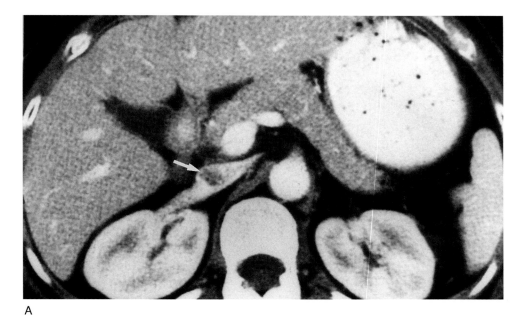

FIGURE 4-5A Inferior Vena Cava (IVC) "Pseudothrombosis." A. Scan early during the renal cortico-medullary phase demonstrates a low attenuation area in the IVC (arrow).

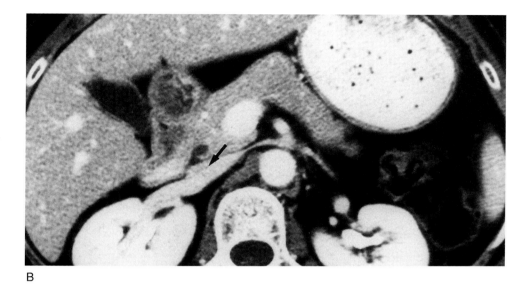

B

FIGURE 4-5 B Delayed scan shows more homogenous mixing within the IVC (arrow). It is important not to mistake mixing artifacts for thrombus.

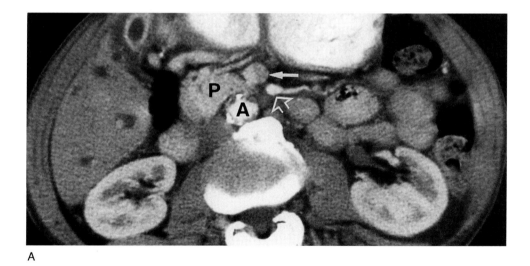

A

FIGURE 4-6A Poor Mixing of Contrast in the Superior Mesenteric Vein Mimicking Thrombus. A. Five mm collimation helical scan of the pancreas was performed using the dual phase technique. The first sections were obtained approximately 40 sec after the beginning of the contrast injection. While excellent opacification of the aorta (A) and superior mesenteric artery (open arrow) is noted, inhomogeneity of the superior mesenteric vein (solid arrow) is also seen. It is common on scans obtained early in the contrast injection to have incomplete opacification of the superior mesenteric vein. Unopacified blood from mesenteric venous branches or from the inferior mesenteric vein may contribute to this appearance. It is important not to mistake inhomogeneity for thrombus (P = uncinate portion of the pancreas).

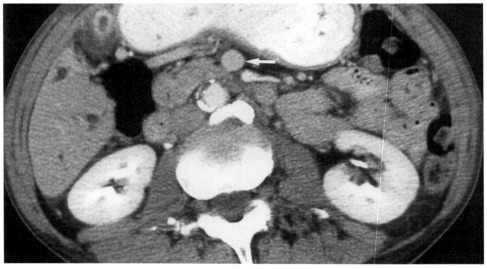

B

FIGURE 4-6B Delayed scan obtained approximately 40 sec later shows more uniform enhancement of the superior mesenteric vein (arrow). Obtaining slightly delayed scans will usually allow differentiation of true thrombus from pseudothrombus. At other levels a pancreatic mass was identified in this patient and was responsible for the biliary dilatation evident on these sections.

extremities produces a central defect within the cava, surrounded by more peripheral opacified blood entering via both renal veins. When this occurs, the appearance can be quite confusing, but is readily clarified by several delayed nonhelical views at this level. These are not routinely needed, but scans at two to three minutes can be useful; clot shows persistent low attenuation, while mixing artifacts become more uniform in appearance over time.

The kidney also poses a problem in terms of optimizing the scan timing. The renal cortex enhances early in the arterial phase, but the medulla may not be enhanced even as late as two minutes after initiation of the contrast injection. Because of its low attenuation, medullary tissue may be mistakenly called a mass. More commonly, the unenhanced medulla may hide low attenuation real masses (see Figure 4-29). The kidney must be scrutinized carefully even on routine screening studies. If there is any suspicion of a mass in the medulla, delayed, nonhelical scans should be obtained.

Reconstruction of overlapping sections is not only useful in recognition of pathology, but also in visualizing normal anatomy (Figure 4-7).[2] Small structures which follow a very horizontal (in-plane) course such as the pancreatic duct or renal arteries are frequently subject to partial volume averaging on nonoverlapping scans. Without overlap it may also

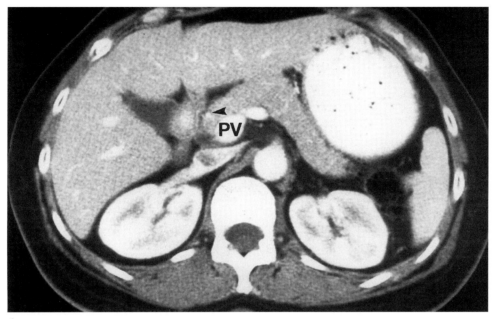

A

FIGURE 4-7A Use of Overlapping Sections to Delineate the Pancreatic Duct. A. This five mm collimation section obtained through the pancreas shows normal appearing parenchyma. The pancreatic duct is not identified. The portal vein (PV) and gastroduodenal artery (arrowhead) are identified.

be difficult to visualize these structures in their entirety. By reconstructing overlapping sections, the ability to see small structures is improved. In our recent series, the normal pancreatic duct was seen on overlapping sections in 87 percent of patients. Even structures that run perpendicular to the scan plane, such as the bile duct, are better evaluated with overlapping sections. We now visualize at least one segment of normal-sized extrahepatic bile ducts in nearly 100 percent of patients.

EVALUATION OF THE LIVER

The focused evaluation of the liver is one of the most common indications for helical CT. Before presenting our scanning protocol and the unique features of helical CT of the liver, we must discuss the evolution of contrast enhancement strategies. Early in the history of CT it was appreciated that intravenous contrast enhancement was valuable. It improved the confidence in detecting lesions, the ability to identify increased numbers of lesions,

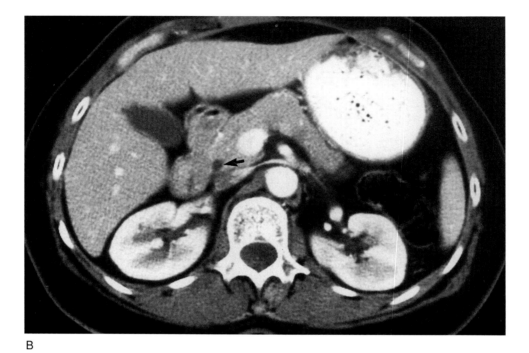

B

FIGURE 4-7B On this section five mm below that of 7A, the pancreatic duct is not seen. The normal common bile duct (arrow) is identified just above the ampulla.

and also the specificity of the examination.[8] Unfortunately, the road to determining the optimal method of hepatic contrast enhancement has been convoluted and controversial.

Contrast Administration in Hepatic CT: An Historical Perspective

Burgener and Hamlin defined what is now the classical three phases of contrast enhancement.[9] The bolus phase occurs when the difference between the aorta and inferior vena cava enhancement is greater than 30 Hounsfield units (H). A second phase, the nonequilibrium phase, is present when the aortic-vena cava attenuation difference drops to 10 to 30 H. This occurs one minute after a contrast bolus or early during a rapid drip infusion. The final or equilibrium phase corresponds to a less than 10 H difference, occurring two minutes after the bolus or following drip infusion. Burgener and Hamlin's results have been incorrectly extrapolated by some to mean that a drip infusion of contrast allows an indefinitely sustained nonequilibrium phase. This is not true. In fact, their work suggested that scanning in clinical practice should not be performed during a drip infusion or during the equilibrium phase.

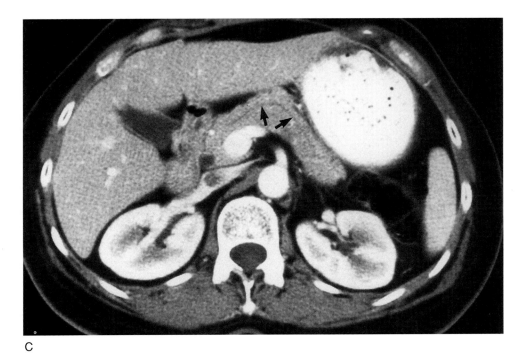

C

FIGURE 4-7C By reconstructing the sections using three mm spacing, this section was reconstructed two mm above that which is shown in Figure 4-7B. On this section the normal sized pancreatic duct (arrows) is identified. Altering the scan spacing is useful for detecting small anatomic structures as well as subtle pathology. While it is possible to specifically prescribe the location of reconstructed scans, we usually find that this is not necessary, and reconstruction of 40 to 60 percent overlapping scans will provide sufficient images. *(Courtesy of Zeman et al.[2])*

Young et al. specifically studied the bolus technique versus drip infusion technique for the detection of liver neoplasms.[10] They found that the best-quality images were obtained immediately after the bolus of contrast. Since contrast rapidly diffuses from vessels into the extravascular and interstitial spaces, these authors correctly identified the need to scan rapidly in order to optimally detect lesions in a clinical setting. Any delay in scanning resulted in lesions enhancing to a similar degree to the surrounding liver tissue and becoming isodense. They concluded that drip infusion should be avoided in hepatic scanning since lesions tended to become isodense three to five minutes after a bolus of contrast. This is the so-called phenomenon of the "disappearing lesion" (Figure 4-8). It is easy to miss lesions late after a bolus, on drip infusion scans, and on drip infusion scans following a loading bolus.[11] Equilibrium phase images can be readily identified when contrast is present within the collecting system of the kidneys and when there is little difference in attenuation between the aorta and inferior vena cava. This indicates that the scan is suboptimal for detecting liver pathology.

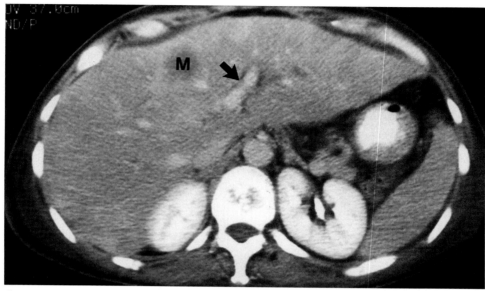

A

FIGURE 4-8A Contrast Equilibration Masking Hepatic Metastases Due to Breast Cancer. A. This scan was obtained nonhelically during a drip infusion of contrast material at another institution. Although contrast material is identified within the left portal vein (arrow), there is no significant difference in attenuation between the aorta and the inferior vena cava. Cortico-medullary differences in renal attenuation are also not identified. This signifies that we are likely to be within the equilibrium phase of contrast enhancement. There is evidence of hepatic inhomogeneity, and a solitary mass (M) on this section. No additional masses were identified at other levels. Incidental gastric wall thickening is also suspect for metastatic involvement in this patient with known breast cancer.

Despite mounting evidence in favor of using a bolus administration of contrast, a survey of members of the Society of Body Computed Tomography performed by Zeman et al. in 1988 indicated 41 percent of members scanned the liver during a drip infusion following a loading bolus.[12] This was deemed necessary since scanners could still not adequately image the entire liver during the nonequilibrium phase, and the drip portion of the examination allowed the continued administration of contrast while scanning other body parts. Since the time of that survey, faster conventional scanners and helical scanners have made this suboptimal method of administering contrast obsolete.

Our recent understanding of contrast dynamics comes from Foley et al. who have more accurately defined the three phases of contrast enhancement.[13] As a result of their work, it has generally been accepted that the bolus phase occurs during the time at which aortic enhancement is rapidly increasing. It lasts for approximately one minute. Aortic enhancement increases progressively during the bolus phase and then rapidly falls after the injection

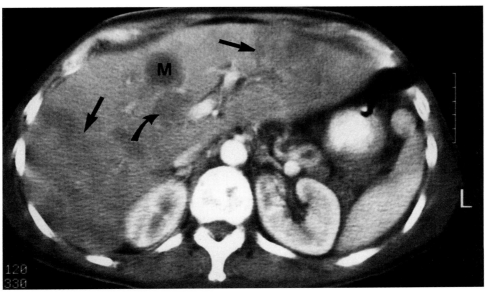

FIGURE 4-8B Because the patient was being considered for surgery, a repeat helical scan was performed two days following the scan shown in Figure 4-8A. The helical scan shows extensive replacement of the liver by tumor. The originally seen mass (M) is again noted. A second, more posterior mass (curved arrow) is also seen. Diffuse replacement of the posterior segment of the right lobe and lateral segment of the left lobe (arrows) is present. This case illustrates how important it is to scan during the nonequilibrium phase of contrast enhancement.

is concluded. A progressive rise in liver enhancement occurs during the bolus phase, representing both vascular and extravascular contrast material. The nonequilibrium phase follows the bolus phase and is of brief duration. During nonequilibrium, vascular enhancement declines rapidly, while hepatic parenchymal enhancement rises and reaches a plateau. Peak liver enhancement is maintained until late in the nonequilibrium phase even as the portal venous enhancement begins to diminish. The third phase of contrast enhancement, the equilibrium phase, is characterized by a slow decline in enhancement of the liver at a rate predicted by renal filtration. As defined by Foley and colleagues, this point occurs when the aortic and liver enhancement curves become parallel and decline at an equal rate (Figure 4-9).[13] It is possible to avoid scanning the liver during the equilibrium phase because liver enhancement maintains a rather broad enhancement plateau during nonequilibrium. Although there is a significant "optimal temporal window" for scanning of the liver, the duration of this window for both conventional and helical CT continues to be debated and may be shorter than originally thought.[14]

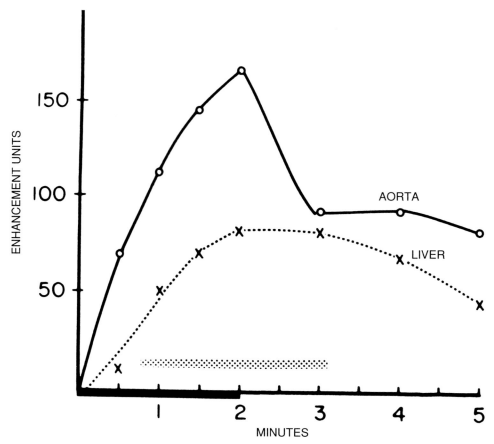

FIGURE 4-9 Aortic and Hepatic Enhancement Curves. During rapid contrast injection, the aorta rises rapidly in attenuation, while the liver undergoes a prolonged increase and sustained plateau. The stippled interval represents the nonequilibrium phase. Since helical scanning is best performed near the plateau of the hepatic curve, the early nonequilibrium phase is best not used for routine scanning. *(Courtesy of Foley et al.[13])*

Uniphasic Versus Biphasic Contrast Administration

Scanning is optimized through the use of a power injector. The power injector provides a reliable and reproducible means of administering contrast at rates that cannot be effectively achieved by any other mechanical means. Its safety and efficacy have been established based on many years of clinical experience.[15] There are two methods for injecting contrast material: uniphasic (monophasic) and biphasic. Each method has its advocates.

The most widely utilized technique for scanning the liver is a simple, uniphasic injection of contrast. Uniphasic implies injecting contrast at a constant rate (such as two mL/sec) for the entire volume. Most investigators have employed a dose equivalent of 150 mL of 60 percent contrast material. Those who use a biphasic injection will use an initial rate of three to five mL/sec for approximately 50 mL, followed by a much slower one mL/sec injection rate for a total of 150 mL. Proponents of a uniphasic injection state their technique is simpler, and with faster scanners allows the entire liver to be scanned while it is at approximately 70 percent or greater peak enhancement.[16] The uniphasic proponents also cite that their enhancement curve shows a higher peak enhancement than that achieved with biphasic injections (Figure 4-10). When we scan helically, we usually use a uniphasic injection.

The advocates of a biphasic injection rightfully claim that their technique provides a longer duration of hepatic enhancement and a wider temporal window for scanning (Figure 4-10).[17,18] The biphasic protocol has a distinct advantage in the case of slower scanners or when examinations of multiple body parts in addition to the liver are required on scanners with significant delays between helical and nonhelical image acquisitions. Since a helical scan of the liver requires only one-fourth to one-sixth of the time required

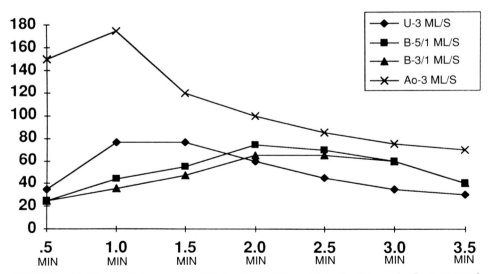

FIGURE 4-10 Hepatic Enhancement Utilizing Three Different Injection Protocols. Contrast may be injected uniphasically or biphasically. A uniphasic injection at a rate of three mL/sec (U-3 ml/sec) results in slightly greater enhancement than a biphasic injection utilizing a first phase of five mL/sec followed by one mL/sec (B-5/1 ml/sec) or a first phase injected at three mL/sec followed by one mL/sec (B-3/1 ml/sec). The hepatic enhancement plateau is of shorter duration for the uniphasic injection than for the biphasic injection. All three techniques allow excellent hepatic enhancement. (Ao-3 mL/sec = aortic enhancement during a uniphasic injection at a rate of three mL/sec).

for a conventional scan, sustaining nonequilibrium via a biphasic injection is not necessary on most helical scanners.

Practical Approach to Contrast Administration and Scanning Strategies for Helical CT

In our practice, evaluation of suspected metastatic disease is the most common indication for hepatic CT. Exclusion of other space-occupying masses, especially hepatoma, is also a common indication. We tailor our exam approach based on the clinical setting. Cases will be protocolled ahead of time so there is little confusion or delay once the patient is in the CT suite.

It has been suggested that metastatic lesions due to breast cancer or hypervascular primary tumors such as renal cell carcinoma may be seen better in some patients on noncontrast studies.[19,20] While this may be true, the previously published reports in this area did not use current contrast administration or scanning methodology. We are currently studying the role of noncontrast scans in patients with metastatic breast cancer and hypervascular tumors. Until those results are clear, performing noncontrast, nonhelical cluster scans through the liver prior to performing the helical scans in this group of patients is prudent. We use 7 to 10 mm collimation for these nonhelical scans. For patients with lesions that are likely to be hypovascular, such as metastatic colorectal cancer, we do not routinely perform noncontrast scans.

The liver is scanned helically from top to bottom, unless the study is performed in conjunction with CT of the thorax (Table 4-3). In that case, the liver will be scanned from bottom to top. If noncontrast scans were not performed, the top of the liver will be localized for the helical acquisition by the technologist viewing the "scanogram." The contrast is uniphasically injected at a rate of two to three mL/sec up to a total of 150 mL, depending on the patient's weight. We tend to use the higher injection rates in patients with potentially hypervascular lesions and in whom placement of a 20-gauge intravenous catheter is technically possible. At two mL/sec we find that a 70-sec delay between the initiation of the contrast injection and the start of the scan is ideal. This allows the liver to be near its peak enhancement. The vessels will also be well opacified and, therefore, not mistaken for small lesions. At three mL/sec, scanning can be initiated slightly sooner, at approximately 55 sec.

Most of our hepatic exams will be conducted as a single 30- to 32-sec helix through the liver. A number of centers are now studying the value of doing an early *and* late helix through the liver (also called dual phase scanning). It is believed that by doing two "passes" in this fashion, the sensitivity for detecting lesions will be improved, especially those that are hypervascular. Using this approach and injection rates as described above, the first helix should be done starting at 25 to 35 sec and the second helix at 60 to 70 sec. Each helix will be of 20 sec duration with at least a seven- to ten-sec breathing interval between the helices. We will discuss our experience with this technique later in this chapter.

When scanning the liver we would recommend use of seven to eight mm collimation. There is no clinical data showing that this results in statistically greater lesion detection than 10 mm collimation, but small lesions are definitely easier to see with the thinner collimation. It is best to use 1:1 pitch if that is available on your device. The milliAmperage should also be adjusted based on the patient size and the allowable duration of the helical exposure. On the GE HiSpeed we use approximately 300 mA. One hundred twenty kVp is used. The images are reconstructed without overlap, but in selected cases a set of images with 40 to 50 percent overlap will also be reconstructed. We photograph our images using a 350 H window width and a level of 20 to 40 H. We no longer find routine filming of liver windows at a 200 to 250 H window width necessary.

Before we leave our scanning strategy, a word of caution is in order about attempting to reduce contrast material volume. Cost considerations have become a major driving force in CT. We prefer to use nonionic contrast to avoid motion artifacts (due to nausea and vomiting) on helical scans and in cases potentially considered for 3-D reconstruction. A number of studies have attempted to answer the question: Can less than 150 mL of 60 percent contrast (or its equivalent) be used for liver imaging without significant compromise of the examination? We and others believe the answer is *no*. Unlike other organs, increased enhancement of the liver seems to directly translate into improved detection of lesions. Chambers et al. have found that when 100 mL of nonionic contrast was compared to 150 mL at various rates within the same patient, the use of 100 mL caused a significant decrease in hepatic enhancement, and thus may have a direct effect on tumor conspicuity.[21] Dupuy et al. found that with a 40 percent reduction in contrast material, they suffered a 25 percent decrease in attenuation of the liver which could compromise lesion detection.[22] In smaller patients (less than 60 Kg) less contrast, such as 125 mL, may be utilized with satisfactory results and savings of contrast. This can translate into a savings of $25 per patient study. In larger patients, however, a full contrast load should be used.

Primary and Metastatic Tumors of the Liver

Accurate detection of hepatic lesions is dependent on a number factors; most important among these is the difference in enhancement between the lesion and the surrounding liver. Since most lesions (cysts and metastases) are hypovascular when compared to the hepatic parenchyma, the optimal time to scan the liver is near the peak liver enhancement. As we indicated earlier, when contrast is injected at two mL/sec, we begin scanning 70 sec after the initiation of the contrast injection. Since there has been much debate regarding the optimal delay, we studied a large number of metastatic liver lesions using *both* a 40- to 50-sec and 60- to 70-sec delay. We found that about 85 to 90 percent of lesions are better seen with the longer delay (Figure 4-11). Almost all the lesions in our series were hypovascular, and metastatic breast cancer or gastrointestinal adenocarcinoma dominated our population. Only 10 to 15 percent of hypovascular lesions were better seen on early scans. This occurred because they became isodense and "filled-in" with contrast on the later scans (Figure 4-12). For most hypovascular metastases, the increased yield of routinely doing early and late scans is probably not worth the effort. We will, however, continue to use the dual-phase approach if we are evaluating a patient for the first time, and they are a potential liver resection candidate.

When evaluating the liver for metastases from tumors with a propensity to be hypervascular (melanoma, islet cell tumors of the pancreas, renal and thyroid carcinomas, and

(Text continues on page 182)

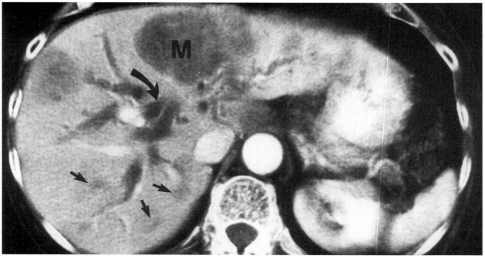

A

FIGURE 4-11A Better Visualization of Hepatic Metastases on the Late Phase of a Dual-Phase Liver Study. A. On this seven mm collimation section obtained during the first phase of a dual-phase liver study, multiple hepatic lesions are identified in this patient with breast cancer. In addition to the large mass (M) bridging the medial and lateral segments of the left lobe, subtle tumor deposits also appear present in the posterior segment of the right lobe (arrows). (Curved arrows = dilated biliary ducts).

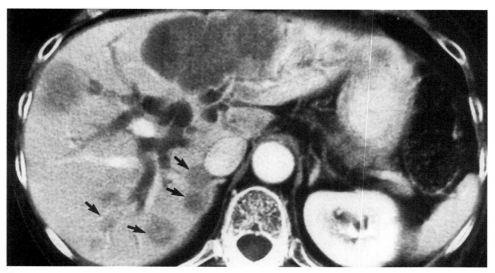

B

FIGURE 4-11B During the second phase of this dual-phase study, the lesions within the posterior segment of the right lobe (arrows) are better seen. This has probably occurred because of greater overall enhancement of the liver parenchyma during the later scans. Detection of hypovascular metastases appears superior on the second phase of dual-phase hepatic studies in most patients.

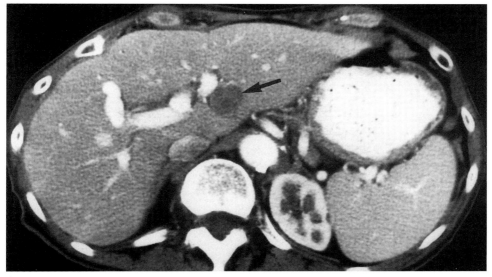

A

FIGURE 4-12A Early Versus Late Helical Scans of Hepatic Metastasis of Colorectal Origin. A. Scan obtained 50 to 60 sec after start of injection of contrast medium (two mL/sec) shows well-defined metastasis (arrow) in lateral segment of the left lobe of the liver.

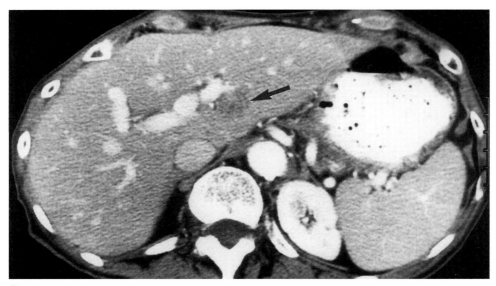

B

FIGURE 4-12B Scan obtained 30 sec after Figure 4-12A, but well within nonequilibrium phase, shows partial "fill-in" of metastasis (arrow) during equilibration of contrast material. A second lesion was actually seen better on delayed scan. Speed of helical scanning makes it possible to evaluate liver in early and late stages of nonequilibrium phase. *(Courtesy of Zeman et al.[1])*

sarcomas), the dual-phase study probably will prove to be advantageous in the future. On images obtained during the first phase of the helical study (early in the contrast injection), hypervascular lesions may be seen as enhancing nodules surrounded by less enhanced hepatic parenchyma (Figure 4-13).[23] The tumor, who's blood supply is generally via the hepatic artery, will reach its peak enhancement 20 to 30 sec earlier than the liver, which derives its blood supply from the portal vein. Scans early in the contrast injection may, therefore, be superior for seeing vascular metastases because these lesions quickly become isodense as the liver enhances. The dual phase approach also may be useful in the detection of hepatomas, which are commonly hypervascular.

Unlike conventional "stop and go" CT, helical CT represents a continuous volume set of data that can be reconstructed as overlapping sections. In one study in which eight mm thick scans were reconstructed with an overlap of four mm, seven percent more lesions were detected simply as a result of the data being processed in this manner.[24] Importantly, almost one-fourth of lesions (22 percent) were more confidently diagnosed with this added information. This is beneficial when the lesions are small, and may also be helpful in distinguishing low attenuation tumors from small, benign cysts. This technique can also

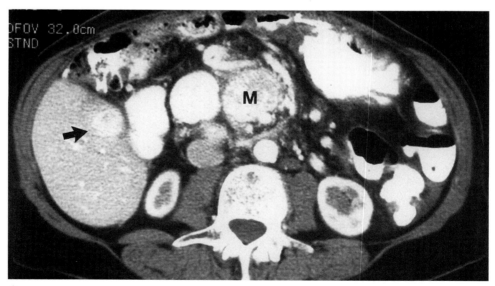

A

FIGURE 4-13A Hypervascular Metastases from Islet Cell Carcinoma Better Seen on the First Phase of a Dual-Phase Liver Study. A. This five mm collimation scan was obtained during the first phase of a dual-phase liver study. The patient has a known islet cell tumor infiltrating the pancreas (M). A small hypervascular hepatic metastases (arrow) is identified on this section because of its greater attenuation than the surrounding parenchyma.

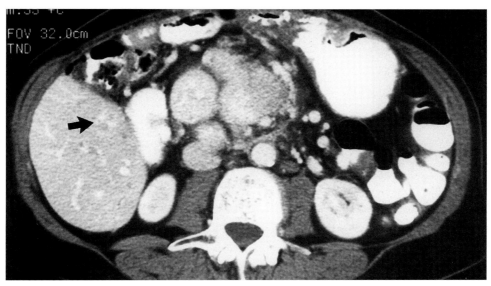

B

FIGURE 4-13B On the second phase of this dual-phase study, it is more difficult to identify the metastatic tumor deposit. The attenuation of the lesion (arrow) has rapidly declined, and it is barely perceptible on this late phase image. For patients with known hypervascular primary tumors, the early phase of a dual-phase study may improve detection of metastases.

be used in solving problems related to partial volume averaging of vascular structures (Figure 4-14). In general we have found that the overlapping of slices of up to 50 percent or slightly greater can be useful, but as further overlap is performed, there are diminishing returns. It would not be practical to review the large number of images that would be produced with overlapping reconstruction in all patients; but when detection of a small lesion may have a significant impact on the patient's clinical treatment, we will use this technique.

It is usually possible to accurately localize hepatic masses on axial sections. At times, our surgeons find it helpful to see the relationship of tumors to the major hepatic vessels, should resection be contemplated. Using a dual threshold method which includes the attenuation of the mass and the major vessels, tumor and vascular anatomy may be displayed in a single model (Figure 4-15).

Benign Hepatic Lesions

There is not yet enough data to provide convincing evidence that helical CT results in diagnostic advantages over conventional CT for characterizing benign lesions such as

(Text continues on page 187)

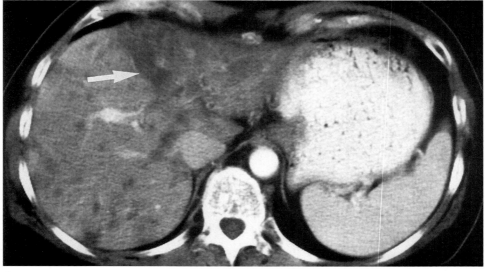

A

FIGURE 4-14A Left Portal Vein Thrombus Identified on Overlapping Sections. A. This seven mm collimation helical scan shows evidence of extensive hepatic metastases due to breast carcinoma. The metastatic deposits appear to be diffusely infiltrative, as well as giving rise to multiple small (approximately one cm) lesions. The left portal vein could not be identified in its usual position (arrow).

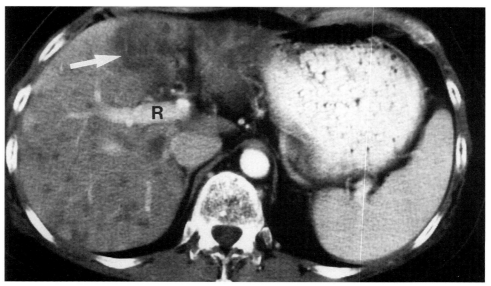

B

FIGURE 4-14B This section, seven mm below that shown in Figure 4-14A, also fails to show the left portal vein (arrow). The right portal vein (R) is identified.

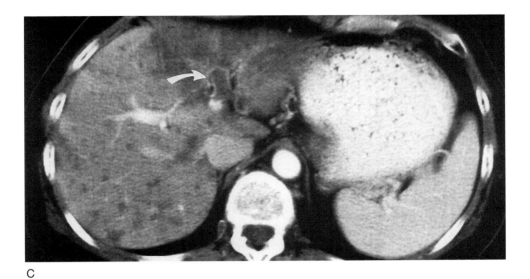

C

FIGURE 4-14C Using overlapping reconstruction, this section was reconstructed between those of Figures 4-14A and 4-14B. On this section, the thrombus-filled left portal vein is clearly identified (curved arrow). When small lesions or anatomic structures follow a horizontal (in-plane) course, overlapping reconstruction may boost our diagnostic confidence. This patient ultimately developed thrombosis of the main portal vein.

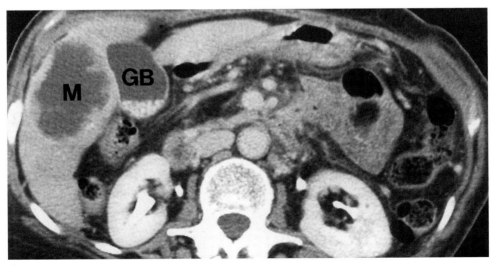

A

FIGURE 4-15A Use of 3-D Rendering for Anatomic Localization of Hepatic Metastases. A. This potentially operable patient with hepatic metastases was evaluated by helical CT. A large necrotic metastasis (M) is present at the tip of the right lobe. It is often difficult to localize lesions in this area because the hepatic veins (which form the segmental boundaries of the liver) are usually not well seen this caudad within the liver. Another lesion was seen cephalad to the lesion depicted in this section (GB = gallbladder).

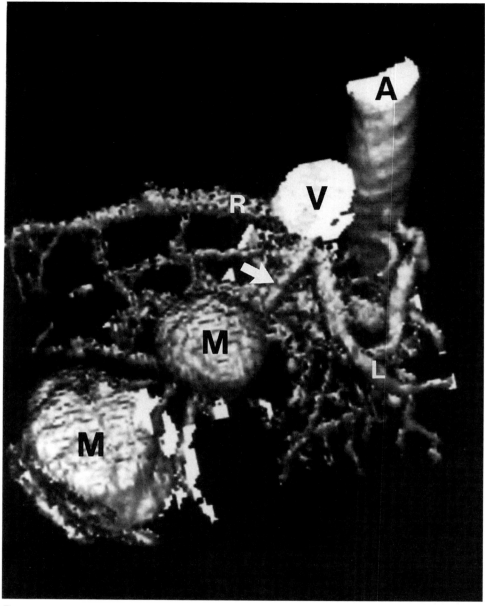

B

FIGURE 4-15B This three-dimensional model rendered from the helical CT data shows two large metastases (M). They are within the plane of the middle hepatic vein (arrow). This vein acts as the boundary between the right and left lobes of the liver. The location of these lesions would, therefore, not be amenable to lobectomy. For demonstration of vascular anomalies and helping surgeons plan hepatic resection, three-dimensional views may be valuable (R = right hepatic vein, L = left hepatic vein, V = inferior vena cava, A = aorta).

focal nodular hyperplasia, adenomas, or hemangiomas. Adenomas and focal nodular hyperplasia may be better seen on early dual-phase scans, but this has yet to be confirmed in large series. In the case of hemangiomas, high-quality, conventional, dynamic CT has been extremely effective in characterizing these lesions when they meet the criteria of initial peripheral pooling of contrast and centripetal isodense fill-in.

Diffuse Liver Disease

Fatty infiltration of the liver is most commonly associated with alcohol abuse, hyperalimination, diabetes, chemotherapy, obesity, steroid use, and Cushing's syndrome. Most often the involvement is diffuse or involving segmental areas of the liver. Rarely, it can be geographic or even focal, and can mimic metastases. Fatty infiltration has a predilection for the region adjacent to the falciform ligament, or near the gallbladder fossa. Helical CT with its excellent definition of vascular structures and high levels of enhancement of the liver has resulted in increasing recognition of focal fatty infiltration in our practice.

Hepatic Vasculature

The identification of clot in the main portal vein or smaller portal venous radicals has been well recognized using bolus dynamic CT. With appropriate timing, helical CT can often better demonstrate a clot because of the high contrast levels within vascular structures. The ability to "center" the section right on an area of suspected clot (by overlapping reconstruction) is helpful in confidently establishing the diagnosis (Figure 4-14). Caution should be exercised if using the dual-phase technique. Helical scanning during the early phase frequently causes inhomogeneous enhancement of the liver and portal vein due to poor mixing of opacified and unopacified blood. This should not be confused with the appearance of vascular thrombosis. The later phase scans will usually clarify the findings. On rare occasions, complimentary examination with sonography or magnetic resonance can also be used as a problem solver.

PANCREATOBILIARY APPLICATIONS

Helical CT is resulting in dramatic improvement in our ability to evaluate the pancreas as compared to conventional CT. CT is currently the best method for screening the pancreas and biliary tract for neoplasm. New modalities such as endoscopic ultrasound (EUS) and magnetic resonance imaging (MRI) have stirred considerable debate as to whether or not CT can visualize fine pancreatic detail and accurately stage pancreatobiliary tumors.[25-28] In gastroenterology circles, the claim has been repeatedly made that EUS is superior to CT in assessing vascular invasion and for TNM staging of pancreatic cancer.[27] While no large scale comparison with helical CT has been made, there is no question that refinements in CT evaluation of the pancreas would be most welcome in this modality horserace.

The speed of helical scanning allows the pancreas to be scanned during maximum contrast enhancement. Since most tumors are of lesser attenuation than the pancreatic parenchyma, it stands to reason that they will be more apparent if the normal parenchyma is well enhanced. Similarly, if the vessels are well enhanced, vascular encasement will be more readily recognized. More work is needed to establish the contrast dynamics for pancreatic scanning, but we believe high levels of contrast are beneficial.

Strategy for Helical CT Evaluation of the Pancreas

As with any new technology, there is controversy as to the optimal way to study the pancreas (Table 4-4). There are also considerable differences in the approach to contrast administration for helical versus conventional CT. When we are evaluating the pancreas in patients with suspected tumors, we usually do not administer oral contrast, but prefer to distend the duodenum with water and a gas-producing agent, or 24 oz of a carbonated beverage. This approach allows us to accurately see tumor invasion of the duodenal wall (Figure 4-16). By avoiding oral contrast, 3-D rendering of the peripancreatic vessels is also made much easier. Identifying vascular encasement on a 3-D model is difficult if the vessels are insinuated between barium-filled small bowel loops of similar attenuation. Using water and gas as a bowel contrast agent eliminates this problem. In the setting of pancreatitis, we still tend to administer dilute oral barium because it can be difficult to differentiate small pseudocysts from negatively (fluid and gas) opacified bowel loops.

For the pancreas we administer intravenous contrast in a similar fashion to that for our routine abdominal screening study and focused liver exams. A rate of at least two mL/sec is recommended and two to three mL/sec is preferable. We will generally use the lower injection rate if a 22 gauge intravenous catheter has been placed. If it was possible to safely place a 20 gauge catheter, three ml/sec will be used. There is nothing magical about these rates, but in our experience they produce adequate pancreatic enhancement. We prefer to use 300 mgI/mL concentration nonionic contrast because of previously stated reasons, but 60 percent ionic contrast also results in acceptable studies in most patients. We inject the contrast uniphasically. We believe a biphasic injection may be necessary to prolong the bolus for conventional scanners,[29] but is not necessary when scanning helically.

A conservative approach should be taken before considering a substantial reduction in contrast dose for evaluation of the pancreas. Dupuy et al. have shown that the speed of helical CT allows a "cosmetically appealing" exam of the pancreas to be performed with as little as 90 ml of contrast.[30] While we agree with this observation, we worry about the impact of the lower contrast dose on tumor recognition and identification of vascular encasement in patients that prove to have pancreatic carcinoma. Since the liver must also be evaluated in the same sitting, in patients who prove to have pancreatic tumors, reduction in contrast dose could also adversely affect the detection of hepatic metastases. When we study the pancreas we will use a full 150 mL dose of contrast for the initial staging study. If the tumor grossly enlarges the gland and proves unresectable, follow-up studies to check for radiation or chemotherapy response may be performed with a lower contrast dose.

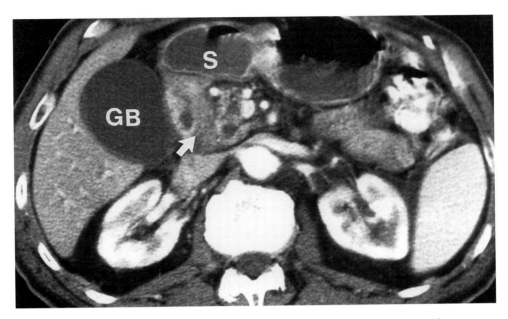

FIGURE 4-16 Use of a Carbonated Beverage to Assess Duodenal Invasion by Pancreatic Carcinoma. A carbonated beverage or water and a gas-producing agent may be used to distend the stomach and duodenum for abdominal CT. High levels of circulating contrast material and a negatively opacified duodenum allows detection of asymmetric duodenal wall thickening due to tumor. In this patient the tumor can be seen infiltrating the medial wall of the duodenal sweep (arrow). There is hyperemia of the opposing wall, probably due to vascular stasis and mild duodenitis. While evaluation of the duodenum effects tumor staging, this entire portion of the duodenum would be excised if Whipple procedure is performed (S = stomach, GB = Courvoisier gallbladder).

When should the helical scan be performed in relation to the contrast injection? Data on this topic is still evolving. When using conventional CT, Megibow has suggested that scanning in the setting of pancreatic cancer should begin 45 sec following the start of the contrast injection.[29] This allows completion of the entire scan prior to the equilibrium phase, when hepatic metastases could be missed. For helical scanning however, scanning this early in the contrast injection is not optimal. The portal vein or superior mesenteric vein may not be opacified when using such a short injection delay (Figure 4-17). There is increasing evidence that the portal vein enhancement may not peak until 70 sec or longer using two to three mL/sec contrast injections.[14,18] Scanning the portal vein at its peak enhancement is important and will assure recognition of encasement of this vessel when present.

Scanning the pancreas both early and late may offer some benefit for recognition of small tumors and staging.[31] Scanning as early as 20 to 40 sec may show tumors not evident

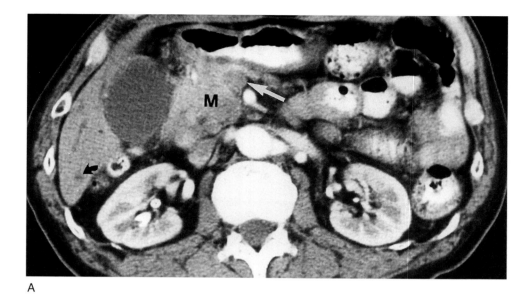

FIGURE 4-17A Early Phase of a Dual-Phase Pancreatic Exam Fails to Show Opacification of the Superior Mesenteric Vein. A. Five mm collimation helical scan through the pancreas was performed during the first phase of a dual-phase pancreatic study. The patient's pancreatic carcinoma (M) is clearly identified. Although there is opacification of the superior mesenteric artery, the superior mesenteric vein (arrow) is not enhanced with contrast material. This could be mistaken for thrombosis of this vessel. A lesion suspicious for hepatic metastasis (curved arrow) is also identified.

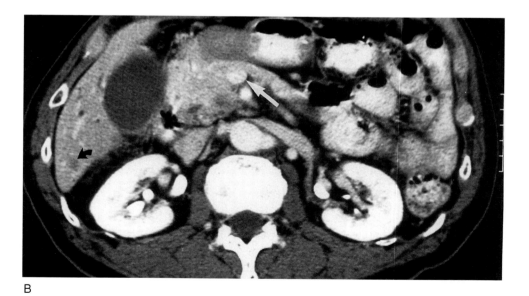

FIGURE 4-17B Scan obtained 30 sec after Figure 4-17A shows normal enhancement of the superior mesenteric vein (arrow). The additional delay has allowed for opacification of this vessel. Notice that with the longer delay, the hepatic metastasis (curved arrow) is also better identified.

later in the contrast injection. We now have seen several very small tumors which showed progressive "filling-in" with intravenous contrast over time (Figure 4-18). This made the tumors harder to recognize and of apparently smaller size, analogous to the behavior of liver metastases during equilibration of the contrast material. We are not yet sure if early scanning will result in a statistically significant improvement in tumor recognition, but late scans (60 to 90 sec) to assess possible venous encasement will also be needed.

Prior to helically scanning the pancreas, a few noncontrast, nonhelical localizing scans should be performed to properly position the helical acquisition. After proper positioning, the helical scan may be performed "top-down" or "bottom-up" through the pancreas. We usually scan from the bottom-up so that the pancreas is scanned before the liver. If the

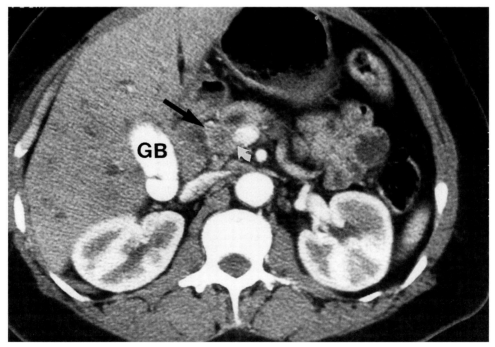

A

FIGURE 4-18A Improved Visualization of a Small Pancreatic Carcinoma on the First Phase of a Dual-Phase Study. A. Five mm collimation helical scan of the pancreas was performed during the first phase of a dual-phase pancreatic study. A small, low attenuation mass (arrow) is identified within the pancreatic head. The mass is approximately one and one-half cm in diameter. Despite the small size of this tumor, there appears to be irregularity to the lateral contour of the superior mesenteric vein (curved arrow). This irregularity was also seen on adjacent sections and is suspicious for vascular involvement. (GB = gallbladder opacified during previous ERCP).

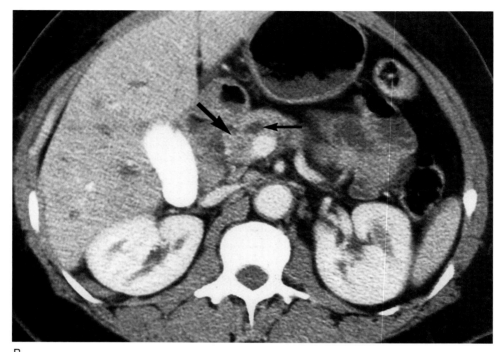

B

FIGURE 4-18B On the second phase of this dual-phase study, the small pancreatic mass (large arrow) has increased in attenuation and is nearly isodense with the surrounding pancreas. In some patients, the first phase of a dual-phase study may show small pancreatic masses better. At surgery, adenocarcinoma with adherence to the superior mesenteric vein was identified. (small arrow = dilated pancreatic duct).

patient has difficulty holding their breath at the end of the helix, the upper liver images may be degraded, but at least the critical pancreatic portion of the study will be salvaged. The images should be acquired using four or five mm collimation. On the GE HiSpeed we use approximately 300 mA but this will vary for different devices. One hundred twenty kVp is used.

If a single helical "run" is to be made, an exposure length of 30 sec should cover the pancreas and liver. If an early and late "run" are made, the first helix will be limited to approximately 20 sec through the pancreas. After a breathing interval, the second run will be made starting at 60 to 70 sec to include the pancreas and liver. Some scanners accomplishing these two-pass helical studies of the pancreas will require reduction in milliAmperes or use of increased pitch. For the initial assessment and staging of pancreatic cancer, five mm collimation scans are reconstructed at both five mm and three mm (40 percent overlap) intervals. Overlap can help recognition of small tumors (see Figure 4-23).

Pancreatic Tumors

On CT, pancreatic adenocarcinoma commonly produces a contour abnormality or frank enlargement of the pancreatic head.[32,33] Because helical CT results in excellent pancreatic enhancement, small tumors which do not enlarge the gland are increasingly being recognized (Figure 4-18). The tumor is usually of soft-tissue attenuation and frequently enhances less than the pancreatic parenchyma. Areas of necrosis may be present (Figure 4-19). Since two-thirds of pancreatic adenocarcinomas are in the pancreatic head, obstruction of the bile duct and pancreatic duct occurs commonly (Figure 4-19). At times, the

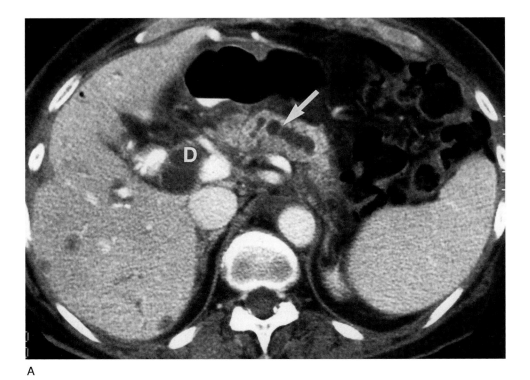

A

FIGURE 4-19A Obstruction of the Pancreatic Duct and Bile Duct by Pancreatic Carcinoma. A. Five mm collimation helical scan of the pancreas shows dilatation of the pancreatic duct (arrow) and bile duct (D). When both the pancreatic duct and bile duct are obstructed, the most likely etiology is pancreatic carcinoma. Chronic pancreatitis is much less likely to produce obstruction of both ducts.

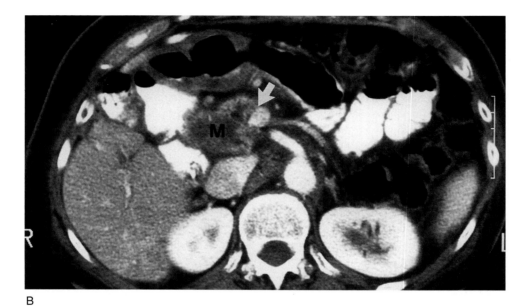

B

FIGURE 4-19B On this section one cm below that of Figure 4-19A a necrotic pancreatic carcinoma is present (M). There is flattening of the lateral edge of the superior mesenteric vein (arrow). The tumor was adherent to this surface of the vessel at surgery.

dilated ducts are more easily recognized on the second pass of the dual-phase study. When both ducts are obstructed by a mass it is suggestive, but only about 80 percent specific for malignancy.[34] Chronic pancreatitis can produce similar changes. In our institution between 10 and 20 percent of pancreatic adenocarcinomas are resectable.

When a mass is identified which does not have benign features (see below), it must be staged. While the TNM staging scheme is gaining popularity, we tend to be more descriptive, but as specific as possible in describing nodal involvement, vascular encasement, and distant disease to our surgical colleagues. The peripancreatic tissue must be carefully scrutinized for nodes and tumor infiltration in the mesentery. While pancreaticoduodenal nodes may be excised en bloc at the time of pancreatic resection, enlargement of most other nodal groups implies nonresectability. This includes the celiac, porta hepatis, mesenteric and para-aortic chains (Figure 4-20). Involvement of the transverse mesocolon or posterior wall of the transverse colon does not by itself preclude resection, but obtaining margins free of tumor may be surgically difficult.

The greatest nemesis of the radiologist in determining resectability of pancreatic cancer is vascular invasion. This is one of the most common causes of nonresectability, yet has been inconsistently identified on standard, conventional CT scans. Freeny and colleagues, in a careful study comparing dynamic CT and angiography, showed vascular involvement on CT in 15 of 16 patients in whom it was surgically confirmed.[32] In a similar surgical

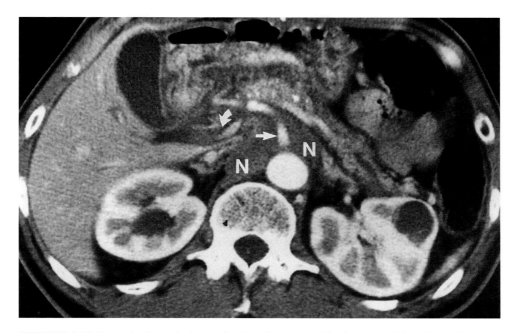

FIGURE 4-20 Extensive Lymphadenopathy From Pancreatic Carcinoma. In this patient with pancreatic carcinoma, there is extensive mesenteric and para-aortic lymphadenopathy (N). The adenopathy surrounds the superior mesenteric artery (arrow). The adenopathy also has an infiltrative component extending up into the porta-hepatis. This has resulted in flattening of the normally rounded contour of the portal vein (curved arrow). Extensive tumor infiltration such as this is common in the late stages of pancreatic carcinoma.

series, Vellet et al. identified vascular invasion on CT in only 31 of 39 patients, and portal venous invasion in 37 of 40 patients.[25] In this same series MR fared better, identifying 34 and 37 patients respectively in each of these categories. Warshaw and associates reported correct identification of vascular encasement on CT in only 21 of 35 patients with pancreatic head neoplasms.[35] These authors suggested that angiography played a complementary role in assessing vascular invasion. It correctly identified 25 of 35 patients with vascular involvement, many of whom did not have vascular invasion on CT. Muller found similar results with CT missing small tumors and understaging T3 (vessel involvement) lesions.[36]

Against this confusing backdrop, helical CT appears ideally suited to detect vascular invasion. The lack of misregistration and the ability to produce overlapping scans allows recognition of subtle caliber changes in both arteries and veins (Figures 4-21, 4-22). Overlapping scans also may show small tumors and encasement of peripancreatic vessels not evident on nonoverlapping scans (Figure 4-23). We find our accuracy approaching 85 percent in detection of vascular encasement when using overlapping sections.

(Text continues on page 199)

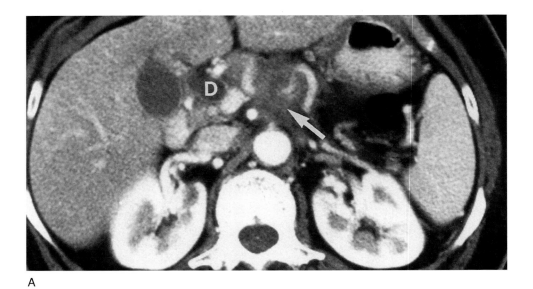

A

FIGURE 4-21A Infiltrative Pancreatic Carcinoma. A. Five mm collimation helical scan shows a large pancreatic carcinoma in the pancreatic body (arrow). There appears to be encasement of both the splenic and hepatic arteries distal to the celiac bifurcation. The bile duct (D) is dilated and obstructed by the tumor mass.

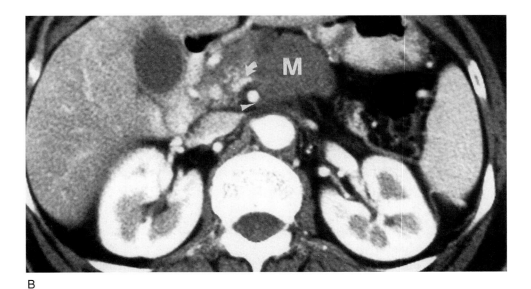

B

FIGURE 4-21B Section obtained 1 cm below Figure 4-21A shows further extension of the mass (M) with involvement of multiple vessels. The tumor has infiltrated posteriorly around the left lateral margin of the superior mesenteric artery (arrowhead). There also is early infiltration of the fat just anterior to the left renal vein as it crosses in front of the aorta. The portal vein caliber is narrowed and slitlike at this level (curved arrow). When vascular encasement such as this is identified, tumor resection is not possible.

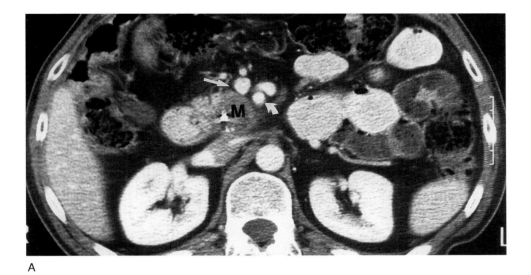

A

FIGURE 4-22A Subtle Encasement of the Superior Mesenteric Vein by Pancreatic Carcinoma. A. Five mm collimation helical scan shows a pancreatic mass (M) within the pancreatic head and uncinate portion of the gland. At this level the superior mesenteric artery (curved arrow) appears normal. A preserved fat plane (arrow) is identified separating the mass from the superior mesenteric vein.

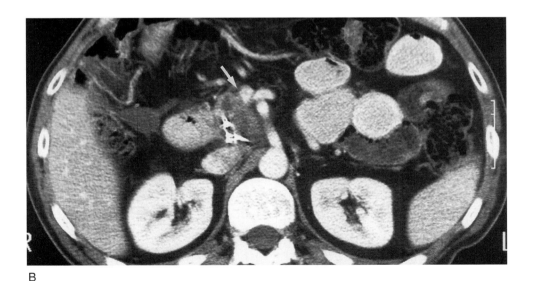

B

FIGURE 4-22B This section was obtained one cm above Figure 4-22A. At this level the normal, rounded shape of the superior mesenteric vein has been lost (arrow), and there is no distinct fat plane between the tumor and the vessel. In order to detect vascular involvement, it is important to closely scrutinize the vessel caliber and shape as it is followed from section to section. In this patient, tumor adherence and encasement of the superior mesenteric vein was confirmed at surgery. We find that these subtle changes in vessel caliber are more readily detected using 3-dimensional rendering (see Figure 6-16 for 3-D view of this same patient).

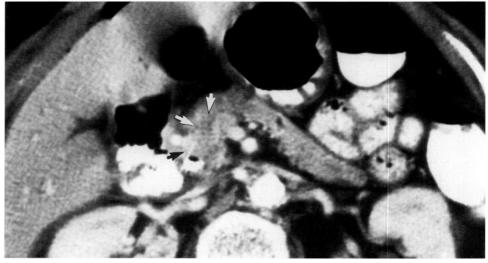

A

FIGURE 4-23A Improved Definition of Cholangiocarcinoma by Retrospectively Shifting Slice Location of the Helical CT Scan. A. Helical CT scan obtained with five mm collimation reconstructed every five mm shows questionable fullness of the pancreatic head compared with caliber of rest of gland. The gland contour is irregular and of slightly lower attenuation (arrows). Biliary stent is present.

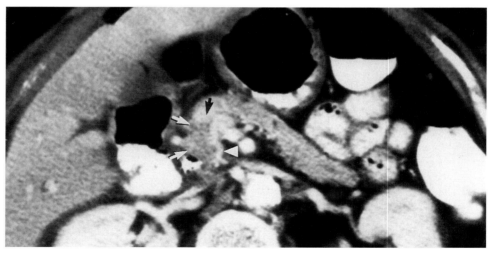

B

FIGURE 4-23B After retrospective overlapping reconstruction of the scans at three mm spacing, this slice was located one mm cephalad to Figure 4-23A. Despite the slice location looking quite similar to that of Figure 4-23A, note how the low attenuation of the mass (arrows) is accentuated and encasement of the pancreaticoduodenal vein branches draining into gastrocolic trunk (arrowhead) is better defined. Slight changes in scan location can greatly affect appearance of small tumors. This patient had an unresectable cholangiocarcinoma of the distal bile duct infiltrating pancreatic head. *(Courtesy of Zeman et al.[1])*

When overlapping sections are used in concert with 3-D renderings of the peripancreatic vessels, our accuracy increases further. These techniques will be discussed in detail in chapter 6. Three-dimensional models are especially appreciated by the surgeon who must decide whether the vascular involvement which is present precludes resection or not.[37] In general, involvement of the portal vein, superior mesenteric vein, celiac axis, or superior mesenteric artery implies nonresectability (Figure 4-24). If the lesion does appear resectable, arterial anomalies that might affect creation of a biliary-enteric anastomosis

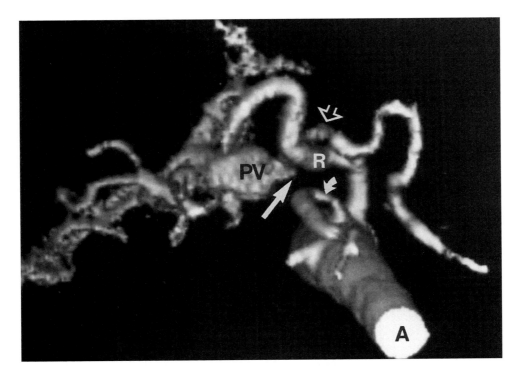

FIGURE 4-24 Three-Dimensional Model Demonstrating Vascular Encasement by Pancreatic Carcinoma. This shaded-surface display viewed obliquely from below was rendered from five mm collimation helical sections reconstructed with three mm spacing. The portal vein (PV) exhibits a bird-beak narrowing (arrow) due to encasement by tumor. The superior mesenteric vein is not identified because the tumor has produced total thrombosis of this vessel. Because the vessel did not enhance with contrast material it is not seen in this model which depicts only those vessels with attenuation of greater than 120 H. The origin of the superior mesenteric artery (curved arrow) is also involved by tumor. The more distal superior mesenteric artery, beyond the area of narrowing, appears of normal caliber. In this patient the right hepatic artery (R) appears to have a separate origin from the left hepatic artery (open arrow). On other views there also is slight narrowing of the origin of the right hepatic artery due to tumor. All of the changes described represent extensive tumor involvement of the arterial and venous structures (A = aorta).

can be seen on the 3-D views (Figure 4-25). If short segments of the portal venous system are involved, they may be grafted at the time of tumor resection, but this entails substantial morbidity and is technically difficult. Most often the 3-D models have acted as one more piece of evidence against resectability in patients with advanced tumors. Multiplanar reformatting may also be used to provide this type of information.[38] Eliminating needless surgery results in significant cost-savings and may improve the quality of life in patients with advanced disease.

Other tumors of the pancreas are far less common than adenocarcinoma. Neuroendocrine tumors, such as islet cell carcinoma, are frequently malignant but tend to have a

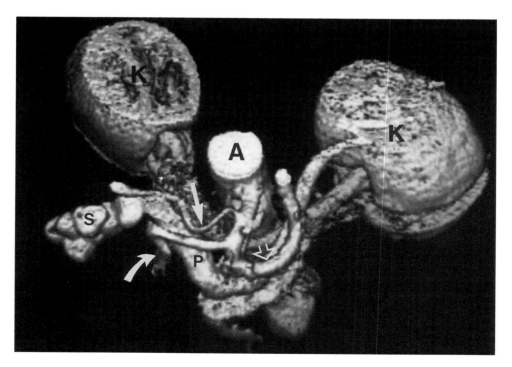

FIGURE 4-25 Aberrant Origin of the Hepatic Artery. Surface model created from helical CT data, viewed from above, shows the hepatic artery (straight solid arrow) arising from the proximal part of the celiac axis and coursing behind the portal vein (P). This location is unusual: the artery normally passes anterior to portal vein. As the celiac axis bifurcates in this patient, it gives rise to the splenic artery (open arrow) and gastroduodenal artery (curved arrow). Ability to recognize anomalous branches of the hepatic artery is important for surgical planning, as these branches commonly supply arterial blood to the common hepatic duct. (K = kidneys, S = radiopaque gallstones of attenuation similar to that of enhanced vessels, A = aorta.) *(Courtesy of* AJR[37] *with permission.)*

slightly better prognosis than adenocarcinoma. As a general rule, the functional tumors tend to be smaller than the nonfunctional tumors at presentation. This is because of systemic, hormonally related symptoms causing the patient to seek medical care earlier. Angiography, venous sampling, and intraoperative ultrasound all remain useful in detection of these small tumors, but we are increasingly seeing them on helical CT (Figure 4-26). Partly because of achieving better vascular opacification and scanning prior to significant contrast equilibration, the tumors more often reveal their hypervascular nature than on conventional CT. While this is encouraging, large series looking at helical CT in patients with islet cell lesions will be needed to prove if CT is a viable screening technique.

Thus far, we have seen solid and papillary epithelial neoplasms, microcystic adenomas, and mucinous cystic neoplasms with helical CT. Their appearance, however, has not substantially differed from that expected on conventional CT. The hypervascular rim of the papillary epithelial group of tumors shows better enhancement and definition on helical CT than on conventional CT. Similarly the enhancing septa in patients with cystic neoplasms are better seen, but thus far this has not yet resulted in significant clinical implications.

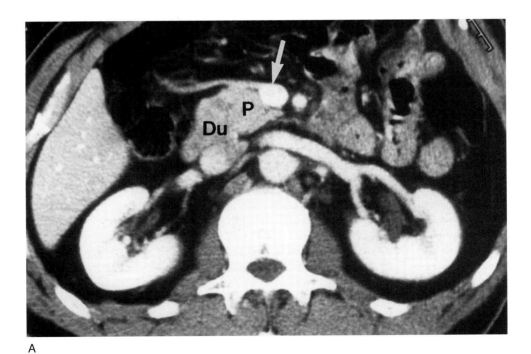

A

FIGURE 4-26A Malignant Islet Cell Carcinoma. A. This five mm collimation section shows a normal uncinate portion of the pancreas (P). The superior mesenteric vein (arrow) is identified in its usual position. (Du = duodenum).

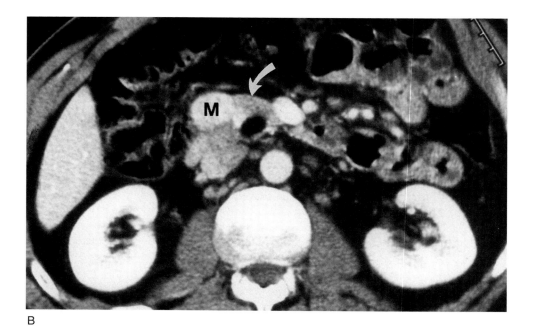

B

FIGURE 4-26B This section five mm below Figure 4-26A shows a small hypervascular mass (M) extending inferiorly from the uncinate. A small amount of normal pancreatic tissue (curved arrow) is seen interposed between the mass and the normal superior mesenteric vein. At surgery this proved to be a resectable malignant islet cell carcinoma.

Pancreatitis

There is no published experience, thus far, in the evaluation of pancreatitis using helical CT. Based on our experience, the hyperemia associated with acute pancreatitis is readily apparent on helically acquired scans. Devascularized phlegmonous change is also impressively low in attenuation when surrounded by a densely enhancing gland. Recognition, however, of peripancreatic fluid collections seems a bit easier on delayed scans. Pseudocysts and postinflammatory fluid does not show "filling-in" or delayed enhancement based on our experience to date. Recognition of vascular complications such as pseudoaneurysm formation or portal and splenic vein thrombosis requires high levels of vascular opacification. Because of this, we will usually scan pancreatitis patients with our usual 70-sec contrast administration delay. We then add delayed nonhelical scans one to two minutes later to study suspected peripancreatic fluid collections.

Biliary Obstruction

Helical scanning does offer some unique attributes which result in improved evaluation of the patient with biliary obstruction. Overlapping reconstruction and scanning with high levels of contrast contribute to improved recognition of the normal extrahepatic bile duct, and help us better appreciate the level and etiology of biliary obstruction. This is especially true when obstruction is due to subtle abnormalities that have not produced significant mass effect. When we scan the biliary tract, we use a similar protocol to that for the pancreas, but make sure to include as much of the intrahepatic biliary tree as possible.

The two etiologies of biliary obstruction where we have found helical scanning to be most helpful are cholangiocarcinoma and choledocholithiasis. Using conventional CT we find cholangiocarcinoma frequently more difficult to diagnose than the literature would suggest.[39,40] Of the last 10 cholangiocarcinomas which we have seen, only one was larger than two cm at presentation. Helical scanning has helped us recognize and stage these lesions in several ways. First, many cholangiocarcinomas are hypervascular when scanned with high levels of circulating contrast (Figure 4-27). Seeing this hypervascularity really

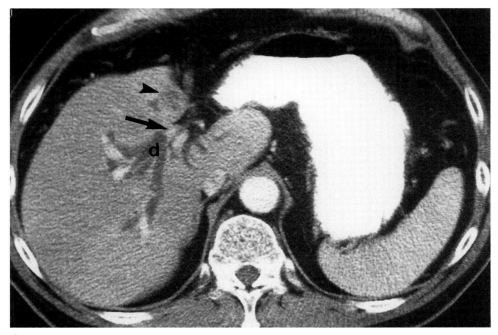

A

FIGURE 4-27A Klatskin Tumor (Cholangiocarcinoma) Producing Biliary Obstruction. A. Five mm collimation helical scan reveals the presence of a small hypervascular mass (arrow) producing dilatation of the intrahepatic bile ducts (d). There appears to be isolation of the right and left ducts. An area of mixed attenuation (arrowhead) is also seen and is worrisome for metastatic disease. Although unlikely, the possibility that the small high attenuation mass could represent partial volume averaging of the portal vein must be considered. On a section five mm below this, only the normal portal vein was identified.

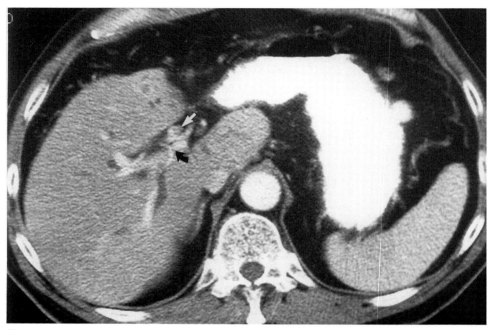

B

FIGURE 4-27B Reconstruction of overlapping sections using three mm spacing resulted in this image two mm below Figure 4-27A. This section demonstrates the lower extent of the tumor (arrow). It lies just anterior to the hepatic artery and the normal portal vein (curved arrow). While the tumor does not appear to be encasing the major vessels, the lesion identified in the liver did prove to be metastatic cholangiocarcinoma. By use of overlapping sections, the mass within the porta was more confidently identified. (The caudate lobe is enlarged due to chronic biliary cirrhosis).

helps delineate the mass. If delayed scans are performed immediately after completion of the helical scan, the tumors decline slightly in attenuation and appear similar in attenuation to liver parenchyma. This may be why these lesions may be difficult to identify with conventional CT. If scans are done 5 to 10 minutes later, the decline in tumor enhancement may be slower than that of the liver, and the tumor may actually appear of higher attenuation than liver parenchyma. This feature, although unusual, does appear in a significant minority of cholangiocarcinomas, especially the intrahepatic variety.[41] It is believed to be due to slow blood flow in the interior of the tumor.

Overlapping sections help show the precise transition zone where the bile duct is narrowed. In staging these lesions, only tumors that do not extend up into the bifurcation will be resectable. The overlapping sections allow precise recognition of the upper edge of the lesion in relation to the duct bifurcation. The overlapping sections also allow precise

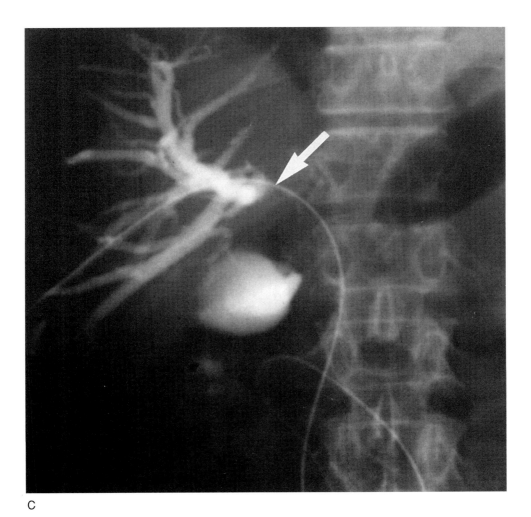

C

FIGURE 4-27C Endoscopic retrograde cholangiogram shows a high-grade stricture of the right hepatic duct (arrow). There has been isolation of the right and left ductal systems. The appearance is suggestive of a Klatskin tumor.

delineation of the relationship between the tumor and adjacent vessels (Figure 4-27). Tumor involvement of the main, right, or left portal vein also implies nonresectability.

Overlapping sections can aid in detection of choledocholithiasis. Partial volume averaging has always been the radiologist's foe in our efforts to recognize common duct stones on conventional CT. If the stone does not lie centered within the section, it may appear of lower attenuation than it really is. When this occurs, the stone may be missed because it blends into the surrounding soft-tissue of the pancreas. A faint halo of bile, analogous to the meniscus sign on cholangiography, may be seen just above the equator of a stone.[42,43] Without overlapping sections, this can be easily missed. Most patients with suspected choledocholithiasis will undergo endoscopic retrograde cholangiopancreatography, but it may be time to revisit the role of CT as a screening exam in this setting.

Using similar techniques as will be discussed for CT angiography in chapter 6, 3-D rendering of the biliary tract may also be performed. This requires software which allows setting of a narrow threshold range which will allow the ducts to be isolated from the surrounding soft-tissue. An alternative approach is to use minimum intensity projections which depict only the lowest pixel values within the model. Once accomplished, these models resemble a cast of the biliary tract and can be quite dramatic when obstruction is present (Figure 4-28).

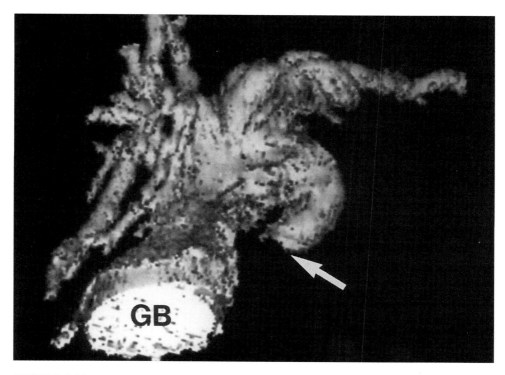

FIGURE 4-28 Three-Dimensional Rendering of the Biliary Tree. This shaded-surface display was rendered from five mm collimation helical scans reconstructed with three mm spacing. A narrow threshold range was used centered at 0 H. In this patient with pancreatic carcinoma, amputation of the bile duct is identified (arrow). The intrahepatic ducts are dilated and a Courvoisier gallbladder (GB) is present. While 3-D rendering of the bile duct may not confer additional diagnostic information as compared to the axial sections, it does allow the surgeon to better visualize the length of bile duct available for anastomosis construction.

There are two uses we find for biliary 3-D rendering. The first is in showing the relationship of tumors such as cholangiocarcinoma to the duct bifurcation. The second use is in showing the length of common hepatic duct above a tumor, which can be used by the surgeon for creation of a biliary-enteric anastomosis. There needs to at least one to two cm of extrahepatic bile duct available to allow surgical biliary diversion. Review of the 3-D images seems to convey this type of information in a more easily understood format than axially displayed images.

EVALUATION OF THE KIDNEY

Helical scanning has improved our evaluation of the renal parenchyma, but will probably not have the far reaching clinical impact as it has for the liver and pancreatobiliary tract. For vascular abnormalities such as renal artery stenosis, however, helical CT has had a dramatic impact, and over time may change the whole approach to renovascular hypertension. We will discuss renovascular disease in chapter 6.

Strategy for Evaluation of the Kidney

As mentioned earlier in this chapter, the focused exam of the kidney is conducted differently than the routine abdominal survey study (Table 4-5). The best way to examine the kidney is controversial and we will present several alternatives to evaluate in your practice.

When a renal mass that does not appear to be a simple cyst is encountered as part of a routine screening study, we will usually add several delayed, nonhelical sections to the exam following completion of the helix. During the helical acquisition, the cortex will be well enhanced but usually not the medulla (Figure 4-29). By waiting one to two extra minutes, the medulla will enhance and the collecting system will become partially opacified. Enhancement of the medulla is important in detecting all types of renal masses (Figure 4-29) and delineating the extent of renal tumors. Visualization of the collecting system is also important in determining whether the mass is transitional cell or renal cell in origin.

The focused exam of the kidney in a patient with a suspected renal mass differs in several ways from our abdominal survey study. Prior to obtaining helical scans, the kidney is evaluated without contrast material. These scans are done nonhelically, using five mm collimation, and at a slightly reduced milliAmperage. The milliAmperage is reduced so heat buildup will not be a problem when we begin our helical scan. If the milliAmperage is reduced by about 30 percent, attenuation measurements will not exhibit an excessive standard deviation, and will allow reliable comparison of pre- and postcontrast values.

For the helical scan, contrast is injected at a rate of two mL/sec. A total volume of 100 to 120 mL is used. An injection delay of 60 to 70 sec is needed to make sure the renal veins are well-opacified. The noncontrast scans are reviewed by the physician or technologist to properly place the helix at the level of the kidneys. The direction of scanning does not matter, but we will usually begin the scan at the bottom of the right kidney, which is

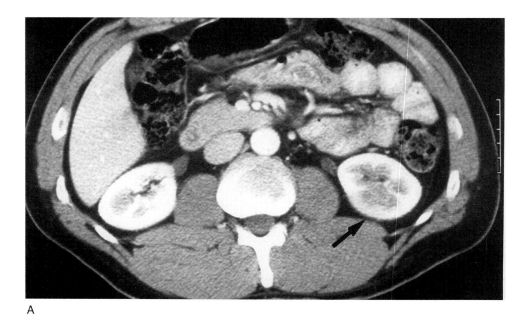

A

FIGURE 4-29A Renal Hematoma Better Seen on Delayed Sections. A. Following a motor vehicle accident, this patient developed hematuria. Seven mm collimation helical scan through the kidney shows a faintly decreased nephrogram in the posterior portion of the left kidney (arrow). The central lucency within the kidney was ascribed to the normal appearance of the medulla.

commonly lower than the left. The scan will be carried up as high in the liver as possible. Using five mm collimation and a 40-sec exposure (with a breathing interval at 20 sec) usually allows sufficient coverage. The liver is evaluated as part of our renal mass study because if the patient proves to have renal cell carcinoma, hepatic metastases must be excluded. We use approximately 300 mA at 120 kVp for exposure factors. We use 1:1 pitch on the GE HiSpeed. If this is not possible on the device in your practice, increasing the collimation or increasing the pitch ratio to 1.5:1 may be necessary. Higher pitch ratio or collimation in excess of eight mm may compromise evaluation of small lesions, especially if it proves necessary to compare pre- and postcontrast attenuation values.

Following completion of the helical scan, delayed sections are obtained. Again, on the GE HiSpeed, these will be preprogrammed to occur approximately 10 sec after completion of the helical scan. A longer delay of up to one minute would be acceptable and may be necessary on some devices due to tube heating or software resets. The delayed scans are performed to better see the medulla (Figure 4-29) and collecting system; do not wait too long because all the vascular contrast will dissipate. For the delayed scans, similar scan parameters are used as for the helical scan, but the delayed scans are performed as nonhelical, cluster scans.

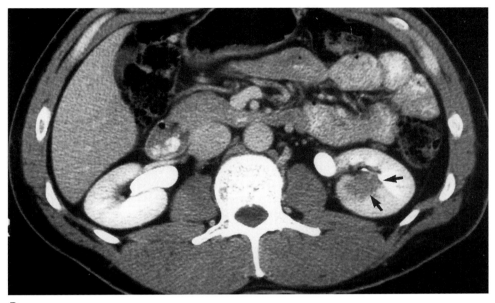

B

FIGURE 4-29B Delayed sections obtained two minutes later clearly show a low attenuation mass (arrows) within the medulla. This proved to be a hematoma. Use of delayed sections plays an important role in identifying masses within the medulla which may not be seen on early views.

We feel this approach optimizes our sensitivity. Unfortunately it means performing three series of images through the kidney. Because of the speed of helical scanners, even when a portion of the exam is nonhelical, the exam goes very quickly. It does entail a slightly higher total radiation dose to the patient. Because the milliAmperes used during our helical and precontrast nonhelical scans is actually less than that used on many conventional scanners, the total radiation dose is not dramatically greater, but this should be considered in scanning younger patients. It does take the radiologist longer to look at the large number of images which are generated. Overlapping reconstruction is added only as a problem solver in selected situations, such as for small indeterminate renal masses. Our approach to renal masses may be excessive in patients that prove to have bulky, advanced tumors. By the same token, detection of small, early tumors and differentiating complicated cysts from small neoplasms requires a meticulous, methodical approach such as this.

Why not just scan the kidney late after contrast administration? Small hypervascular masses, renal artery aneurysms, arteriovenous malformations, and renovascular disease may all be missed with late scans. We have chosen to scan helically in a superior direction from the bottom of the kidney. We do this because it makes entering the starting and stopping location of the scan easy to program. Given that hypervascular hepatic metastases may be better seen early in the contrast bolus, it may make more sense to begin scanning the liver early (30 to 40 sec) and carry the scan down through the kidneys. We plan to evaluate this approach, but do not want to compromise evaluation of the liver or kidney, nor make the exam difficult for the technologist to perform.

Detection and Characterization of Renal Masses

Conventional dynamic CT has been successfully used to image renal masses for many years.[44] The primary advantage of helical CT lies in its potential for improved characterization of indeterminate renal masses.[45] Silverman et al., in 48 patients with indeterminate renal masses less than three cm in diameter on either US or conventional CT, definitively showed seven lesions to be carcinoma and 32 to be benign lesions or complicated cysts. Helical CT was successful in this regard for three reasons: First, the lack of misregistration helps identify small masses that otherwise might be overlooked; second, by scanning when the contrast level is high, subtle enhancement indicative of tumor neovascularity is easily detected; and third, overlapping reconstruction may be used to position small lesions within the center of a section. This serves to reduce partial volume averaging, makes small masses more visible (Figure 4-30), and results in more reliable CT number measurements.

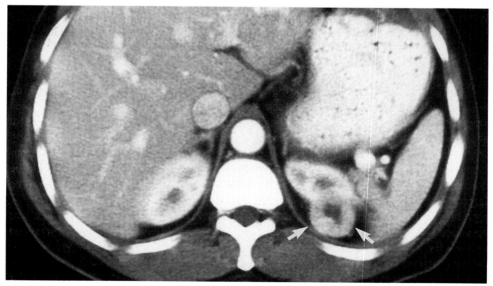

A

FIGURE 4-30A Use of Overlapping Sections to Demonstrate Small Renal Tumor. A. This seven mm collimation helical scan was obtained through the upper pole of the left kidney. There is a protuberance of tissue from the upper pole (arrows) which may represent a mass or possibly eccentric renal tissue with normal corticomedullary enhancement differences.

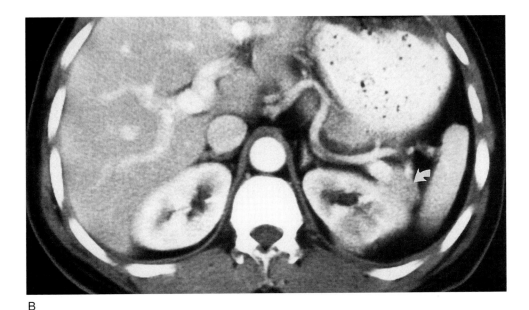

FIGURE 4-30B On this section seven mm below Figure 4-30A, no abnormality is identified. The pancreatic tail (curved arrow) is seen protruding into the section.

Bosniak has reported that renal mass enhancement resulting in a CT number rise of greater than 10 H (postcontrast CT number minus precontrast CT number greater than 10 H) is unlikely to be a cyst.[46,47] While we agree with this principle, there are two caveats relevant to helical scanning to keep in mind. First, using an inappropriately low milliAmpere or pitch ratios in excess of one and one-half can produce inaccurate CT numbers. Most radiologists realize that attenuation measurements should only be taken on lesions whose diameter is greater than the slice thickness. Increased pitch may also contribute to volume averaging. We will not rely on CT numbers of small lesions obtained with a pitch ratio of greater than 1.5:1. Second, it is important to take advantage of the capability of helical CT to "shift" the slice location to center masses within the section. Often the most reliable CT numbers will, therefore, come from the overlapping set of reconstructed images, not the set reconstructed without overlap.

Small hyperdense cysts or masses that are of greater than 20 H to begin with, and show any enhancement beyond the measured CT number standard deviation are suspicious for neoplasm. In elderly patients we may follow these lesions at six month intervals, but in younger patients we recommend surgery. Every radiologist we know has seen one to two cases where slightly hyperdense masses that should have been benign cysts based on CT numbers, proved to be renal cell carcinoma.

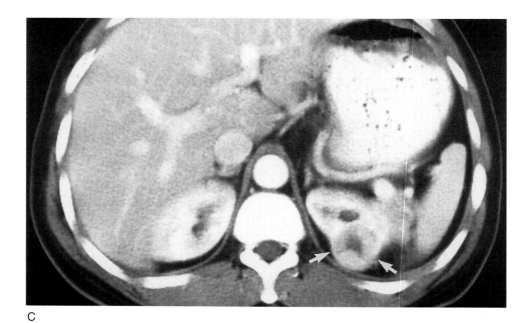

C

FIGURE 4-30C Following reconstruction of overlapping sections, this section is three mm below Figure 4-30A. A well-circumscribed mass (arrows) is better identified than on either of the nonoverlapping sections. Small tumors may more confidently be seen when using overlapping sections. At surgery this proved to be a renal oncocytoma.

Renal Cell Carcinoma

As yet there are no large series studying helical CT in renal cell carcinoma. It is logical that helical methods will allow better detection of small tumors, especially through the use of overlapping sections (Figure 4-30). There is ongoing debate regarding the natural history[48,49] and role of partial nephrectomy for small renal cell carcinomas.[50] There is no debate, however, that more informed decisions and ultimately higher cure rates will result when tumors are detected when they are smaller and at an earlier stage.

In general, CT does an excellent job of staging renal cell carcinoma (Figure 4-31). Stages 1 and 2 are readily differentiated from more advanced stages of tumor. This is important because the surgical approach may be quite different for bulky, vascular tumors (Figure 4-32) or those with frank vascular invasion. Distinguishing stage 1 from stage 2 lesions (spread beyond the renal capsule) is generally not important because the perirenal fat is taken at the time of radical nephrectomy. No imaging technique can detect microscopic tumor spread beyond the capsule better than microscopic examination of the specimen.

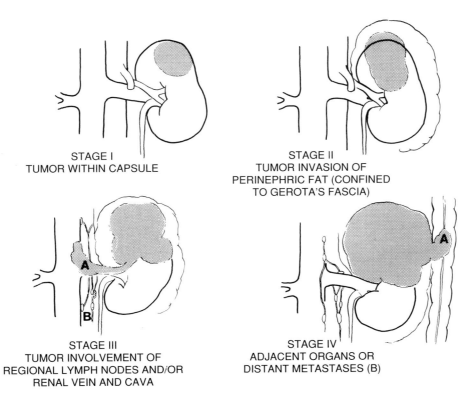

FIGURE 4-31 Staging of Renal Cell Carcinoma.

Tumor invasion into the ipsilateral renal vein or inferior vena cava must accurately be determined preoperatively. If the surgeon cross-clamps the renal vein, not realizing that it harbors tumor thrombus, you can expect a rather unpleasant phone call from the surgical suite. We find that scanning with high levels of contrast allows excellent recognition of vascular involvement. The renal veins will be densely opacified using an injection delay of 60 to 70 seconds before starting the scan. The inferior vena cava above the level of the renal veins will also be well-opacified, although there may be some inhomogeneity at the level of the renal veins due to contrast mixing. Below the renal veins, the cava may not be well-opacified. We therefore must rely on the delayed sections to make certain that there is no caval thrombus below the level of the renal veins. Infrarenal caval thrombosis is very rare in renal cell carcinoma. Usually when inferior vena cava thrombus occurs due to renal cell carcinoma, it results from direct extension via the renal vein. Thus, the tumor thrombus almost always extends superiorly within the cava, not inferiorly. Secondary bland thrombus may occur below tumor thrombus.

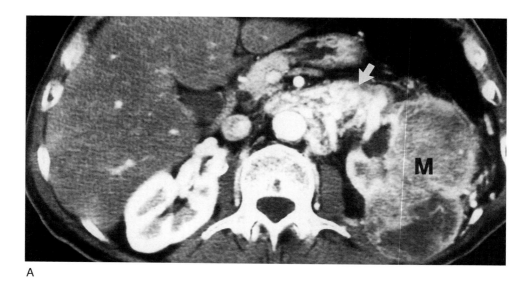

FIGURE 4-32A Renal Cell Carcinoma with Tumor Thrombus in the Inferior Vena Cava. A. A large, hypervascular mass (M) is identified within the left kidney. The appearance of the mass is suggestive of renal cell carcinoma. A normal left renal vein is not identified, however extensive neovascularity (arrow) is seen in the vicinity of this vessel.

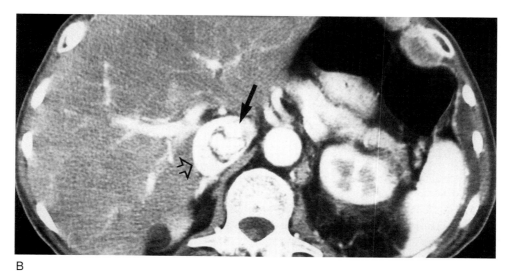

FIGURE 4-32B Section obtained two cm above Figure 4-32A shows extensive arterial collaterals (arrow) within the inferior vena cava. The appearance of enhancing tumor and collateral vessels is very suggestive of tumor thrombus. A small "sliver" of normal inferior vena cava enhancement (open arrow) is also identified.

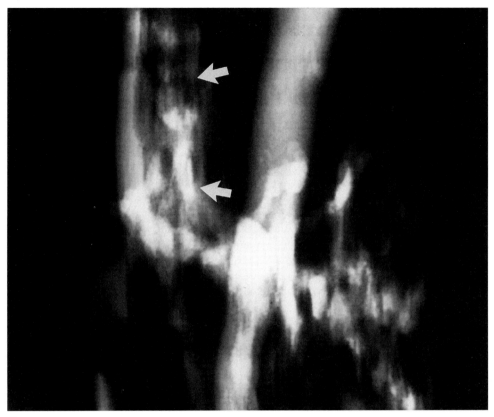

C

FIGURE 4-32C Ray-sum 3-D view shows the extensive collateral arteries (arrows) within the inferior vena cava. This view is not necessary for diagnostic interpretation, but it does better show the surgeon the vascular anatomy to expect in the operating suite.

It has been claimed that MRI may be more sensitive than CT for staging renal cell carcinoma.[51] Even with the addition of gradient echo MR angiography sequences, MR and CT are probably comparable in their ability to detect vascular invasion. In patients with renal failure or contrast allergies, MR can play an important staging role. Both MR and CT can detect vascularized tumor thrombus in the renal veins or inferior vena cava (Figure 4-32). When highly vascularized thrombus is present, multiple collateral vessels (usually arteries) will be seen within the enlarged lumen of the renal vein or inferior vena cava. The thrombus itself may show profound enhancement. Three-dimensional rendering is usually not needed for diagnosis, but it can dramatically show the vascular anatomic relationships to the surgeon (Figure 4-32).

In some advanced renal cell carcinomas, it may be difficult to determine whether or not adjacent organ invasion is present. In this setting, multiplanar reformatting can be useful.

It is best to create the reformatted images from overlapping scans. This will result in minimal stairstepping artifacts. Any viewing orientation may be selected which maximizes detection of fat planes between adjacent structures. MR also offers multiplanar display, and can thus also be helpful in selected cases.

PELVIS

Helical CT has not yet offered a clear advantage for scanning the pelvis. We are beginning to realize that contrast enhancement of pelvic organs seen on CT may be analogous to that which has been reported on MR using paramagnetic contrast. Even in patients in whom the chest and abdomen were scanned prior to scanning the pelvis, high levels of circulating contrast may be identified.

During helical CT we have observed differential enhancement within the uterine endometrium and myometrium. Similarly, the uterine body appears to enhance more than the cervical region. It is not clear whether or not this will prove to be diagnostically useful. Most fibroids during helical scanning have a hypervascular element, but also may contain areas of necrosis (Figure 4-33). On delayed scans, fibroids exhibit contrast equilibration and appear of similar soft-tissue attenuation to the remainder of the uterus (Figure 4-33).

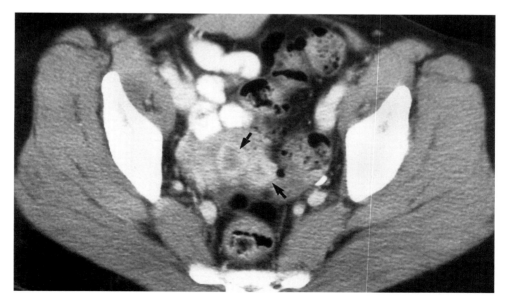

FIGURE 4-33A Enhancing Leiomyomas of the Uterus. A. Ten mm collimation helical scan through the pelvis shows enhancing masses (arrows) within the uterus. Leiomyomas may exhibit varied appearances, but should be considered when areas of increased vascularity are identified.

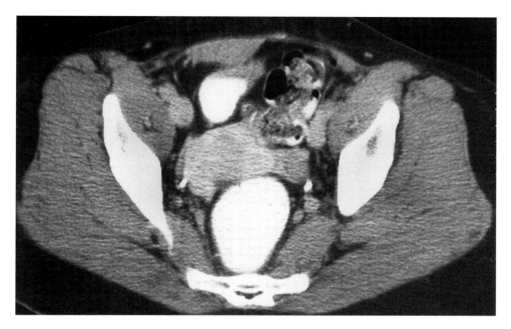

FIGURE 4-33B On this delayed scan, the leiomyomas are not clearly identified. Inhomogeneity within the uterus, however, is seen. In the future, scanning the uterus while there is a high level of circulating contrast may provide diagnostic information regarding tumors, the endometrium, and myometrium analogous to MR.

The ovaries also exhibit "filling-in" and equilibration of contrast over time. The diagnostic significance and implications of these observations are unknown, but are being studied.

CONCLUSION

Helical scanning methods represent a major refinement in abdominal CT. The combination of speed and volumetric data acquisition offer specific advantages for evaluating the abdominal organs. The impact of these advantages has included improved tumor recognition, tumor staging, and surgical planning.

REFERENCES

1. Zeman RK, Fox SH, Silverman PM, Davros WJ, Carter LM, Griego D, Weltman DI, Ascher SM, Cooper CJ. Helical (spiral) CT of the abdomen. *AJR* 1993; **160**:719–725.
2. Zeman RK, Zeiberg AS, Davros WJ, et al. Routine helical CT of the abdomen: image quality considerations. *Radiology* 1993; **189**:395–400.

3. Silverman PM, Wechsler RJ, Griego D, Cooper C, Davros WJ, Zeman RK. Cluster scanning in body CT. *Abdom Imaging* 1994; **19:**210–212.
4. Gore RM, Levine MS, Laufer I, eds. *Textbook of gastrointestinal radiology.* Philadelphia: Saunders, 1994.
5. Freeny PC, Stevenson GW, eds. *Alimentary tract radiology.* 5th ed. St. Louis: Mosby-Year Book, 1994.
6. Lee JKT, Sagel SS, Stanley RJ, eds. *Computed body tomography with MRI correlation.* 2nd ed. New York: Raven Press, 1989.
7. Moss AA, Gamsu G, Genant H. *Computed tomography of the body.* 2nd ed. Philadelphia: WB Saunders, 1989.
8. Moss AA, Schrumpf J, Schnyder P, Korobkin M, Shimshak RR. Computed tomography of focal hepatic lesions: a blind clinical evaluation of the effect of contrast enhancement. *Radiology* 1979; **131:**427–430.
9. Burgener FA, Hamlin DJ. Contrast enhancement of hepatic tumors in CT: comparison between bolus and infusion techniques. *AJR* 1983; **140:**291–295.
10. Young SW, Turner RJ, Castellino RA. A strategy for the contrast enhancement of malignant tumors using dynamic computed tomograph and intravascular pharmacokinetics. *Radiology* 1980; **137:**137–147.
11. Paushter DM, Zeman RK, Scheibler ML, Choyke PL, Jaffe MH, Clark LR. CT evaluation of suspected hepatic metastases. Comparison of techniques for IV contrast enhancement. *AJR* 1989; **152:**267–271.
12. Zeman RK, Clements LA, Silverman PM, et al. CT of the liver: a survey of prevailing methods for administration of contrast material. *AJR* 1988; **150:**107–109.
13. Foley WD, Berland LL, Smith DF, Thorsen MK. Contrast enhancement technique for dynamic hepatic computed tomographic scanning. *Radiology* 1983; **147:**797–803.
14. Silverman PM, Griego D, Davros WJ, Cooper C, Zeman RK. *Determining the optimal temporal window for helical liver CT: evaluation with time-density analysis* presented at society of computed body tomography and magnetic resonance. 16th Annual Course. Orlando, FL., Jan., 1993.
15. Zeman RK, Clark LR, Silverman PM et al. *The use of a mechanical power injector for CT contrast enhancement: reflections after 3500 patients.* 88th Annual Meeting of the American Roentgen Society. Paper #134, San Francisco CA, May 1988.
16. Walkey MM. Dynamic hepatic CT: how many years will it take 'til we learn? *Radiology* 1991; **181:**17–24.
17. Foley WD. Dynamic hepatic CT. *Radiology* 1989; **170:**617–622.
18. Heiken JP, Brink JA, McClennan BL, Sagel SS, Forman HP, DiCroce. Dynamic contrast-enhanced CT of the liver: comparison of contrast medium injection rates and uniphasic and biphasic injector protocols. *Radiology* 1993; **187:**327–331.
19. Dubrow RA, David CL, Libshitz HI, Lorigan JG. Detection of hepatic metastases in breast cancer: the role of nonenhanced and enhanced CT scanning. *J Comput Assist Tomogr* 1990; **14:**366–369.
20. Bressler EL, Alpern MB, Glazer GM, Francis IR, Ensminger WD. Hypervascular hepatic metastases:CT evaluation. *Radiology* 1987; **162:**49–51.
21. Chambers TP, Baron RL, Lush RM, Dodd GD, Miller WJ. Hepatic CT enhancement: comparison of ionic and nonionic contrast agents in the same patients. *Radiology* 1994; **190:**721–725.
22. Dupuy DE, Costello P. Can spiral CT allow effective imaging of the liver with smaller contrast media volumes? *Radiology* 1992; **185**(P):110.
23. Oliver JH. *Optimal CT of the liver: use of contrast, CT portography, and CT angiography.* Presented at the 23rd Annual Meeting and Postgraduate Course of the Society of Gastrointestinal Radiology, Maui HI, February, 1994.
24. Urban BA, Fishman EK, Kuhlman JE, Kawashima A, Hennessey JG, Siegelman SS. Detection of focal hepatic lesions with spiral CT: comparison of 4- and 8-mm interscan spacing. *AJR* 1993; **160:**783–785.

25. Vellet AD, Romano W, Bach DB, Passi RB, Taves DH, Munk PL. Adenocarcinoma of the pancreatic ducts: comparative evaluation with CT and MR imaging at 1.5T. *Radiology* 1992; **183**:87–95.
26. Semelka RC, Kroeker MA, Shoenut JP, Kroeker R, Yaffe CS, Micflikier AB. Pancreatic disease: prospective comparison of CT, ERCP, and 1.5-T MR imaging with dynamic gadolinium enhancement and fat suppression. *Radiology* 1991; **181**:785–791.
27. Tio TL, Tytgat GNJ, Cikot RJLM, Houthoff HJ, Sars PRA. Ampullopancreatic carcinoma: preoperative TNM classification with endosonography. *Radiology* 1990; **175**:455–461.
28. Semelka RC, Ascher SM. MR imaging of the pancreas. *Radiology* 1993; **188**:593–602.
29. Megibow AJ. Pancreatic carcinoma: designing the examination to evaluate clinical questions. *Radiology* 1992; **183**:297–303.
30. Dupuy DE, Costello P, Ecker CP. Spiral CT of the pancreas. *Radiology* 1992; **183**:815–818.
31. Fujii M, Itoh K, Togashi K, Nakano Y, Itoh H, Konishi J. Spiral CT with a bolus of contrast material: efficacy in the detection of small pancreatic cancer (abstr). *Radiology* 1993; **189**(p):230.
32. Freeny PC, Marks WM, Traverso LW. Pancreatic ductal adenocarcinoma: diagnosis and staging with dynamic CT. *Radiology* 1988; **166**:125–133.
33. Ward EM, Stephens DM, Sheedy PF. Computed tomographic characteristics of pancreatic carcinoma. An analysis of 100 cases. *Radiographics* 1983; **3**:547–565.
34. Ralls PW, Halls JM, Renner I, Juttner H. Endoscopic retrograde cholangiopancreatography (ERCP) in pancreatic disease. A reassessment of the specificity of ductal abnormalities in differentiating benign from malignant disease. *Radiology* 1980; **134**:347–352.
35. Warshaw AL, Gu Z, Wittenberg J, Waltman AC. Preoperative staging and assessment of resectability of pancreatic cancer. *Arch Surg* 1990; **125**:230–233.
36. Muller MF, Meyenberger C, Bertschinger P, Schaer R, Marincek B. Pancreatic tumors: evaluation with endoscopic US, CT, and MR imaging. *Radiology* 1994; **190**:745–751.
37. Zeman RK, Davros WJ, Berman PM, et al. Three-dimensional models of the abdominal vasculature based on helical CT: usefulness in patients with pancreatic neoplasms. *AJR* 1994; **162**:1425–1429.
38. Fishman EK, Wyatt SH, Ney DR, et al. Spiral CT of the pancreas with multiplanar display. *AJR* 1992; **159**:1209–1215.
39. Zeman RK, Silverman PM, Garra BS, Burrell MI, Buck JL. CT of the gallbladder and bile ducts: a practical approach to biliary disorders. [In] *Contemporary issues in computed tomography: CT and MRI of the liver and biliary system.* Silverman PS, Zeman RK, eds. New York: Churchill Livingstone. 1990; 183–221.
40. Nesbit GM, Johnson CD, James EM, et al. Cholangiocarcinoma. Diagnosis and evaluation of resectability by CT and sonography as procedures complementary to cholangiography. *AJR* 1988; **151**:933–938.
41. Itai Y, Araki T, Furui S, Yashiro N, Ohtomo K, Iio M. Computed tomography of primary intrahepatic biliary malignancy. *Radiology* 1983; **147**:485–490.
42. Pedrosa CS, Casanova R, Lezana AH, Fernandez MC. Computed tomography in obstructive jaundice: II. The cause of obstruction. *Radiology* 1981; **139**:635–645.
43. Baron RL. Common bile duct stones. Reassessment of criteria for CT diagnosis. *Radiology* 1987; **162**:419–424.
44. Zeman RK, Cronan JJ, Rosenfield AT, et al. Renal cell carcinoma: dynamic thin-section CT assessment of vascular invasion and tumor vascularity. *Radiology* 1988; **167**:393–396.
45. Silverman SG, Seltzer SE, Adams DF, Tumeh SS, Allegra DP, Mellins HZ. Spiral CT of the small indeterminate renal mass: results in 48 patients (abstr). *Radiology* 1991; **181**(P):125.
46. Bosniak MA. The current radiologic approach to renal cysts. *Radiology* 1986; **158**:1–10.
47. Bosniak MA. The small (≤ 3.0 cm) renal parenchymal tumor: detection, diagnosis, and controversies. *Radiology* 1991; **179**:307–317.
48. Curry NS, Schabel SI, Betsill WL Jr. Small renal neoplasms: diagnostic imaging, pathologic features, and clinical course. *Radiology* 1986; **158**:113–117.

49. Amendola MA, Bree RL, Pollack HM, et al. Small renal cell carcinoma: resolving a diagnostic dilemma. *Radiology* 1988; **166:**637–641.
50. Provet J, Tessler A, Brown J, Golimbu M, Bosniak M, Morales P. Partial nephrectomy for renal cell carcinoma: indications, results, and implications. *J Urol* 1991; **145:**472–476.
51. Hricak H, Demas BE. Williams RD, et al. Magnetic resonance imaging in the diagnosis and staging of renal and perirenal neoplasms. *Radiology* 1985; **154:**709–715.

Chapter 5

Musculoskeletal System

Bradford J. Richmond

INTRODUCTION

The musculoskeletal applications of helical/spiral CT provide an exciting new horizon which will revolutionize and greatly enhance the ability to diagnose complex musculoskeletal problems. This is a relatively new technology, but one which has rapidly disseminated. There are currently over 400 spiral scanners in the United States. Although many centers use spiral methodology for musculoskeletal applications, the literature has not kept up with this rapidly expanding field. The majority of information that exists is either anecdotal or in the form of scientific abstracts from regional or national radiology meetings. This chapter will discuss the current status of musculoskeletal spiral CT including its advantages, limitations, protocols and role of multiplanar and 3-D reformations.

ADVANTAGES OF SPIRAL CT

Spiral CT has many advantages applicable to the musculoskeletal system. One of the chief advantages is rapid acquisition of volume image data. The volume data can then be reconstructed in traditional axial images with resolution equaling that of conventional CT in most cases. Additionally, 2-D multiplanar and 3-D reformations can be rendered at the CT console, CT workstation, or on an independent workstation. Rapid volumetric imaging is important especially in the trauma patient, pediatric patient, and patients experiencing significant pain who would have trouble remaining immobile for conventional CT.

Trauma

Trauma patients can be rapidly assessed, minimizing additional risk to the patient who is unstable and requires close monitoring. Additionally, some scanners can perform extended spiral scans with the capability of changing scan techniques so that multiple organ systems can be evaluated with minimal interscan time delays. Musculoskeletal scanning is less dependent on breath-holding than other organ systems to obtain diagnostic images. The speed, however, of spiral scanning improves image quality in the trauma patient because the patient is not required to lie still for long periods. Miller et al.[1] demonstrated the utility of spiral CT scanning in trauma. Spiral CT was able to cover articulations in less than 40 sec with minimal table speed and collimation. Multiplanar reformations of pelvis, tibial plateau, ankle, and calcanial fractures were equal to or superior to conventional CT. Two-dimensional multiplanar reformations can be rapidly processed (usually in a minute or less) in the trauma patient to aid in surgical planning.[2] True 3-D rendering is more time consuming, but can easily be accomplished by a trained technologist in 10 to 15 minutes.

Pediatrics

Spiral scans of pediatric patients can usually be accomplished without sedation.[3] This is especially true in toddlers. The spiral CT "experience" for this patient population, as well as for adults, is far more tolerable, and patient compliance is greater should additional CT scans be required. The pediatric patients find spiral scanning less threatening. Short scan times allow for frequent contact with the child, providing a calm atmosphere.

Absence of Misregistration Artifacts

Use of spiral scanning virtually eliminates misregistration artifacts. Patients who have difficulty lying still for a sustained spiral exposure can be scanned with short 10 to 15 sec spiral acquisitions. While there is some risk of misregistration between each of the short spirals, this can be minimized by careful patient coaching. The patient may be afforded a rest period between scans, if necessary. The need for repeat scans because of motion or other artifacts is greatly reduced through the use of spiral scanning.[4]

Radiation dose

Radiation dosage is less with spiral CT. There are several reasons for reduced radiation dosage. Spiral scanners use lower milliAmperage than conventional scanners in order to limit heat accumulation. While image noise may be slightly increased with current interpolation methods (such as 180° linear interpolation), this is not of great concern for high contrast objects such as bone. Less need for repeat scans also serves to reduce the radiation exposure. Finally, spiral CT does not require overlapping images for multiplanar and 3-D image reformation. This results in a marked reduction in exposure because the same volume of tissue is not exposed twice to the x-ray beam.

Radiation surface dose was measured for 100 percent and 150 percent spiral scanning with single- and multiple-section scans. Average surface dose was 34 percent less than conventional CT for the 150 percent spiral scan and equal to conventional CT for the 100 percent spiral scan.[5] The results of this study are interesting since all manufacturers contacted state the radiation dose is lower for spiral CT than conventional CT, the result of low milliAmperes and short scan techniques. Obviously, scanning techniques will vary, and radiologists are urged to optimize their techniques based on the lowest radiation dose that will yield diagnostic images. The reader is referred to the appendix for current CTDI (Computed Tomography Dose Index) values for the major manufacturers.

Multiplanar (2-D) Reformation and 3-D Rendering

Three-dimensional rendering from spiral CT data results in higher quality models than those rendered from conventional CT data. Two-dimensional multiplanar reformations are also better. The multiplanar reformations have smoother edges with greater clarity, but may result in banding artifact which can be corrected by mathematical algorithms (spiral interpolators). There are two reasons why 3-D models and reformations look so good. One reason is thin collimation. Using extended spiral scanning, it is possible to maintain excellent coverage while using one to two mm collimation through small structures such as the physis or joint surface. It is also possible to reconstruct spiral images with high degrees of overlap. The greater the overlap, the better the fidelity of the model. In practice, 50 to 60 percent overlap is ideal for musculoskeletal applications.

In the early spiral CT experience, many radiologists felt that the broader section sensitivity profile of spirally acquired sections would result in a clinically significant reduction in spatial resolution. This could also affect the quality of multiplanar reformation. This has not proven, however, to be the case. Kasales et al. used a specially designed z-axis resolution phantom to compare spiral CT with conventional CT reformatted images.[6] Two mm axial image reformations from conventional CT were compared with two mm standard and extended spiral CT reformations. Reformations were made at one, two, and four sections (spacing) per incrementation occurring during 360° tube rotation. The z-axis resolution of spiral CT was better than conventional CT and improved when increasing the number of sections per rotation. Kalender and Polacin[7] measured spatial and contrast resolution for conventional and spiral CT. Section thickness and spiral pitch were varied. Contrast resolution was dependent on the reprocessing algorithms used for spiral CT. Contrast for small lesions on spiral CT scans can be improved twofold. Conventional and spiral CT in-plane spatial resolution is the same; spiral CT 3-D spatial resolution was superior.

Reynolds, Heuscher, and Vembar[8] used CATPhan (AAPM New York, NY) and a special z-axis resolution phantom to evaluate conventional and spiral CT. Two mm spiral-scan z-axis resolution equaled conventional two mm with one mm overlap scans. In-plane spiral spatial resolution was equivalent to conventional axial CT. Greater than 20 line pairs per centimeter resolution was achieved, but pixel noise increased with higher resolution. Kasales et al.[9] used a 14- to 21-line-pair resolution phantom varying y-axis coordinates and using half water techniques. Their findings agree with those of Reynolds; there is no difference in x-y (in-plane) resolution between standard spiral, extended spiral, and conventional CT.

Extended Scan Capability

Extended spiral scanning covers large areas in a short time, often with minimal interscan delay. Several manufacturers provide protocols which provide the ability to change collimation on sequential spirals with essentially no delay. This allows for effective evaluation of specific anatomic areas of interest. Setup of individual scans, which add to overall patient time on the scan table, were found predominantly on earlier versions of spiral software.[10] Most vendors have or are in the process of addressing unacceptable delays between spiral acquisitions. For musculoskeletal applications, a minimum of 32 sec of scan time, optimally 40 to 60 sec, is required since thin collimation is used. Tube heating, a factor with extended scan times, is avoided by using reduced milliAmpere techniques (120 to 210 mA). This is acceptable for most musculoskeletal work because the extremities do not require high milliAmperes.

More Efficient Use of Contrast Material

Contrast is frequently not needed for evaluation of bone lesions. Contrast may be used when evaluating soft-tissue lesions. There is increasing interest in the use of spiral CT for evaluation of musculoskeletal tumor extent, and the relationship of soft-tissue components to adjacent blood vessels for surgical planning. Rapid scan techniques with reduced contrast have the potential to establish these relationships. With proper timing of the scan, there will be optimal visualization of the bolus for visualization of arterial anatomy. A repeat scan through the area of interest after a short delay can provide information on venous flow. This application is just emerging, but may be used in conjunction with display of the vessels and bony structures in a single reformatted plane or 3-D model.

Smaller volumes of contrast will be necessary compared to conventional CT. It has been noted in chest and body applications that contrast dose is reduced when using spiral CT. Foley[11] demonstrated several examples of the use of variable-mode helical CT (GE HiSpeed Advantage) which resulted in reduced IV contrast dose for chest and abdominal studies. Sagel, Fishman, and Sheedy[12] concur that IV contrast load is reduced with spiral CT.

LIMITATIONS OF SPIRAL CT FOR MUSCULOSKELETAL EVALUATION

Earlier versions of reconstruction software for spiral CT had reduced z-axis resolution. Recent improvement in protocols and software have improved z-axis resolution to equal or better than that of conventional CT.[13-16] Manufacturers are presently working on software applications which will further improve z-axis resolution beyond that of conventional CT. X-y resolution may be decreased due to smoothing algorithms;[17] however, newer algorithms have also improved x-y resolution.[18] Certain scanners presently oversample due to a large number of detectors optimizing focal spot and detector aperture widths which results in improved x-y resolution.

For some scanners, reconstruction of spiral data requires significant computer time, during which additional scanning cannot be performed. This ultimately extends the overall time the scanner is not available.[19] The vendors are working to reduce reconstruction delays, or at the very least to prioritize reconstruction so that the user may select the images that are to be viewed first. Additionally, if reformation is attempted in addition to active image reconstruction, scanning may be slowed down even further. The use of a workstation networked to the CT scanner or an independent workstation can help eliminate the latter cause of slow throughput. This is particularly true for 3-D rendering, which we strongly recommend not be performed on the operator's console or a console with a shared processor with the main system. Limited image raw data storage capability on some first generation spiral CT scanners limited their utility, especially in larger joints which required a 32-sec or longer scan. Most scanners now do not have this limitation (see appendix, Table 7).

Volume measurements using 3-D models is highly dependent on the scan, reconstruction, and rendering parameters. Hopper et al.[20] demonstrated that estimation of volume by spiral CT was best limited to four mm collimation, and eight mm collimation overestimated volume of a phantom by up to 20 percent. Reconstruction at one, two, and four sections per tube revolution resulted in no significant improvement in volume estimates. Extended spiral scans with two overlapping slices per revolution did not adversely affect volume measurements. Davros, Carter, and Zeman[21] state that the use of thin-beam collimation comparable to the size of the objects being rendered best estimated the volume of acrylic spheres using a General Electric 9800 HiSpeed scanner. Jerjian et al.[22] concluded that conventional CT phantoms were not adequate for characterizing the performance capabilities of spiral CT. He states phantoms specific for the characteristics of spiral CT (e.g., volume image data, z-axis resolution) need to be developed.

All scanners are not capable of rapid sequential spiral scans without the technician entering the technique prior to each scan acquisition. This may be a problem in the trauma patient or the patient with severe pain since it prolongs the time the patient is physically in the scanner. Even though the overall time of scanning may be less than conventional technique, the ability to preprogram sequential and different protocol spiral CT scans further enhances the utility of this technology in the difficult patient.

INDICATIONS AND RECOMMENDED SCANNING TECHNIQUES

The most common indications for spiral CT of the musculoskeletal system include evaluation of trauma, demonstration of the relationship of benign or malignant pathologic processes to the joint or growth plate, and for surgical planning in the setting of neoplasm.

In most clinical settings for which spiral CT is used, 3-D or multiplanar reformation should be considered as an important adjunct, because of the ease with which these images communicate anatomic relationships to the orthopedic surgeon.

Each manufacturer has standard protocols for extremity and spine which are presently utilized by their spiral CT users. Table 5-1 provides protocol information provided by manufacturers and radiologists from centers performing high-volume spiral CT examinations. The protocols all share common features. Thin collimation is essential. The milliAmperes must be carefully adjusted to appropriately image the body part being studied. The lumbar spine poses the greatest challenge to musculoskeletal spiral scanning, because high milliAmperes are necessary. If a sustained exposure at adequate milliAmperes cannot be achieved on the scanner in your practice, consider reducing the duration of the spiral, achieving adequate coverage by increasing the pitch, breaking the spiral into several shorter duration spirals with a tube-cooling interval in between, or scanning the lumbar spine nonspirally. Increasing the kiloVolt peak is another alternative which boosts exposure, while not increasing tube heating.

Optimizing 2-D reformation and 3-D rendering technique goes hand-in-hand with optimizing the scan acquisition parameters.[23] There is no question that spiral 3-D renderings are equal to or better in quality than those from conventional CT. This is due to better z-axis resolution.[24] There is not uniform agreement, however, on the optimal collimation and spacing to use. For fine bony detail, our experience suggests that three to five mm collimation is most appropriate. We and others reconstruct three mm scans at one mm intervals.[25] When using five mm collimation, scans are reconstructed at two mm spacing. This provides sufficient overlap to produce high quality reformation and rendering. Murakami et al.[26] reported that for 3-D surface-rendered images, a five to seven mm or less section thickness is optimal. This is a thicker collimation than most experts in the field would use. Prokop et al.[27] scanning spherical and tubular phantoms concluded that for 3-D applications table increments of greater than five mm should not be used. Small objects are particularly prone to distortion. Bandlike distortion was also found in the z-axis. Most investigators and manufacturers contacted agree with Hopper et al.[28] that 3-D reconstructions are best reformatted from spiral CT with thin collimation.

Scans of 32- to 60-sec duration are usually required to adequately cover the area of interest. Shorter duration scans can be adequate if the exam is limited to a single joint surface. Sequential scans maybe needed for very large areas of interest. Sequential scans using protocols for the chest and abdomen may be performed in conjunction with musculoskeletal scans in the trauma patient and for evaluation of metastatic disease. It may be necessary to obtain additional thin collimation, nonspiral sections in areas not optimally evaluated using routine body-scanning parameters. Reconstruction after applying a bone algorithm is also helpful in selected cases.

There is considerable debate over the merits of scanning with increased pitch. Posniak et al.[29] report 1.5:1 pitch has several advantages: reduced radiation dose per volume of irradiated tissue, a shorter scan duration, and reduction of IV contrast dose. The disadvantages of 1.5:1 pitch are also significant and include: decreased image contrast resolution

TABLE 5-1 Recommended musculoskeletal protocols

Vendor	Area of Interest	mA	kVp	Collimation[a]	Scan Time	Reconstruction Algorithm[b]
General Electric HiSpeed CT[c]	Cervical spine	240	120	3 mm	1 sec	Bone
	Lumbar spine	340	120	5 mm	1 sec	Bone
	Facial Bones	240	120	3 mm	1 sec	Bone
	Extremity	240	120	3 mm	1 sec	Bone
	Hip	280	120	3 mm	1 sec	Bone
	Hand/foot	160	120	1 mm	1 sec	Bone
Siemens Somatom Plus S[d]	Cervical spine	165	120	5 mm	1 sec	High/Ultra
	Lumbar spine	165	120	10 mm	1 sec	High/Ultra
	Facial Bones	165	120	2–3 mm	1 sec	High/Ultra
	Extremity	165	120	2–3	1 sec	High/Ultra
	Hip					
	Hand/foot					
Picker PQ 2000, V 4.2 Software[e]	Cervical spine	175	130	4 mm	1–2 sec	Sharp/Extra
	Lumbar spine	175	140	4 mm	2 sec	Sharp/Extra
	Facial Bones	125	130	2–4 mm	1 sec	Sharp/Extra
	Extremity	125	130	2–4 mm	2 sec	Sharp/Extra
	Hip/Pelvis	200	140	5 mm	1–2 sec	Sharp/Extra
	Hand/foot					
Philips SR 7000[f]	Cervical spine	250–300	120	3 mm	1 sec	
	Lumbar spine	300	140	5 mm	1 sec	
	Facial Bones	200–250	120	3 mm	1 sec	
	Extremity	200	120	5 mm	1 sec	
	Hip	300	140	5 mm	1 sec	
	Hand/foot	150–200	120	3 mm	1 sec	
Elscint CT Twin[g]	Bone	280	120	2.7	1 sec	High/Concurrent
	Spine	250	120	3.2	1 sec	
Toshiba X-press[h]	Lumbar spine	250	135	3 mm	1 sec	FC 11, 180^a
	Bony pelvis	250	135	5 mm	1 sec	FC 11, 180^a
	Extremity	150	120	2 mm	1 sec	FC 11, 180^a
	Joints	150	120	2 mm	1 sec	FC 30, 180^a

[a]All vendors recommend use of 1:1 pitch ratios with the exception of Picker

[b]For abnormalities which involve the soft-tissues, both bone and soft-tissue reconstruction algorithms should be used

[c]Courtesy of Stan Fox, Ph.D., GE Medical Systems. Collimation and pitch may be adjusted in sequential helices to optimize coverage

[d]Adapted from Siemens Clinical Protocols and courtesy of Lisa Reid, Siemens Medical Systems

[e]Courtesy of Greg Powell, Ph.D., Picker International. For musculoskeletal applications a pitch ratio of 1.25:1 is recommended.

[f]Courtesy of Chris Talbot, Philips Medical Systems

[g]Courtesy of Esther Medved, Elscint Inc.

[h]Courtesy of Bryan Westerman, Toshiba Medical

and image blurring secondary to a broad section sensitivity profile. Our impression has been that use of increased pitch is an effective tool only in conjunction with thin collimation. Scanning with two mm collimation and a pitch of 1.5:1 will result in greater coverage than use of 1:1 pitch. Two mm collimation and 1.5:1 pitch will produce the same coverage, but better resolution than three mm collimation and 1:1 pitch. In order to use this strategy, however, the scanner must be capable of producing sufficient milliAmperes so that the thin collimation images are not excessively photopenic.

Bone images should be reconstructed with a detail or bone algorithm. Soft-tissue components of bone lesions can be reconstructed both using algorithms for soft-tissues, and an ultrahigh bone algorithm. This postprocessing allows for optimal evaluation of both components, soft tissue and bone when assessing musculoskeletal tumors. Remember that raw data is needed for reconstruction using this additional algorithm. Bone and soft-tissue windows should be routinely photographed.

Postprocessing in planes other than axial is best performed on a networked or independent workstation so as not to hinder scanning and to preserve patient throughput. Most vendors are trying to increase their system multitasking capabilities. For the present, reformation and rendering are more efficiently performed on a freestanding workstation. Since volume data is obtained, a cookbook approach to multiplanar reconstruction is not realistic. Each 2-D reconstruction must be tailored to the disease, anatomy, or injury being evaluated including curved reconstructions. An example of tailored reformatting would be an occult facet fracture. An oblique reformation in the plane of the facets at one mm reformations would provide the most diagnostic information. Selecting the appropriate curve and obliquity for the reformation is easily accomplished from review of the axial source images and a preliminary sagittal reformation. Since a volume image data set is acquired, fractures in any plane may be demonstrated by thin reformations. A potential drawback to such flexibility and reformations of complex anatomy in nonorthogonal planes is the difficulty in image interpretation by the clinician/surgeon. A close working relationship between the radiologist and her/his clinical colleagues is essential for optimal utilization of image information.

Many musculoskeletal radiologists feel that the information provided by 2-D multiplanar reformations may compare favorably in selected clinical settings to that of direct acquisition by MR. Bone detail is better for cortical and trabecular bone than with MR. Bone marrow involvement by infection, neoplasm, and edema is best evaluated by MR. Two-dimensional reformations using spiral CT can demonstrate fractures which are masked by 3-D surface rendering techniques. To demonstrate the utility of spiral CT scans for musculoskeletal evaluation, several specific applications and case histories will be presented.

NEOPLASM, INFECTION, AND BONE ARCHITECTURE

The patient whose images are shown in Figure 5-1 is an adolescent female who presented with knee pain. Plain films demonstrated a lytic lesion on the lateral side of the tibia in the

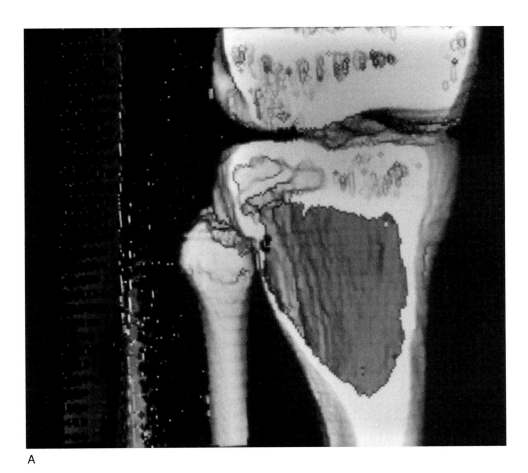

A

FIGURE 5-1A Coronal (A) 3-D reformation, cut away, made on a Voxel Q workstation. The image shows extension of the lytic giant cell tumor through a partially fused physis.

metaphysis. The physis was visualized; however, it was difficult to determine whether the physeal plate was in the process of fusing or not. Multiplanar reformations of spiral CT data demonstrated the lateral side of the physis to have fused. At the site of fusion, the lytic lesion crossed the physis, and thus was not a purely metaphaseal lesion. The relation to the physis was not seen on the axial sections alone. The reformatted images allowed us to suggest the diagnosis of giant cell tumor. Pathology confirmed the diagnosis from intraoperative tissue.

Benign exophytic lesions of bone density are readily demonstrated by 3-D rendering of spiral CT data (Figure 5-2). This occurs because they are of similar attenuation to the

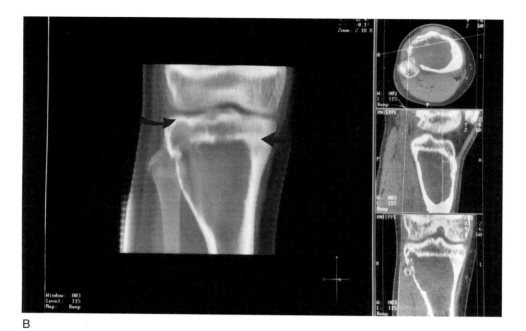

FIGURE 5-1B In this case the (B) 2-D coronal image better represents the anatomy. The physeal (arrow) and subchondral (curved arrow) plates are better visualized. The exam was performed on a Picker PQ 2000 CT scanner. *(Reprinted with permission from Picker International)*

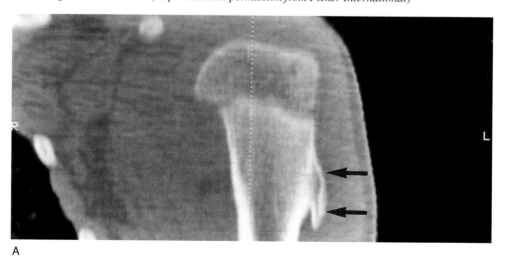

FIGURE 5-2A A benign bony exostosis (arrow) of the humerus is well delineated on both (A) reformatted coronal multiplanar image and the (B) 3-D reformation. *(The case was provided by Dr. Lawrence Tanenbaum, New Jersey. The exam was performed on a GE HiSpeed Advantage CT scanner.)*

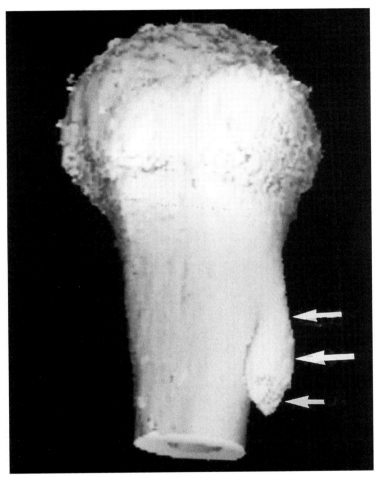

B

FIGURE 5-2B *(continued)*

normal bony structures. Depiction of benign exostoses and their anatomic orientation is readily apparent on shaded-surface displays. The image of bony attenuation lesions can be further enhanced by transparency display through compositing on the workstation. This capability allows for projection of image data with transparency of a pixel defined by its intensity. Transparency display would demonstrate the relatively transparent soft-tissue relationships to the relatively opaque exostosis.

Surface models are not useful for analysis of intracortical lesions. The overlying cortex obscures the underlying abnormality. Intracortical lesions are best seen on reformatted images (Figure 5-3). In the illustrated case, a lytic component with a central area of sclerotic bone is exquisitely shown. The differential of this type of lesion is osteoid osteoma versus Brodie's abscess.

Spiral CT readily shows the bony destruction of osteomyelitis. The patient shown in Figure 5-4 has extensive osteomyelitis/discitis and soft-tissue, paraspinal, and abdominal/pelvic abscess involvement due to Pott's disease. The images were reconstructed with bone and soft-tissue algorithms and displayed at appropriate window settings. The extent of paraspinal abscess was shown with comparable clarity to MR in this patient.

TRAUMA

Trauma is the major indication for spiral CT of the musculoskeletal system. With thin collimation and adequate milliAmperage, it is possible to produce images free of artifact even

(Text continues on page 235)

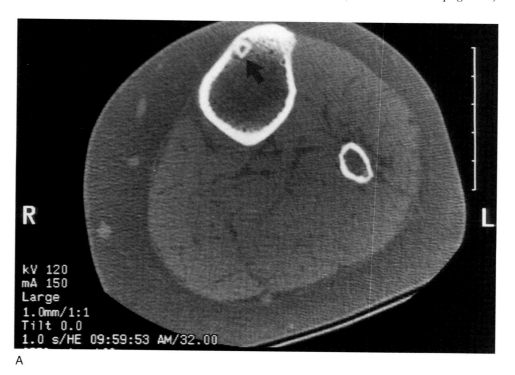

FIGURE 5-3 Axial (A) and nonorthogonal (B) 2-D reformations of an obviously intracortical lesion (arrow). Note the low 150 mA and 120 kV used for this scan. *(Case provided by Dr. Lawrence Tanenbaum, New Jersey. The exam was performed on a GE HiSpeed Advantage scanner.)*

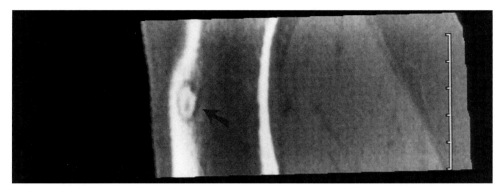

B

FIGURE 5-3B *(continued)*

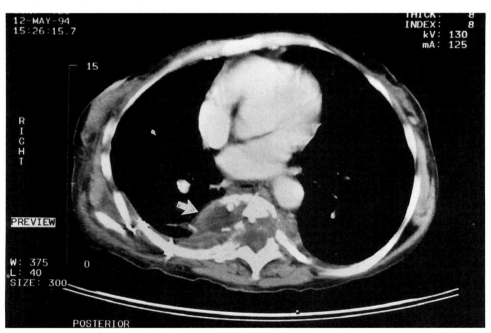

A

FIGURE 5-4A Pott's disease, tuberculous vertebral osteomyelitis-discitis. (A) Axial spiral image in the chest with vertebral involvement and a paraspinal abscess (arrow). Axial views of the abdomen (B, C) demonstrating axial reconstructions using soft-tissue and bone algorithms. Note the large psoas abscesses present (arrows) in conjunction with the vertebral osteomyelitis. A gadolinium-enhanced (D) T1 MR image is provided for comparison. *(The case was provided by Dr. Kenneth D. Hopper, Hershey Medical Center. The scan was performed on a Picker PQ 2000 scanner.)*

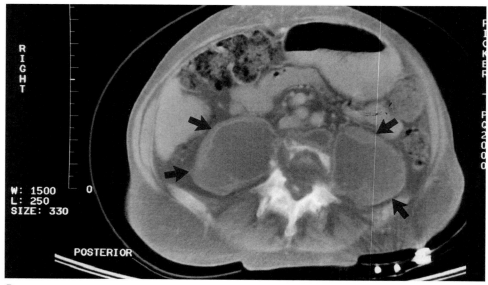

FIGURE 5-4B *(continued)*

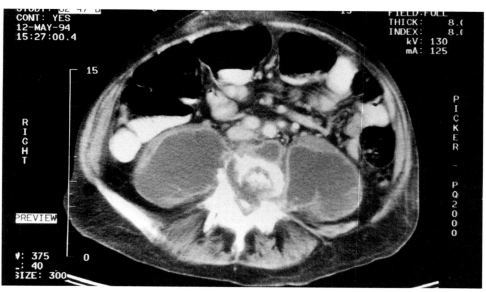

FIGURE 5-4C *(continued)*

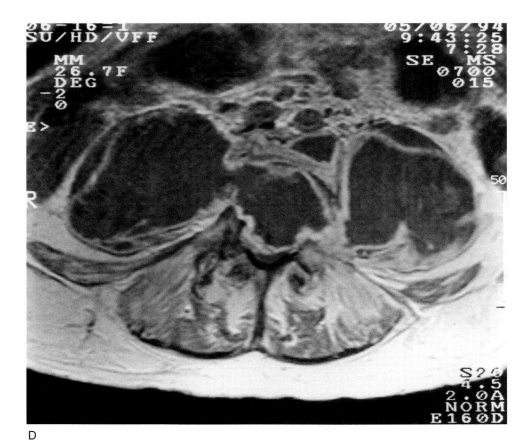

FIGURE 5-4D *(continued)*

when metal fixation devices are present. In the patient shown in Figure 5-5, plain films and tomography failed to demonstrate a suspected trochanteric fracture and femoral neck fracture. The patient has a medullary rod in place for a midshaft femoral fracture (Figure 5-5). A spiral CT performed with two mm collimation at one mm reformations demonstrated the femoral neck fracture with extension into the intertrochanteric area and down the diaphysis. This case is remarkable because cortical bone was adequately demonstrated around a metal rod, and with minimal artifact. Use of spiral CT in this setting is worthy of further evaluation.

Cadaver tibial plateau fractures and phantoms were studied to assess fracture displacement were performed by McEnery et al.[30] They found a table speed of two mm per sec was

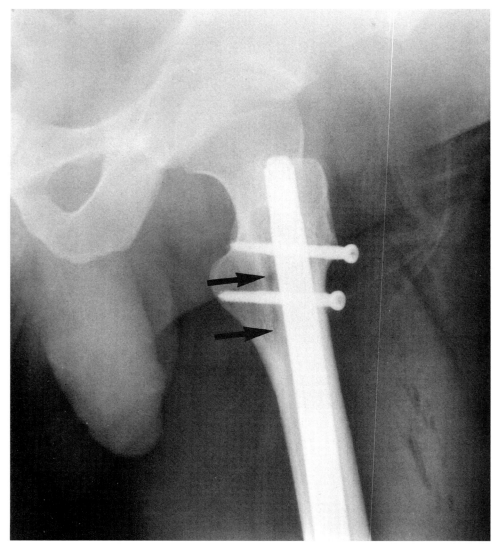

A

FIGURE 5-5A Lateral plain film image (A) of the proximal femur suggest a fracture in the intertrochanteric area (arrow). Conventional axial CT (B) demonstrated a small area of fracture. Spiral CT reformatted in (C) 2-D nonorthogonal and (D) 3-D images demonstrates the extent of the fracture in the femoral neck (long curved arrow) and down the diaphysis (short curved arrows). *(The case was provided by Dr. Marc Kaye, Cleveland Clinic Florida. The exam was performed on a Picker PQ 2000 scanner.)*

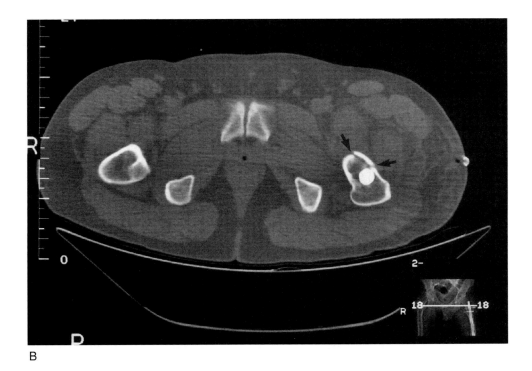

FIGURE 5-5B *(continued)*

optimal for fracture displacements of two mm or less. Multiplanar reconstructions from images with spacing or collimation greater than three mm were unacceptable for fracture fragment displacements of less than two mm.

Facial trauma may be clearly depicted by spiral CT. The 3-D and multiplanar reformations shown in Figure 5-6 demonstrate multiple fractures, fluid and gas in the sphenoid sinus, gas in the orbit, and maxillary, ethmoid, and frontal sinus fractures. There are fractures of the posterior wall of both maxillary sinuses. A fracture of the nasion is also identified. Edema of orbital fat and herniation of the inferior rectus/oblique muscles of the orbit was present (Figure 5-6). The images provide excellent information and a much better overview than plain radiographs for presurgical planning. A nondepressed, anteriorly displaced inferior orbital rim fracture using 3-D reformations is demonstrated (Figure 5-7).

Odontoid fractures can be difficult to identify on conventionally acquired axial sections. The fracture may be in the axial plane and may be missed if it traverses two adjacent sections. Figure 5-8 demonstrates a coronal view of a 3-D model, which has been shown as a ray-sum display. This image simulates a radiograph, however, with greater clarity and

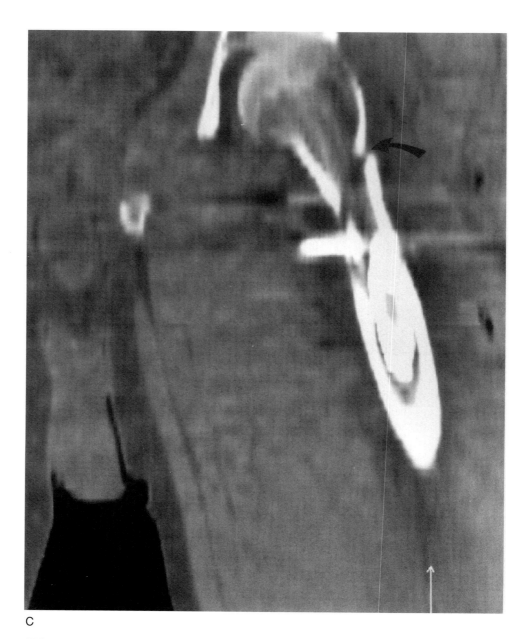

FIGURE 5-5C *(continued)*

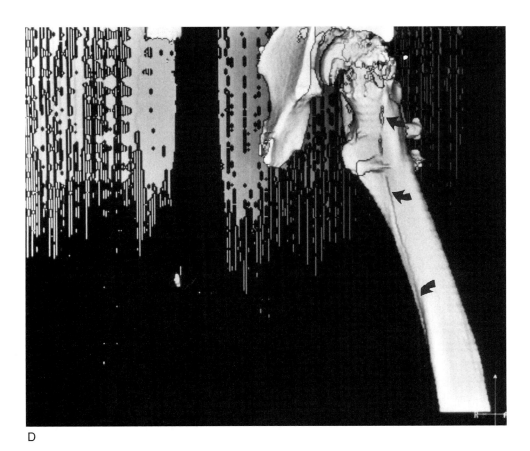

D

FIGURE 5-5D *(continued)*

contrast resolution. The fracture at the base of the odontoid is easily seen on this view. Spiral CT was used to evaluate sequentially 408 patients with neck trauma by Ahmad et al.[31] The scans were compared to plain films. Spiral CT correctly demonstrated all 27 fractures of the cervical spine. Sixteen of the 27 fractures were missed on plain films. One traumatic subluxation in the cervical spine was identified on plain film but missed on spiral CT. This study suggests spiral CT may be the optimal diagnostic study for cervical spine trauma.

Surgical management of ankle fractures depends largely on congruity of joint surfaces and displacement of fragments. Figure 5-9 demonstrates the use of spiral reformations in assessment of a tibial plafond fracture with minimal displacement of the fracture fragment

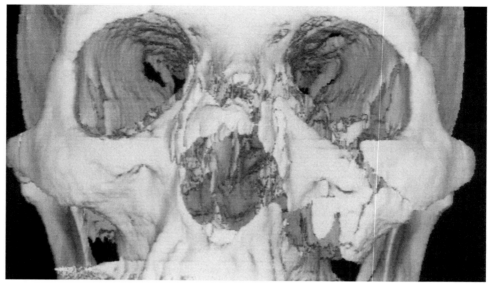

A

FIGURE 5-6A Complex facial trauma. (A, B) 3-D images demonstrate fracture of the nasion, inferior wall of the left orbit and left maxilla. (C) 2-D axial reformation demonstrates maxillary sinus fracture of the nasion. Note the gas and fluid present. (D) Coronal reformation and (E) sagittal reformation help define maxillary and orbital fracture extent. Note the edema of orbital fat and inferior herniation of muscle at the floor of the orbit. *(Case provided by Dr. Lawrence Tanenbaum. Images from a GE HiSpeed Advantage CT scanner.)*

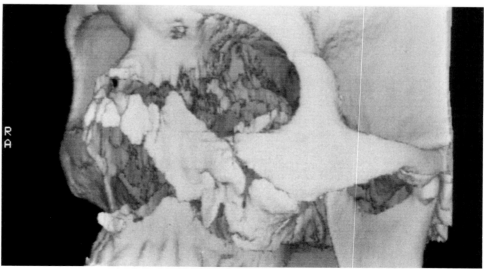

B

FIGURE 5-6B *(continued)*

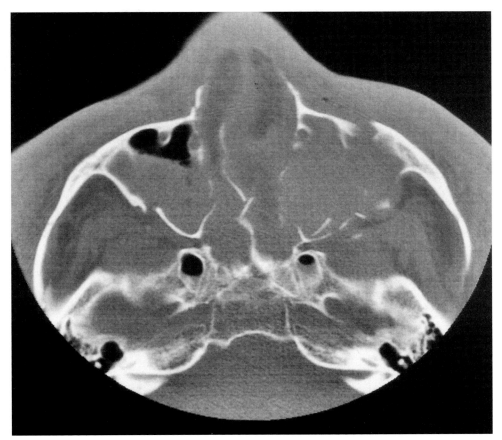

C

FIGURE 5-6C *(continued)*

resulting in discontinuity of the subchondral plate. The reformatted image convincingly suggests the need for surgical reduction.

A comminuted posterior fracture of the acetabulum is demonstrated in Figure 5-10. The displacement of the comminuted fracture fragments is readily assessed. Bone fragments in the hip joint are present. Integrity of the femoral head is established. A comminuted transverse fracture of the acetabulum is shown in Figure 5-11. The information from spiral CT provides excellent resolution images which aids the surgeon in planning fixation. Martinez et al.[32] provide an excellent review of acetabular fracture classification.

The utility of CT of the wrist for trauma, post surgical follow-up, and bony lesions has been recently reviewed.[33] Spiral CT has been demonstrated by McEnery, Wilson, and

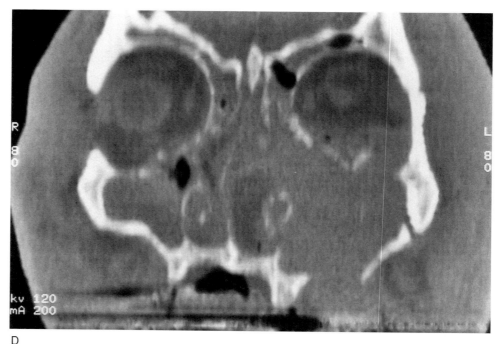

D

FIGURE 5-6D *(continued)*

Murphy[34] to reduce examination time, radiation dose, and to simplify positioning with the use of multiplanar reformations in the wrist examination.

In general, there is far greater experience using multiplanar reconstruction in trauma than true 3-D rendering. The potential for masking fractures with volume-rendered 3-D images is a pitfall that has not yet been studied in large series. We worry that thresholding may influence our ability to see fractures on shaded-surface displays. Maximum intensity projection views may also hide significant fractures because of superimposed normal bone. For the time being we would encourage use of 2-D reformations in all cases of trauma, with selective use of 3-D views.

OTHER APPLICATIONS OF MUSCULOSKELETAL SPIRAL CT

Spiral CT may be helpful in achieving more accurate and rapid localization of lesions during biopsies. We have used 10 mm collimation spiral scans with five mm axial reformations to localize an appropriate area for biopsy. This technique does result in lower

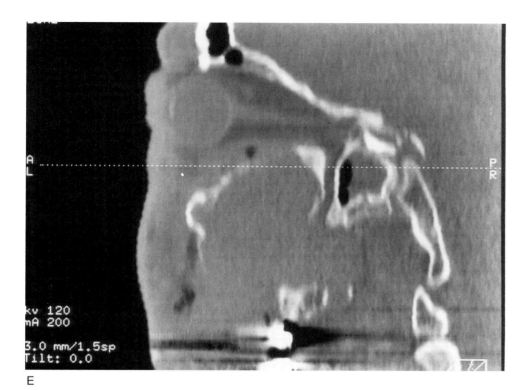

FIGURE 5-6E *(continued)*

resolution images; however, the overall time of biopsy decreases since multiple localization scans need not be performed (Figure 5-12). This technique is best used for lesions covering a large area. Conventional images can then be used for needle introduction.

Another exciting use of spiral CT is for spiral CT arthrography. The ability to evaluate the glenoid labrum with multiplanar reformations has greatly improved the detection of labral tears.[35] A heightened ability to discriminate between labrum and glenohumeral ligaments is provided with spiral reformations. Large patients who are unable to be examined for shoulder pathology may benefit from spiral CT arthrography (Figure 5-13). Other joints are easily examined for cartilage defects or other pathology of articulations and their surrounding soft tissues (Figure 5-14). The general protocol used is two mm collimation with one mm reformation. Relatively high milliAmperes (210 mA) is recommended to allow adequate penetration through the abundant soft tissues surrounding the shoulder.

Spiral CT has been demonstrated to be useful for a broad spectrum of musculoskeletal disorders. Cases of infection, neoplasm, arthrography, and trauma have been

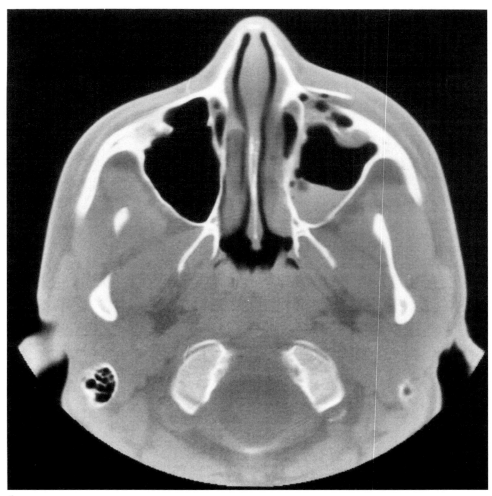

A

FIGURE 5-7A A minimally anteriorly displaced fracture of the inferior rim of the orbit is best appreciated on 2-D reformations (A). 3-D reformations are useful to demonstrate the anterior wall fracture (B) but the displacement is not demonstrated well. *(The case was provided by Dr. Lawrence Tanenbaum. Images from a GE HiSpeed CT scanner.)*

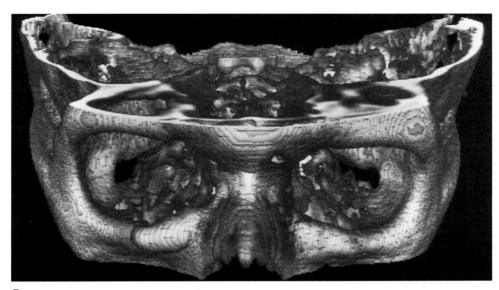

B

FIGURE 5-7B *(continued)*

demonstrated. Protocols are relatively simple and similar. Diagnostic information is most effectively provided with the use of 2-D multiplanar reformations. Three-dimensional reformation is useful when reviewed at the workstation with the surgeon/clinician. Potential limitations of 3-D using surface-rendering technique must be recognized, especially in trauma, and underscores the need for multiplanar reformations in nonorthogonal planes to demonstrate occult fractures.

PITFALLS

Multiplanar reformations allow for evaluation of anatomic orientations not previously utilized routinely. This capability, while impressive, is useful only if the clinician/surgeon can use it in a manner beneficial to the patient. The reformatted image orientation may be inherently obvious to the radiologist performing and analyzing the exam but requires appropriate review with the clinician/surgeon to facilitate therapy. Lulling oneself into a sense of providing useful image data without the appropriate consultative interaction is the biggest pitfall of reformations from spiral CT.

Lesions which are of similar density to surrounding tissue or less than collimation thickness in size can be missed. This was demonstrated by Davros, Carter, and Zeman[21]

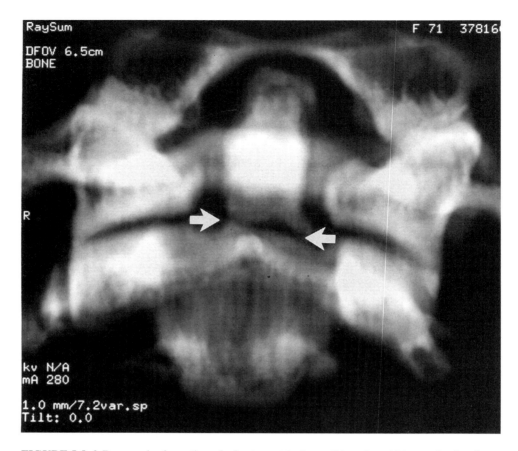

FIGURE 5-8 2-D coronal reformation of a fracture at the base of the odontoid (arrows) using the postprocessing Ray-sum feature has the appearance of a radiograph. *(Dr. Lawrence Tanenbaum provided the case. Images from a GE HiSpeed Advantage CT scanner.)*

using four acrylic spheres scanned by spiral CT. Small image plane reconstruction spacing with thin-beam collimation most accurately estimated volumes of the spheres. Davros also noted the collimation must be at least equal to or larger than the lesion being evaluated to optimize contrast. Hu and Fox,[36] in assessing visibility of phantom tumors, further indicated the need to collimate to the size of the radius of the tumor, use a pitch of one, and use overlapping reconstructions to improve contrast uniformity in tumor evaluation. Jacobson, Metz, and Foley[37] demonstrated the potential to miss high-attenuation small objects (BBs) with spiral CT. Conventional CT performed significantly better than the spiral CT at identifying BBs placed at a 15° incline in gel with one mm z-axis spacing and four mm x-y axis.

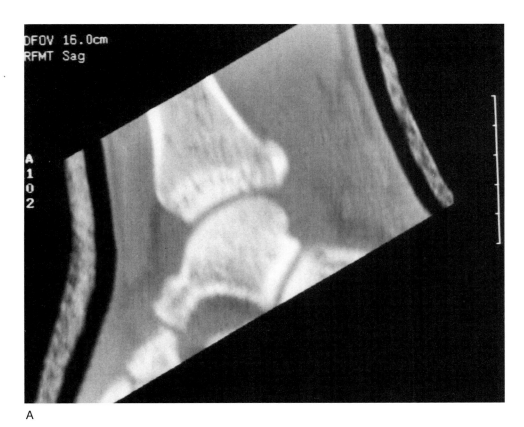

A

FIGURE 5-9A 2-D sagittal reformation demonstrating displacement of a distal tibial fracture (A) and incongruity of the subchondral plate (B). *(Dr. Lawrence Tanenbaum provided the case. Images from a GE HiSpeed Advantage CT scanner.)*

FUTURE APPLICATIONS

What can be expected in the future for musculoskeletal spiral CT? Future developments include more powerful processors. This will result in larger raw image data storage allowing for more extended scans and reduction in the need for sequential scans. Z-axis resolution will also be improved. Scanners with broader detector plates will allow increased coverage with greater parity of in-plane and z-axis resolution. This will improve detection of small lesions and further enhance the ability to visualize trabecular structure and detect matrix within a lesion.

The potential to use spiral CT for bone mineral analysis is now under investigation, and may eliminate the need to scan a reference phantom. The technique involves the analysis of fat and soft-tissue CT numbers as reference tissues of the patient on the same scan.[38]

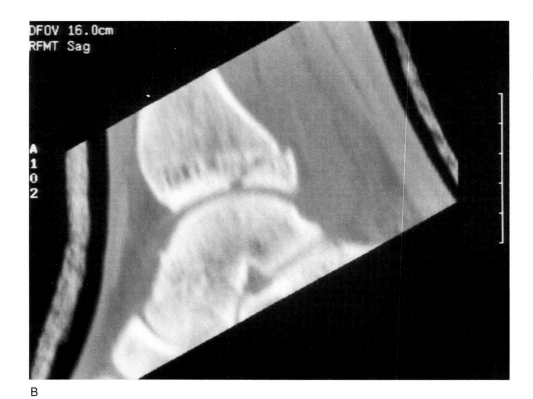

B

FIGURE 5-9B *(continued)*

Since the volume of bone can be reconstructed at any level within the vertebral body or for the whole vertebral body, technical error of reproducibility of position may be less of a problem. Scanner performance is variable within the scan circle; i.e., beam hardening, scatter, and volume averaging all occur. This variation can be minimized by using a reference tissue closer to the vertebral body and which provides more consistent sequential measurements of CT numbers.

Z-axis resolution is excellent at present at pitch ratios of 1:1 and 1.5:1. Further improvements are needed to minimize sampling artifacts for more accurate 3-D reformations of contoured bone surfaces. This improvement can be achieved in spiral sampling by reducing the pitch factor (e.g., 0.5 or 0.75) and/or applying a spiral interpolator minimizing the "banding"[26] or "stairstepping"[39] artifact (Figure 5-15). The radiation dose may be held constant by reducing milliAmperes when scanning with reduced pitch factors. Wider

(Text continues on page 260)

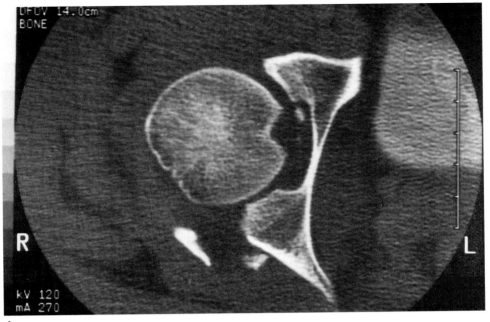

A

FIGURE 5-10A A comminuted posterior column fracture (A) of the acetabulum with displaced (B) and intraarticular fragments (C). *(Dr. Lawrence Tanenbaum provided the case. Images from a GE HiSpeed scanner.)*

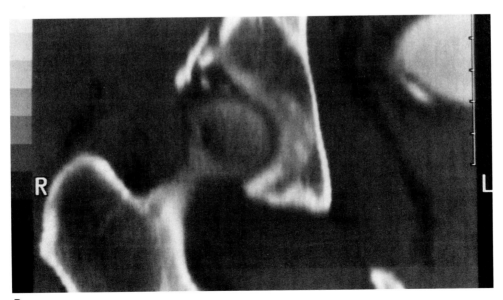

B

FIGURE 5-10B *(continued)*

249

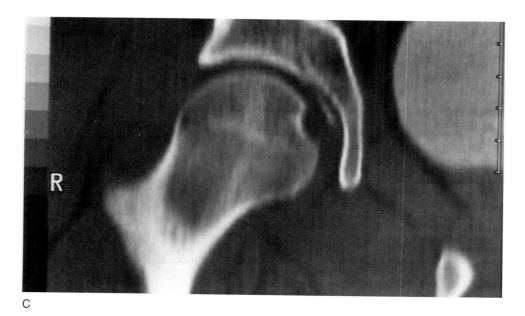

FIGURE 5-10C *(continued)*

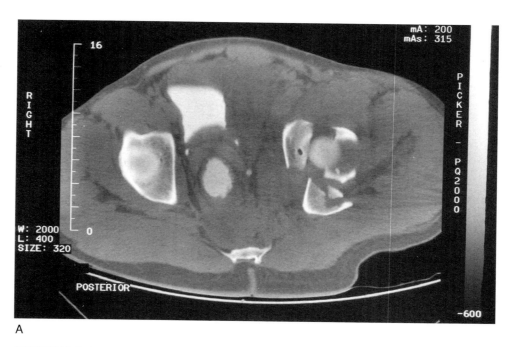

FIGURE 5-11A Axial reformations of a transverse fracture of the acetabulum (A, B). *(Dr. Kenneth Hopper provided the case. Images from a Picker PQ 2000 CT scanner.)*

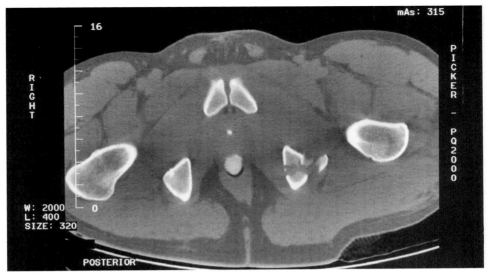

B

FIGURE 5-11B *(continued)*

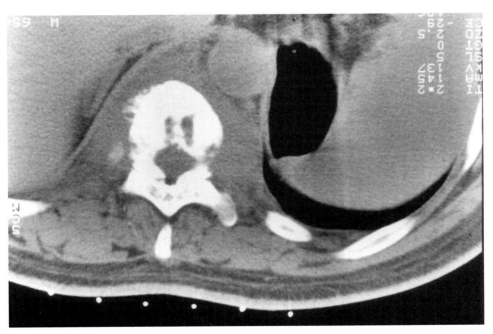

A

FIGURE 5-12A Axial reformations for biopsy localization of the thoracic spine (A) after a 30-sec scan. Subsequent conventional CT biopsy needle placement (B). *(Images from a Siemens Somatom Plus CT scanner.)*

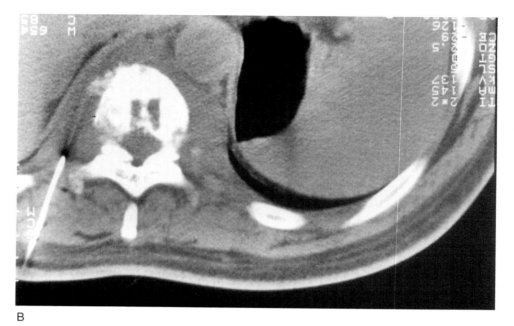

B

FIGURE 5-12B *(continued)*

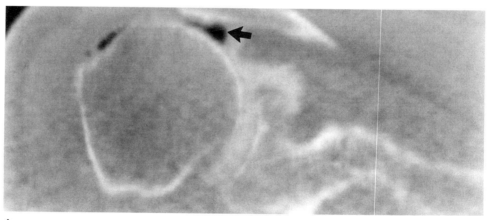

A

FIGURE 5-13A Coronal (A, B) and sagittal reformations (C) of a spiral CT arthrogram show a complete rotator cuff tear (arrow). The sagittal reformation demonstrates a glenohumeral ligament (curved arrows). The patient weighed 250 pounds. *(Dr. Joseph Busch provided the case. Images are from a Siemens Somatom Plus CT scanner.)*

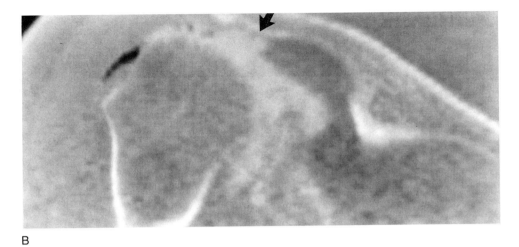

B

FIGURE 5-13B *(continued)*

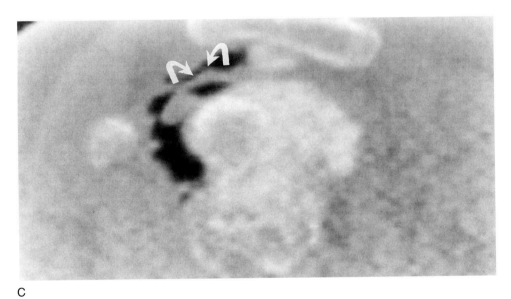

C

FIGURE 5-13C *(continued)*

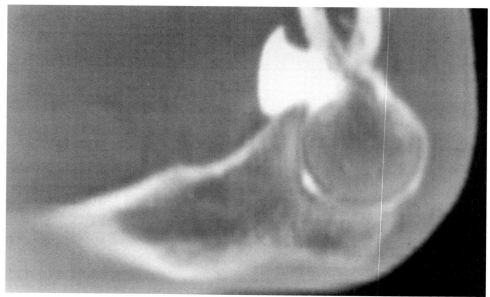

A

FIGURE 5-14A Reformatted sagittal and coronal images of the ulnar trochlear joint (A) and radial capitellar joint (B, C). Sclerosis (arrow) in the capitellum is secondary to a previous osteochondral defect. *(Dr. Joseph provided the case. Images from a Siemens Somatom Plus CT scanner.)*

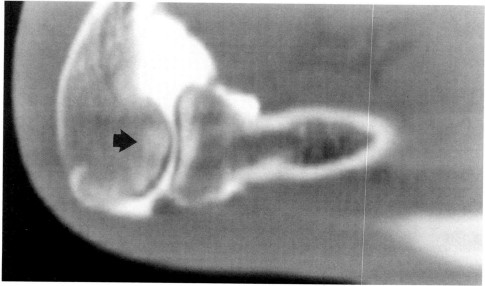

B

FIGURE 5-14B *(continued)*

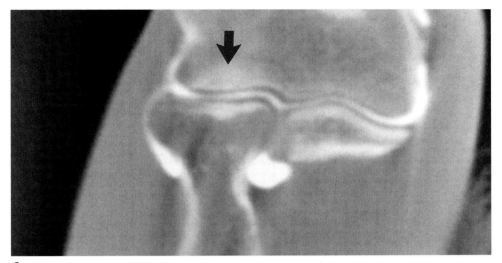

C

FIGURE 5-14C *(continued)*

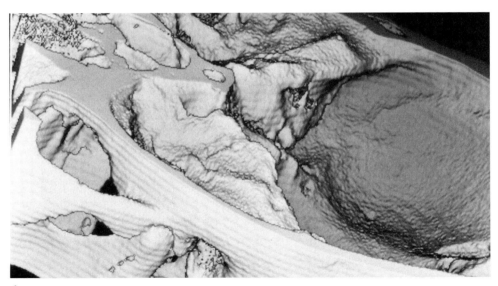

A

FIGURE 5-15A 3-D images constructed using spiral data acquired using a pitch factor of one, an image index of 0.5 mm and a slice thickness of two mm but processed using two different spiral interpolators. The first maximizes z-axis resolution (A) and the second minimizes the "banding" artifact (B). Data gathered using a pitch factor of one and a standard (180° linear) spiral interpolator (C) is compared with a 3-D image created using data gathered with a pitch factor of 0.75 and processed using an appropriate high order spiral interpolator (D). In each case, the slice thickness was two mm and image index was 0.5 mm. *(Dominic Heuscher from Picker International CT (Highland Heights, Ohio) provided the phantom images and data.)*

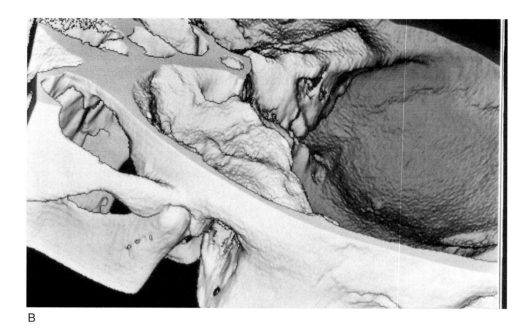

B

FIGURE 5-15B *(continued)*

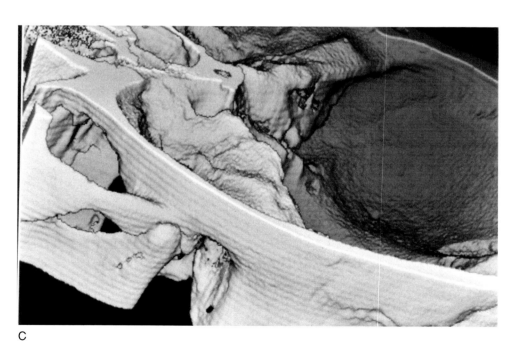

C

FIGURE 5-15C *(continued)*

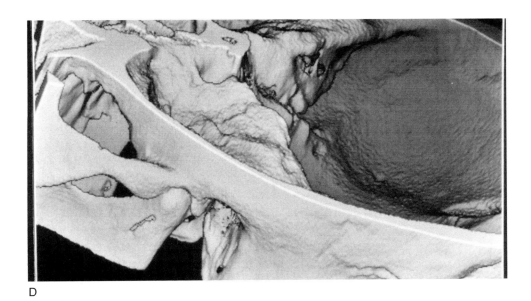

D

FIGURE 5-15D *(continued)*

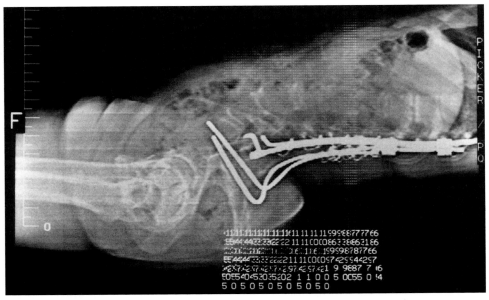

A

FIGURE 5-16A Metal artifact removal. (A) Scout of the patient showing the degree of spinal fixation. (B) Axial reformatted scan with metal artifact. (C) Axial reformatted scan after postprocessing metal artifact removal program. (D, E) Sagittal and coronal reformatted scans demonstrating solid bone graft and no fractures. *(Images from a Picker PQ 2000 CT scanner.)*

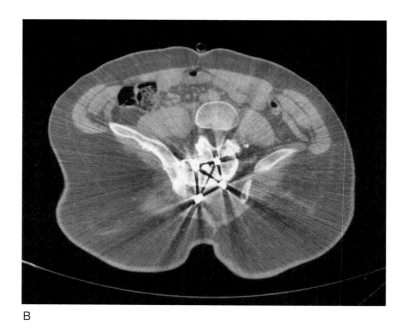

B

FIGURE 5-16B *(continued)*

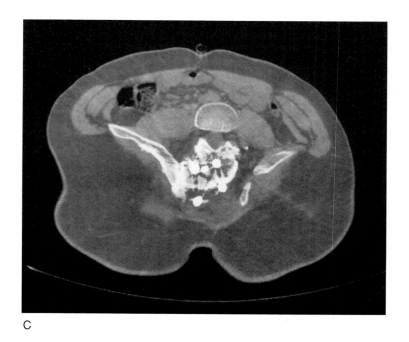

C

FIGURE 5-16C *(continued)*

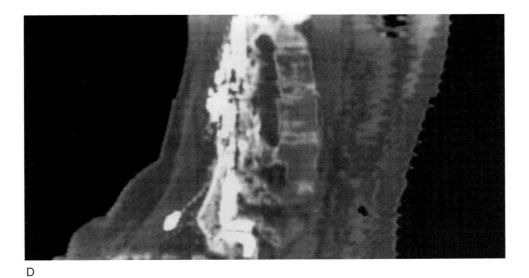

FIGURE 5-16D *(continued)*

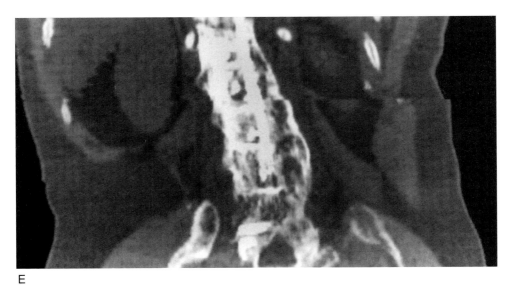

FIGURE 5-16E *(continued)*

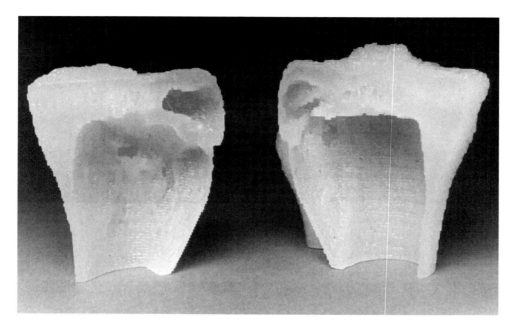

FIGURE 5-17 Solid model from a spiral CT scan of a giant cell tumor of the proximal tibia (see Figure 5-1) made from spiral CT data, Picker PQ 2000 CT scanner by photolithography. *(The model was provided by Joel P. Epstein, President, Spectra Group Limited, Inc., Maumee, Ohio).*

interpolators are used to reconstruct spiral data. Image reconstructions will have the same image quality and noise statistics as the original reconstructions but without the 3-D artifacts.

Presently, no data has been provided to determine the use of contrast for evaluation of neoplasms and vascular integrity in musculoskeletal trauma. There is indication, however, in other body applications that contrast load is reduced with the use of spiral CT. The use of contrast for presurgical assessment of vascular integrity in trauma and displacement/involvement by neoplasm is warranted. Automated bone removal for optimal visualization of vessels from spiral CT 3-D angiography can be performed on an independent workstation by Wunderlich et al.[40] Although this was not a commercial software program, there is great potential for application in musculoskeletal imaging of neoplasms, trauma, and vascular malformations. Subtraction 3-D CT angiography is soon to be available on both Siemens and GE workstations.

The ability to evaluate cortical bone around straight metal orthopedic devices has been demonstrated. Metal artifact is a problem with complex contours (screws, prosthesis, etc.). Heang K. Tuy of Picker CT (Highland Heights, Ohio) has developed a postprocessing metal artifact removal program which is compatible with spiral CT images.[41] This post-processing application is demonstrated in the case of a young male who underwent posterior fusion using metal fixation for correction of scoliosis (Figure 5-16). A fracture of the lumbar spine posterior elements was suspected. Metal from the fixation precluded plain film diagnosis, and metal artifact degraded the CT image on both conventional and spiral CT. The metal artifact program allowed us to detect the fracture. Not all artifact was removed; however, a large reduction in artifact allows for the improved diagnosis.

Piraino, et al.[42] demonstrated anatomic models made from conventional and spiral CT (Figure 5-17). The models are made from a polymer by laser photolithography. Davros et al.[43] also demonstrated the utility of spiral CT-generated models for surgical planning. Pre-surgical planning can be performed with these models, and the material can be used to practice the surgery. Spiral CT and 3-D optical scan of amputee's stumps for CAD/CAE design of limb prosthesis was evaluated by Vannier et al.[44] Spiral CT and 3-D optical scans were found to be accurate to within five percent of caliper measurements for both hard and soft tissue providing important data for custom design of limb prosthesis.

Virtual-reality (VR) simulations using spiral CT 3-D image reformations were recently evaluated by Vining and Shifrin.[45] They demonstrated that this technology allows a viewer to view a volume of data essentially unrestricted. Further work is needed in this area to determine the most clinically useful approach for VR.

CONCLUSION

Spiral CT provides the radiologist with a tool which enhances diagnostic capability in musculoskeletal disorders. Reduced radiation dose, time of scan, contrast load, multiplanar 2-D reformations, 3-D reformations, and comfort of the patient are positive factors for development of further use of this technology in the musculoskeletal system.[46] New applications for evaluation of bone and orthopedic appliances are on the horizon. As long as the cost of this technology is maintained at a reasonable level, its application for bone diagnosis will only grow. Practically, spiral CT is important to the future of musculoskeletal imaging in this ever-changing and cost-conscious healthcare environment.

REFERENCES

1. Miller MA, McEnery KW, West OC, Wilson AJ. Musculoskeletal trauma evaluation with spiral CT. *AJR* 1994; **162**(3):252.
2. Heiken JP. Brink JA, Vannier MW. Spiral (Helical) CT. *Radiology* 1993; **189**:647–656.
3. Luker GD, Lee BC, Erickson KK. Spiral CT of the temporal bone in unsedated pediatric patients. *AJNR* 1993; **14**:1145–11504.
4. Kasales CJ, Hopper KD, Mahraj RM, Heuscher DJ, Grenauer LM, Ariola DN. Linear resolution of spiral and conventional CT in the x-, y- and z-axes. *Radiology* 1993; **189**(P):412.
5. King SH, Reynolds MD, Miller KL. Surface dose comparison for spiral and axial scanning with use of a fourth-generation CT system. *Radiology* 1993; **189**(P):356.

6. Kasales CJ, Hopper KD, Mahraj RM, Heuscher D, Gruenauer LM, Ariola DN. Z-axis resolution of Spiral and extended spiral CT at half- and full-field imaging with one, two, and four reconstructed sections per revolution. *Radiology* 1993; **189**(P):238.
7. Kalendar WA, Polacin A. 3-D spatial and contrast resolution in conventional and spiral CT. *Radiology* 1992; **185**(P):127.
8. Reynolds MD, Heuscher DJ, Vembar M. Resolution evaluation of fourth generation spiral CT. *Radiology* 1993; **189**(P)217.
9. Kasales CJ, Hooper KD, Mahraj, Ariola DN. XY-axis resolution in conventional and spiral CT. *Radiology* 1993; **189**(P):164.
10. Kalendar WA, Seissler W, Klotz E, Vock P. Spiral volumetric CT with single-breath-hold technique, continuous transport, and continuous scanner rotation. *Radiology* 1990; **176**:181–183.
11. Foley WD. Variable mode hHelical CT. *Radiology* 1993; **189**(P):296.
12. Sagel SS, Fishman EK, Sheedy PF. Fast CT scanning clinical applications of spiral and electron-beam CT. *Radiology* 1992; **185**(P):69.
13. Yusuke T, Tochigi J, et al. New reconstruction algorithm in helical volume CT (abstr). *Radiology* 1990. Abstract #121; 177:108.
14. Heuscher D, Mattson R. Volume scanning of a three-dimensional resolution phantom. Radiology 1990; **177**:307.
15. Polacin A, Kalendar WA, Marchal G. Evaluation of section sensitivity profiles and image noise in spiral CT. *Radiology* 1992; **185**:29–35.
16. Vannier M, Wang G. Spiral CT refines imaging of temporal bone disorders. *Diagnostic Imag November* 1993; 116–121.
17. Brink JA, Heiken JP, Balfe DM, Sagel SS, Dicroce, Vannier MW. Spiral CT: decreased spatial resolution in vivo due to broadening of section-sensitivity profile. *Radiology* 1992; **185**:469–474.
18. Polacin A, Kalendar WA, Marchal G. Evaluation of section-sensitivity profiles and image noise in spiral CT. *Radiology* 1992; **185**:29–35.
19 Bieze J. Spiral CT withstands fury over health reform (Market Scan). *Diagnostic Imaging* 1994; **May**:35–39.
20. Hopper KD, Kasales CJ, Van Slyke M, Mahraj RM, Umlaaf MJ, Ariola DN. Comparison of phantom volumes measured with axial, spiral, and extended spiral CT scanning. *Radiology* 1993; **189**(P):164
21. Davros WJ, Carter LM, Zeman RK. Volumetric determination accuracy of spherical targets with helical CT data and 3-D modeling. *Radiology* 1992; **185**(P):126
22. Jerjian KA, Gosham BI, Hendrick RE, Westerman BR, Thickman D. Evaluation of helical volumetric CT scanning. *Radiology* 1991; **181**(P):111
23. Fishman EK, Magid D, Ney DR, Chaney El, Pizer SM, Rosenman JG, Levin DN, Vannier MW, Kuhlman JE, Robertson DD. Three-dimensional iImaging. *Radiology* 1991; **181**:321–337
24. Ney DR, Fishman EK, Magid D, Robertson DD. Comparison of spiral CT with dynamic CT scanning with regard to three-dimensional imaging of musculoskeletal anatomy. *Radiology* 1991; **181**(P):111
25. Tuy HK, Heuscher D, Lindstrom W. Choice of the number of reconstructed sections in helical scanning. *Radiology* 1993; **189**(P):239.
26. Murakami S, Hiramatsu Y, Gomi T, Niomura M, Araki M, Azemoto S. Surface 3-D and simultaneous imaging with spiral CT: effects of technical parameters. *Radiology* 1993; **189**(P):413
27. Prokop M, Schaefer CM, Galanski M, Nischelsky JE, Reimer P, Leppert A. 3-D imaging with spiral CT: experimental evaluation of object distortion. *Radiology* 1992; **185**(P):127
28. Hopper KD, Mahraj RM, Kasales CJ, Mekkstrup JW, Seibert DK, Eggli KD. Quality of 3-D reconstructions from spiral, extended spiral, and axial CT. *Radiology* 1993; **189**(P):120
29. Posniak HV, Olson MC, Demos TC, Pierce KL, Kalbhen CL, Turbin RC. Clinical applications of 1.5:1 pitch helical C. *Radiology* 1993; **189**(P):416
30. McEnery KW, Wilson AJ, Murphy WA, Marushack MM. Spiral CT imaging of the musculoskeletal system: a phantom study. *Radiology* 1992; **185**(P):118

31. Ahmad AAMH, Coin CG, Becerra JL, Nunez D, Soto RF, LeBlang SD. Plain films versus spiral CT in evaluation of cervical spine injuries. *Radiology* 1993; **189**(P):325
32. Martinez CR, DiPasquale TG, Helfet DL, Graham AW, Sanders RW, Ray LD. Evaluation of acetabular fractures with two- and three-dimensional CT. *Radiographics* 1992; **12**:227–242
33. Stewart NR, Gilula LA. CT of the wrist: a tailored approach. *Radiology* 1992; **183**:13–20
34. McEnery KW, Wilson AJ, Murphy WA. Comparison of standard and spiral CT in the evaluation of the wrist. *Radiology* 1993; **189**(P):387
35. Quale JL, Burmeister GE, Smazal SF. Spiral CT arthography of the shoulder. *AJR* 1994; **162**(3):209
36. Hu H, Fox SH. Effect of helical pitch and collimation on tumor contrast: a clinical model. *Radiology* 1993; **189**(P):218
37. Jacobson DJ, Metz SW, Foley WD. Sensitivity for standard and helical CT scanning. *Radiology* 1993; **189**(P):238
38. Boden SD, Goodenough DJ, Stockham CD, Jacobs E, Dina T, Allman M. Precise measurement of vertebral bone densitometry using computed tomography without use of an external reference phantom. *J Digit Imaging* 1989; **2**(1):31–38
39. Wang G, Vannier MW, Yoffie RL. Stairstep Artifacts in spiral CT: a phantom study. *Radiology* 1993; **189**(P):217
40. Wunderlich AP, Lenz MW, Helmberger H, Gross M, Gerhardt P. Spiral CT angiography with automated bone removal. *Radiology* 1993; **189**(P):238
41. Tuy K. A postprocessing algorithm to reduce metallic clip artifacts in CT images. *Eur. Radiol.* 1993; **3**:129–134
42. Piraino DW, Ohman JC, Richmond BJ, Kvach DJ, Schils JP, Belhobek GH, et al. Solid bone model reconstruction for surgical planning and 3-D trabecular architecture. *Radiology* 1993; **189**(P):387
43. Davros WJ, Berman PM, Silverman PS, Cooper C, Zeman RK. Three-dimensional models from helical CT data: impact on surgical planning for 35 patients. *Radiology* 1993; **189**(P): 296
44. Vannier MW, Commean PK, Bhatia GH, Smith KE. Validation of spiral CT and optical surface scanning for use in 3-D design of limb prosthesis. *Radiology*, 1993; **189**(P):218
45. Vining DJ, Shifrin RY. Virtual reality imaging with helical CT. *AJR* 1994; **162**(3):188
46. Fishman EK, Wyatt SH, Bluemke DA, Urban BA. Spiral CT of musculoskeletal pathology: preliminary report. *Skeletal Radiology* 1993; **22**:253–256

Chapter 6

Vascular System and Three-Dimensional CT Angiography

Robert K. Zeman

INTRODUCTION

Because helical scanning allows imaging with very high levels of contrast, it is well suited for evaluation of the vascular system. There are a variety of applications where helical scan methodology in conjunction with three-dimensional (3-D) rendering holds much promise. Four major applications will be specifically addressed in this chapter. They are: (1) evaluation of renal artery stenosis, (2) the abdominal aorta, (3) the thoracic aorta, and (4) the splanchnic circulation. Since the scanning parameters and approach to contrast administration varies for each portion of the vascular system, these will be individually presented in the subsequent sections of this chapter.

There are two distinct philosophical camps for the use of helical CT in the evaluation of vascular abnormalities. One camp dedicates the examination technique to obtaining an optimal three-dimensional model without emphasizing the quality of the axial images that may result. The other camp feels that it is important to optimize the axial images obtained as part of the study in addition to providing data for three-dimensional rendering. We belong to the second camp and firmly believe that it is important to produce high-quality axial sections and a diagnostic study, without necessarily sacrificing the quality of the three-dimensional model. As each of the specific indications for helical CT of the vascular system is presented, this philosophic dichotomy will be highlighted.

EVALUATION OF RENAL ARTERY STENOSIS

As many as ten percent of patients with hypertension will have a renovascular etiology, most commonly renal artery stenosis. Despite the availability of many modalities for renal artery evaluation, renal arteriography has traditionally proven the only accurate means of detecting renal artery stenosis. With the advent of helical scanning, it has been increasingly recognized that axially displayed images as well as three-dimensional renderings may consistently identify hemodynamically significant renal artery stenosis.[1-5]

Helical Scanning and 3-D Rendering Methodology

Helical evaluation of the renal arteries is one of the more straightforward vascular applications. The renal arteries follow a horizontal course and, therefore, do not pose a great challenge with regards to z-direction coverage. For the dedicated evaluation of renal artery stenosis, noncontrast sections will initially be performed to localize the level of the renal arteries. These sections will be done using a low milliAmperage (approximately 150) and five mm collimation. We will specifically look for any evidence to suggest accessory renal arteries which must be included in the subsequent helical acquisition. The nonhelical scans will be performed as cluster scans at a rate of three scans every seven sec on the GE HiSpeed. Using the cluster technique will help to minimize misregistration artifacts, and allow more accurate localization of the arteries prior to helical scanning. The noncontrast scans are also helpful for identifying calcified plaque.

For the helical portion of the exam, we usually inject contrast material at a rate of two and one-half mL per/sec for a total of 120 mL. We find that this is a sufficient rate and dose of contrast material to allow evaluation of the arteries on the axially displayed scans as well as three-dimensional models. The renal artery attenuation can be expected to reach approximately 200 H during the contrast bolus. A 40-sec injection delay between the initiation of the contrast injection and starting to scan results in the renal arteries being near their peak opacification during the scanning interval. Using this injection delay, there will be some enhancement of the renal veins, but this seldom obscures the relevant renal artery anatomy. The renal arteries will appear of much higher attenuation than the adjacent veins.

Even in patients with reduced cardiac output, we find that using a sustained injection at this rate provides sufficient latitude so that the renal arteries are almost always well opacified. An alternative approach suggested by Rubin et al. is to perform much higher injection rates of up to five mL/sec following a low dose test injection to determine the optimal injection delay timing.[1] In our practice, we do not feel comfortable injecting large volumes of contrast into peripheral veins at a rate of five mL per/sec. We similarly find it cumbersome to perform test injections to determine the contrast dynamics before performing helical scans. This adds several minutes of physician time to the examination, which we feel is unnecessary. Using these higher injection rates, the renal artery attenuation appears to be approximately 50 H higher than the attenuation reached using our method. Each radiologist must decide in his or her own practice whether this difference in attenuation is significant with regard to recognition of stenosis.

For the actual helical acquisition, a 30-sec helix acquired during a single breath-hold usually allows sufficient coverage to evaluate the renal arteries. The optimal collimation and pitch ratio remain controversial. Three millimeter collimation and a pitch ratio of 1:1 afford excellent coverage. In our practice it has allowed recognition of stenosis in excess of 70 percent in almost all patients. Many of these patients have atherosclerotic disease with high-grade renal artery stenosis. In patients with lesser degrees of stenosis, branch stenosis, or fibromuscular dysplasia, three mm collimation may not be sufficient. One millimeter collimation would more accurately depict stenosis, but would severely limit the helical coverage. When using one mm collimation we would suggest increasing the coverage by using an increased pitch ratio of 1.5:1. This would increase the coverage during a 30 sec helix to four and one-half cm. Scanners which offer two mm collimation and 1.5:1 pitch may offer the best compromise with regard to resolution and coverage for evaluation of the renal arteries. On the GE HiSpeed we use a tube current of 280 to 300 mA.

The impact of increasing the pitch ratio for evaluation of small structures such as the renal arteries is still unsettled. Polacin[6] has suggested that a pitch ratio of 2:1 increases the section sensitivity profile by 30 percent using 180° linear interpolation. Rubin et al., on the basis of clinical data, has suggested that this is not the case and that it is superior to perform two mm collimation sections using a pitch ratio of 1.5:1 than three mm collimation sections at a pitch ratio of 1:1.[5] This concept has been embraced by many groups, but we would suggest caution in utilizing excessively thin collimation at increased pitch for the following reason. The very thin collimation images may have significantly reduced photon flux and result in photopenia and degradation of the axially displayed scans. This is especially true if the scanner used can only provide marginally sufficient milliAmperage. Assuming the axially displayed scans play an important part in the radiologist's interpretation, it would be a mistake to sacrifice their quality solely for the purpose of generating an arguably better three-dimensional model.

Once the helical data has been acquired, it must be reconstructed with overlap. Approximately 50 percent overlap or greater is sufficient. We generally will reconstruct three millimeter collimation sections at one mm intervals. If one mm collimation was used, the scans will be reconstructed at one-half mm intervals. The nonoverlapping as well as overlapping sections will be reviewed and archived in patients with suspected renal artery stenosis. The overlapping sections will be downloaded to a workstation for three-dimensional and/or multiplanar reformation.

We perform three-dimensional rendering on a GE Windows Advantage workstation. This commercially available workstation uses a SPARC 10 platform (Sun Microsystems, Santa Clara, CA). The workstation uses a traditional volume-rendering technique for generation of three-dimensional models. The volume-rendering approach retains interior pixel values, so that cutting into the model will show interior structure, not just hollow surfaces. After loading the overlapping sections, it takes the computer approximately one minute to produce the initial model. The computer may be instructed to selectively delete specific structures based on their attenuation. We generally set a threshold of approximately 100 H to eliminate structures below this attenuation. This helps remove much of the soft tissue from the model and only leaves residual high-attenuation structures, such as the opacified vessels and the bony skeleton. Use of a threshold which is approximately 50 to 70 percent of the peak vascular attenuation will not result in an eroded model with attenuated or pseudostenosed vessels.

We will electronically disarticulate the unwanted structures from the model. Using an electronic scalpel, the bones are easily dissected from the overlying vessels. Because we use a relatively long injection delay, there will be some opacification of the portal venous system and the renal veins. These unwanted vessels are easily removed when viewing the model obliquely from above or below as they typically lie anterior to the renal arteries.

The model may be displayed as a shaded-surface display, a maximum intensity projection (MIP), or a ray-sum projection (Figure 6-1). The shaded-surface display has opaque

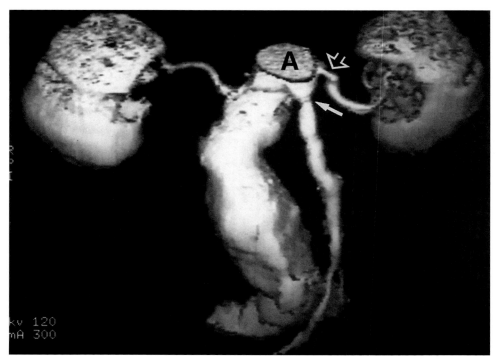

A

FIGURE 6-1A Fusiform aortic aneurysm, left renal artery stenosis, and superior mesenteric artery stenosis. Shaded-surface display shows mild aneurysmal dilatation of the distal abdominal aorta. There is a subtle change in caliber of the left renal artery (open arrow) indicating renal artery stenosis. There also appears to be a narrow bandlike narrowing of the superior mesenteric artery (arrow). (A = aorta).

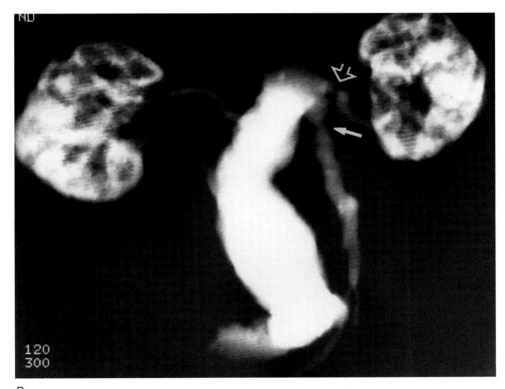

B

FIGURE 6-1B Ray-sum projection is comparable to the shaded-surface display in its depiction of the abnormalities in this patient. Again identified are subtle stenosis of the superior mesenteric artery (arrow) and high-grade stenosis of the left renal artery (open arrow). Stenosis of the renal artery is better seen on the ray-sum view in this patient.

surfaces that obscure the underlying pixel values. It also displays all structures on the surface of the model as a single attenuation. This makes it impossible to differentiate calcification from contrast within the vessel lumen. The MIP view shows only the highest pixel value within the model along the observer's line of sight. This view allows differentiation of calcification from contrast material, because calcification is typically of higher attenuation. The MIP view has opaque surfaces similar to the shaded surface model. We find that the ray-sum projection is the best overall view for visualizing the anatomy as well as being able to discern calcification. The ray-sum view has an appearance very similar to that of a conventional arteriogram and affords relative translucency. This allows vessels to be seen through one another and also prevents calcified plaque from obscuring the underlying vessel lumen.

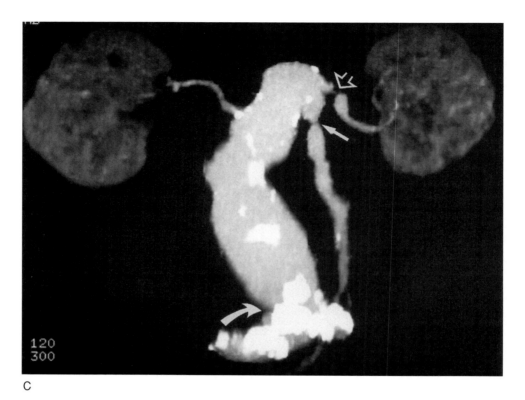

C

FIGURE 6-1C Maximum intensity projection (MIP) view also demonstrates stenosis of the superior mesenteric artery (arrow) and left renal artery (open arrow). We believe this view showed the superior mesenteric artery stenosis best in this patient. Extensive calcification is identified in the iliac region (curved arrow). The stenoses were subsequently angiographically confirmed.

Renal Artery Stenosis: Detection Accuracy

Both the axially displayed images and three-dimensional models allow accurate recognition of renal artery stenosis. Using the axially displayed overlapping images, Galanski et al. correctly identified stenosis in excess of 70 percent in 18 of 19 patients.[3] The diagnosis was facilitated by use of an interactive cine or paging display which is available on most scanners (Figure 6-2). Galanski et al. also found that the ability to detect stenosis was comparable for axially displayed sections versus three-dimensional models. The authors utilized three mm collimation and a 1:1 pitch ratio for scanning. Rubin et al. obtained similar results using three-dimensional rendering in a similar cohort of patients. He found a 92 percent sensitivity and 83 percent specificity for recognition of renal artery stenosis on three-dimensional models. The latter group utilized three mm collimation and pitch ratios varying from 1:1 to 2:1. They also determined that the MIP display more accurately

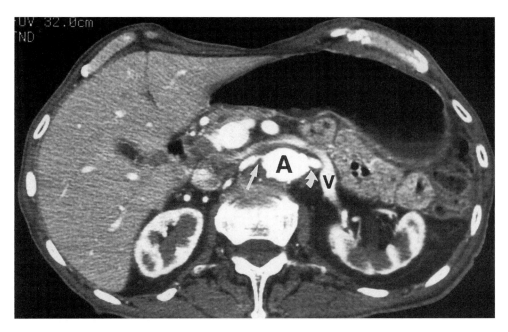

FIGURE 6-2 Identification of right renal artery stenosis on axially displayed section. On helically acquired images reconstructed without overlap, the origin of the right renal artery was not clearly identified. After reconstruction with 40 percent overlap, the origin of the right renal artery is identified (arrow). There appears to be approximately 60 to 70 percent stenosis. The origin of the left renal artery (curved arrow) does not appear stenotic, but has an irregular contour due to the presence of calcification. By using overlapping sections coupled with thin collimation, it is often possible to visualize the entire main renal arteries. (A = aorta, v = normal left renal vein).

assessed the renal arteries because of the ability to differentiate calcified plaque from vessel lumen (Figure 6-3). While we would agree with this observation, we feel the ray-sum view (which was not evaluated in Rubin's series) even offers further advantage in this regard because calcified plaque does not obscure the lumen.

It is difficult to say whether three-dimensional rendering adds diagnostic information to the evaluation of the axially displayed scans of the renal arteries. Creation of three-dimensional models is relatively complex and labor intensive at the present time. It can readily be accomplished by a trained technologist, but it does add to the complexity and potential cost of performing the examination. On the other hand, viewing overlapping axial images on a paging display is quite easy, and allows rapid recognition of significant stenosis. While we would agree that the three-dimensional models provide an important overview, and can dramatically depict the stenosis (Figure 6-4), they may not be necessary

(Text continues on page 274)

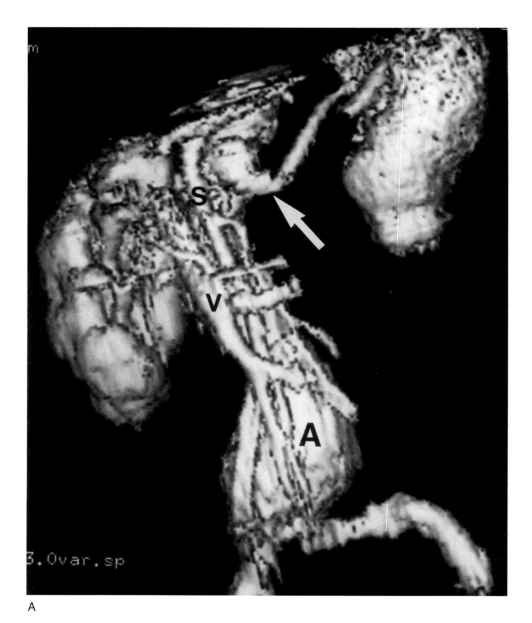

A

FIGURE 6-3A Calcification obscuring left renal artery stenosis on shaded-surface display. This shaded-surface model was reconstructed from overlapping sections acquired with three mm collimation at the level of the renal arteries and seven mm collimation through the distal aorta and iliac arteries. A fusiform aneurysm (A) is identified. The left renal artery has an unusual configuration (arrow), but no definite stenosis is seen. (S = superior mesenteric artery, V = superior mesenteric vein).

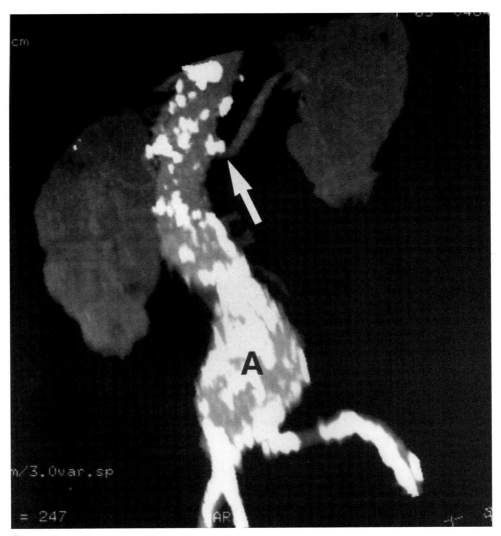

B

FIGURE 6-3B Maximum intensity projection demonstrates extensive calcification of the aorta and abdominal aortic aneurysm (A). At the origin of the left renal artery an eccentric, calcified plaque is present. The MIP view also shows associated stenosis of the left renal artery (arrow). Because calcification and contrast within the vessel cannot be distinguished on the shaded-surface display, the MIP view can be helpful in differentiating a normal caliber vessel from calcification obscuring stenosis. In some patients the ray-sum view may also be helpful in demonstrating a stenotic vessel "through" the calcified plaque.

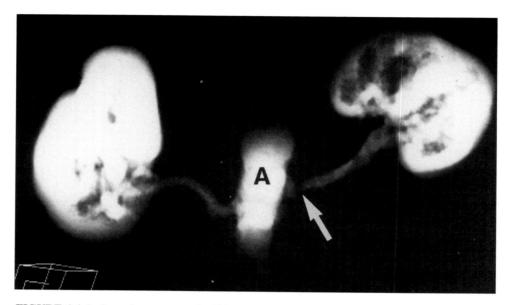

FIGURE 6-4 Left renal artery stenosis. This ray-sum projection rendered from three mm collimation sections demonstrates high-grade stenosis of the left renal artery (arrow). The patient had a history of longstanding hypertension. (A = aorta).

in most patients with renal artery stenosis. We find that vascular surgeons find the 3-D models useful in planning surgery, but in the setting of renal artery stenosis, angioplasty rather than open surgery will usually be performed. The three-dimensional views, therefore, do not play any important role with regard to planning of a subsequent therapeutic procedure in this setting.

ABDOMINAL AORTIC ANEURYSM

To date, we have scanned over 40 abdominal aortic aneurysms. As compared to conventional CT, we believe that axially displayed sections from a helical acquisition, as well as three-dimensional models, may be helpful in further refining our ability to assess aneurysms (Figure 6-5). Many of the technical considerations for scanning the abdominal aorta are similar to those for the renal arteries. Unfortunately, scanning the aorta is not as straightforward because achieving adequate z-direction coverage is a significant challenge. There are several options for meeting this challenge which must be specifically addressed.

The aorta must be scanned at least from the level of the superior mesenteric artery to the iliac bifurcation. Noncontrast scans will be performed to assure proper positioning of

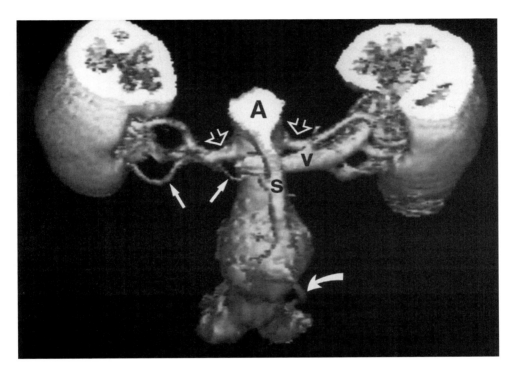

FIGURE 6-5 Infrarenal abdominal aortic aneurysm. Shaded-surface display reveals the presence of an abdominal aortic aneurysm which originates below the level of the renal arteries. A small accessory right renal artery is identified (arrows) just above the neck of the aneurysm. The origins of the right and left main renal arteries (open arrows) are also clearly seen. In most patients the inferior mesenteric artery will be thrombosed when originating from an aneurysm. In this patient, however, the inferior mesenteric artery is patent (curved arrow). (A = aorta, S = superior mesenteric artery, v = left renal vein).

the helical acquisition. If noncontrast scans suggest suprarenal extension of the aneurysm or calcified plaque near the origin of the celiac axis, the scan may be started above the superior mesenteric artery. Approximately 16 cm of z-direction coverage is required. If a 32-sec helical exposure is used, the coverage could be accomplished by any of the three following techniques: five mm collimation and 1:1 pitch ratio; three mm collimation and a 2:1 pitch ratio; or a combination of collimations and pitch ratios. We have found that the latter approach is best to detect stenoses of the superior mesenteric and renal arteries, while providing adequate coverage to evaluate the entire aorta (Table 6-1). We typically will use three mm collimation and 1:1 pitch for the first 16 to 20 sec of the helical acquisition. The patient will then be allowed a short breathing interval of seven sec before completing the remaining 16 to 20 sec of the helix. This latter 16 to 20 sec will

TABLE 6-1 Protocol for focused exam abdominal aorta

Scan mode	Helical[a]
Gantry angulation	None
Scan parameters	120 kVp, 280 mA,[b] 1 sec
Length of helical exposure	30–40 sec
Field of view	30 to 40 cm
Pitch	1:1[c]
Collimation	3, 7 mm[d]
Number of sections	32–40 (approximate)
Area of interest	From diaphragm to symphysis[e]
Patient instructions	Breath-hold in midinspiration[f]
Contrast	Prefer nonionic 300 mgI/mL
Volume	120 mL
Administration route	Intravenous via antecubital vein
Rate	2.5 mL/sec
Scan delay	40–45 sec[g]
Reconstruction algorithm	Standard
Reconstruction spacing	1 mm and 3 mm[h]

[a]Noncontrast, nonhelical scans are used to localize the celiac, mesenteric, renal, and iliac arteries. This is done to make sure the helical scan includes all the major arteries

[b]Minimum suggested mA on GE HiSpeed. Three hundred mA preferable. Adjust appropriately for other scanners. Since using three mm collimation, sections will look photopenic, if less than 280 mA

[c]Alternative is 1.5:1 pitch ratio

[d]Three mm collimation sections from celiac to renal arteries, and seven mm collimation for the distal aorta. These are done as back-to-back helices of 16 to 20 sec duration each. Alternative two then five mm collimation at pitch 1.5

[e]Use noncontrast scans to localize starting location. Scan caudad. Extend helix from celiac artery to iliac bifurcation. Fill in sections through liver and to symphysis as nonhelical cluster scans

[f]Split helix with seven-sec breathing pause after 16 to 20 sec

[g]Optimal for two and one-half mL/sec injection

[h]Overlapping reconstruction at one mm intervals used to evaluate celiac, superior mesenteric, and renal arteries. Use cine/paging controls. Images can be downloaded for multiplanar reformatting/3-D

be acquired using either seven mm collimation with a pitch ratio of 1:1 or five mm collimation with a pitch ratio of 1.5:1. This technique is actually quite easy for the technologist to preprogram into the scanner, assuming it allows mixing of pitch and collimation within a single prescription. A set of images is reconstructed with no overlap and a second set with overlap. When using three mm collimation, we will usually reconstruct the sections every one mm. The seven mm collimation sections will be reconstructed every three mm. The overlapping sections are easily reviewed on a paging display. They also may be downloaded to a workstation for three-dimensional rendering as described above.

Results in Evaluation of Abdominal Aortic Aneurysms

The axially displayed sections from the helical acquisition and three-dimensional models provide complementary information that is useful to both the radiologist and vascular surgeon. Both techniques have strengths and weaknesses in the setting of abdominal aortic aneurysms. Together, both techniques offer a significant advantage over conventional CT scanning of the abdominal aorta.[7] In one of the largest prior series utilizing conventional dynamic CT, Papanicolaou et al. incorrectly assessed the extent of aneurysm in 16 percent of patients.[8] Less than one-third of patients with accessory renal arteries where identified in that series. The ability of conventional CT to diagnose concomitant renal artery stenosis was also low, presumably due to misregistration artifact and partial volume averaging.

Using helical CT, we fare better than conventional CT, but there are still lingering difficulties in determining aneurysm extent on axially displayed images. Among 23 patients we initially studied, there were four errors in determining aneurysm extent. False-positive iliac involvement was the most common cause of error and resulted from aneurysm redundancy mimicking iliac extension (Figure 6-6). While multiplanar reformatting helps alleviate this problem, three-dimensional rendering was best at clarifying the anatomy (Figure 6-6).

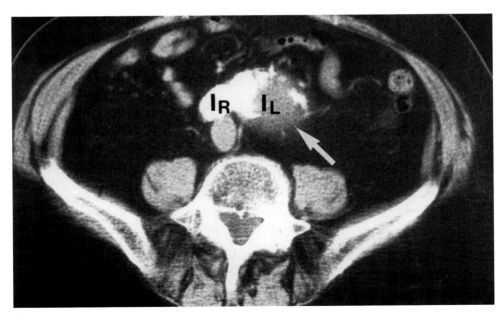

A

FIGURE 6-6A Inability to determine aneurysm extent on axially displayed sections. Axial display of this helical scan appears to show extension of an abdominal aortic aneurysm into the left iliac artery (I_L). Low attenuation clot (arrow) appears to be present within the enlarged iliac vessel. (I_R = right iliac artery).

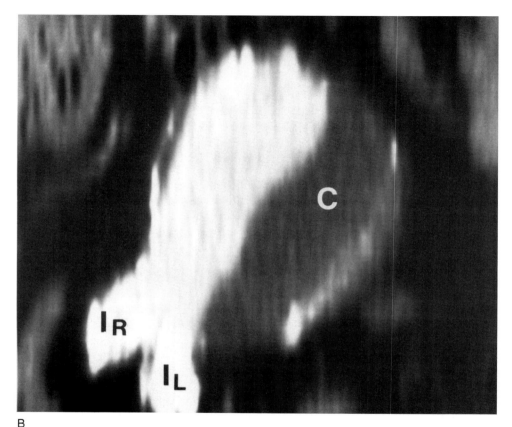

B

FIGURE 6-6B Multiplanar reformation of the aneurysm suggests that extension into the left iliac artery (I_L) is absent. The clot (C) within the aneurysm appears to end at the level of the bifurcation. Use of a multiplanar or true 3-D display is often helpful in determining aneurysm extent. (I_R = right iliac artery).

It is important for the radiologist to recognize vascular anomalies and abnormalities that might affect the surgical plan. We found that axially displayed sections from the helical acquisition depicted renal arteries stenosis or accessory renal arteries in the majority of patients. Three-dimensional rendering, however, improved recognition to eight of nine patients in whom stenosis or accessory renal arteries were present. Accessory renal arteries can be especially difficult to identify on axial sections if they originate close to the origin of the main renal arteries, or closely parallel the course of the main renal artery. Three-dimensional rendering can help visualize accessory renal arteries when they possess this type of anatomy (Figure 6-5). In addition to detection of renal artery stenosis, accessory renal arteries, and aneurysm extent, the radiologist must also be able to identify stenosis of the superior mesenteric artery and anomalies such as retroaortic renal vein. The combination of axially displayed sections and three-dimensional rendering is highly successful in providing this type of complete evaluation of the aorta prior to surgery.

Three-dimensional rendering without reviewing the axially displayed helical sections does not allow complete assessment of the aneurysm, because it is easy to underestimate aneurysm size and in some cases aneurysm extent (Figure 6-7). When viewed alone, three dimensional models convey information very similar to a conventional arteriogram. Only the enhancing lumen of the vessel will be visualized while areas of clot may go unnoticed. At times, calcification at the edge of clot will act as a peripheral marker of the aneurysm; but if calcification is not present, it may be difficult to assess aneurysm size on the basis of three-dimensional models alone. We have seen at least one case where aneurysm extension into the iliacs was not appreciated on three-dimensional views because of extensive clot surrounding a normal-sized opacified lumen (Figure 6-7).

Vascular surgeons are extremely enthusiastic about 3-D rendering because it helps them visualize the anatomy prior to surgery. The two features which they have found most

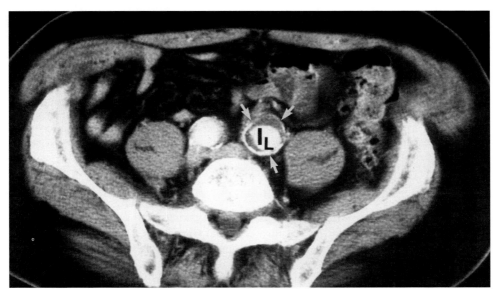

A

FIGURE 6-7A Failure to detect extension of abdominal aortic aneurysm into the iliac artery on three-dimensional views. Axially displayed section from helical scan shows extension of this patient's abdominal aortic aneurysm into the left iliac artery (I_L). There is a rind of clot and calcification (arrows) involving the vessel. The contrast-enhanced portion of the lumen appears of normal caliber.

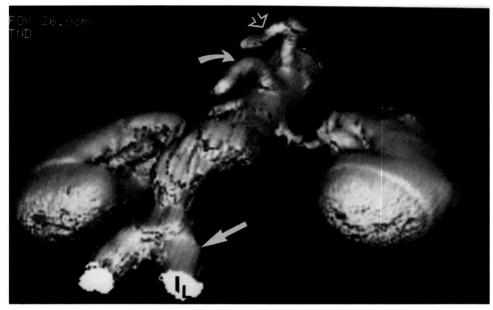

B

FIGURE 6-7B Shaded-surface model demonstrates what appears to be a normal left iliac artery (I_L). The surface of the vessel looks very smooth (arrow) because we are only seeing the outer contour of the flowing contrast-enhanced blood. We are not seeing the calcification which often appears much more irregular on the shaded-surface display. Apparently, the clot and faint calcification was of an attenuation less than the threshold selected for this model. Because of this, these structures do not appear in the model and therefore cause failure to accurately diagnose the extent of aneurysm. Three-dimensional views must be used as an adjunct to the axially displayed sections for accurate diagnosis. (open arrow = celiac axis, curved arrow = superior mesenteric artery).

helpful on the three-dimensional views is recognition of concomitant stenosis and the ability to assess the relative distance between an aneurysm and the major aortic branches. Particularly when aneurysms extend above the renal arteries, the relationship to the superior mesenteric artery will have bearing on whether the aorta can be successfully cross-clamped during surgery. This information could be obtained by counting axial sections to determine the superior-inferior distance, but our surgeons feel much more comfortable obtaining this information by looking at the three-dimensional model. We usually photograph standardized AP and oblique views with 30° of inferior cranio-caudal tilt. Because they may provide complementary information, surface model, MIP, and ray-sum projection views will be displayed for surgical planning. If the three-dimensional anatomy is complex, a rotating display may be videotaped and made available to the surgeon in addition to standard static images.

EVALUATION OF THE THORACIC AORTA

Since scans can be accomplished with such high levels of intravascular contrast, helical CT is beginning to have an impact on the evaluation of the thoracic aorta.[9] Axially displayed sections remain the mainstay of interpretation but three-dimensional views may also help clarify confusing anatomy. Certainly, 3-D views strikingly depict the normal vascular relationships of the aorta and its branches (Figure 6-8). When evaluating the great vessels, there is the opportunity for considerable savings by reducing the dose of contrast material compared to that used for conventional CT.[10] The two most common indications for scanning the thoracic aorta are to exclude an aortic dissection and to evaluate the thoracic aorta for suspected aneurysm.

Scanning Strategy for the Thoracic Aorta

For both suspected thoracic aortic aneurysms and aortic dissections, we essentially use the same scanning protocol. Preliminary nonhelical, noncontrast scans are performed through the chest prior to helical scanning. The nonhelical sections will be performed as cluster scans using 10 mm collimation and relatively low milliAmperes (150 mA). We use the noncontrast scans to look for possible blood in the mediastinum or pleural space, to identify significant intimal calcification, and to localize the great vessels just above the aortic arch prior to helical scanning. For the helical scan, contrast is injected at a rate of two mL/sec for a total of 100 to 120 mL. We use an injection delay of approximately 40 to 50 sec. This delay seems longer than necessary, but it results in excellent aortic opacification with attenuation values approaching 250 H in most patients. By scanning near the end of the contrast injection, contrast levels within the superior vena cava will also be declining, and therefore less prone to produce streak artifacts on the sections through the aortic arch. Some groups advocate using the femoral vein for injection to avoid high-density artifacts from the superior vena cava. This approach works, but usually is not necessary.

We will begin the helical scan through the level of the great vessels, approximately two to three cm above the aortic arch. It is important that the great vessels be visualized should the patient prove to have a dissection, because recognition of extension of the dissection into these vessels is clinically significant. We typically will scan the aorta with a helix of 40 to 50 sec duration. After 20 to 25 sec, the patient is allowed to breath for seven sec prior to continuing the helix. While this breathing interval could introduce misregistration artifact, it usually is at a level well below that of the aortic arch and should not result in failure to diagnose aortic dissection.

The collimation and pitch ratio will vary depending on the device in your practice. On the GE HiSpeed, we use five mm collimation with a pitch ratio of 1:1. A 40- to 50-sec helix allows us sufficient coverage to scan the entire thoracic aorta. Two hundred fifty to 280 mA and 120 kVp provide more than sufficient exposure to result in high-quality images. In thin patients with relatively little subcutaneous fat, the exposure may be reduced further. Increasing the pitch ratio to provide adequate coverage should not be necessary, although a controlled trial

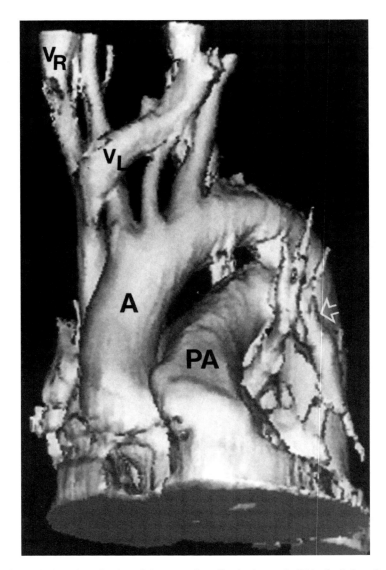

FIGURE 6-8 Shaded-surface display of the normal mediastinal vessels. This shaded-surface display was rendered from five mm helical sections reconstructed using three mm spacing. The ascending aorta (A) and great vessels are clearly identified. The main pulmonary trunk (PA) is also well seen. Because the veins are well-opacified in this patient, the right and left innominate veins (V_R, V_L) are seen within the model. The pulmonary veins are also noted in the background (open arrow). In patients with confusing anatomy or redundant vessels, three-dimensional views may be helpful.

comparing three mm collimation and increased pitch versus five mm collimation and 1:1 pitch is probably justified to study the effect of these combined parameters on spatial resolution and aortic dissection visualization.

There is a potential scanning artifact which has received increasing attention recently in the CT literature. Regardless of whether scans are acquired helically or nonhelically, scanners which acquire images during a one-sec, 360° tube rotation are prone to produce images with aortic pulsation artifacts.[11] These artifacts occur on one-sec scans, because the scan duration closely approximates the duration of a single cardiac cycle. Pulsation is typically not observed with slower scanners utilizing a two-sec or greater scan, or faster electron beam scanners. Pulsation artifacts may very closely mimic the appearance of an aortic dissection (Figure 6-9). The best approach to clarifying these pulsation artifacts is segmenting the scan

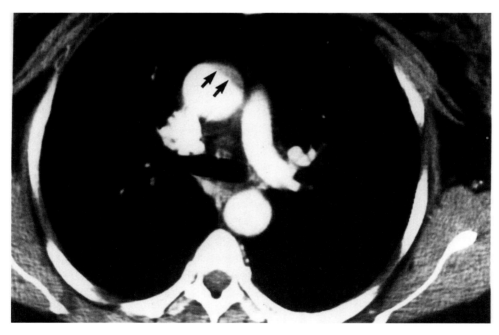

FIGURE 6-9 Pulsation artifact mimicking aortic dissection. This patient with symptoms of aortic dissection was evaluated using five mm collimation helical sections. The sections were reconstructed using three mm spacing. On both the overlapping and nonoverlapping sections, a crescentic region of low attenuation (arrows) was identified at the anterior edge of the ascending aorta. Because of the persistence of this abnormality on several sections, it was suspected to represent clot within the false channel of an aortic dissection. The patient subsequently underwent angiography and magnetic resonance imaging which showed no definite dissection. Presumably, the finding is due to aortic pulsation producing anterior blurring and volume averaging. This is a common artifact when using a scanner whose tube rotates 360° in one sec. Many cases will exhibit frank motion artifact, but in this patient the pulsation produced a convincing appearance mimicking dissection.

data, so that partially reconstructed images can be viewed which represent a fraction of the scan cycle.[12] Not all vendors can do this at the present time, but it should be available on most devices in the future. We typically will segment our one-sec scans into 120°, 330 msec scans. If pulsation is producing the suspected abnormality, it will disappear on either two or three of the segmented images. If the suspected abnormality proves to be a dissection, it will remain present on all the segmented scans. Because the segmented scans represent partial reconstructions, they may appear somewhat noisy compared to completely reconstructed scans, but they are usually of diagnostic quality. Segmenting the images in this fashion is only necessary in a small minority of cases, but it can clarify this potentially confusing artifact.

The helical scans will be reconstructed with and without overlap. The five mm collimation sections will be reconstructed at three mm intervals from just above the aortic arch to just below the main pulmonary arteries. If necessary, any of the reconstructed images can be segmented should an abnormality be identified. Segmenting the image does require raw data, but this usually will be available on the scanner's magnetic disk for several hours. Vendors differ on the availability of raw data; for assessment of the great vessels access to the raw data is not only required for segmenting images, but also for varying the reconstruction spacing or changing the reconstruction algorithm. In looking for a subtle aortic dissection, both the nonoverlapping and overlapping images should be reviewed. For assessment of thoracic aneurysms where dissection is not a consideration, the overlapping scans are seldom necessary.

Results of Helical Scanning in Thoracic Aorta Dissection

Preliminary published experience suggests helical scanning may offer significant advantages over conventional CT and even MRI in the evaluation of aortic dissection.[13] In 16 patients evaluated by Sommer et al., helical CT was found to be equal to MRI in overall accuracy, but superior in depicting carotid or subclavian involvement. In our own experience in screening 12 patients, we have successfully diagnosed seven of seven aortic dissections (Figure 6-10), but incorrectly interpreted one patient with pulsation artifact as having a dissection (Figure 6-9). An intimal flap as short as one cm in length was correctly diagnosed on helical CT. The axially displayed sections satisfactorily showed the relationship between the dissection and the great vessels in five of seven patients. In one instance, progressive development of a dissecting hematoma was followed on serial helical scans (Figure 6-10).

Three-dimensional rendering is usually not necessary for evaluation of aortic dissection, but it may help delineate the relationship between the intimal flap and the left subclavian artery. This was true in two of the seven positive studies in our patients. We find that the various types of three-dimensional displays provide complementary information. Visualization of the intimal flap is dependent upon many factors, but in general the ray-sum projection is best for this purpose. The intimal flap will be seen on surface displays only if the flap extends all the way to the surface of the vessel in the particular viewing projection. If it does not, the aorta may look entirely normal. Similarly, on a MIP view, the

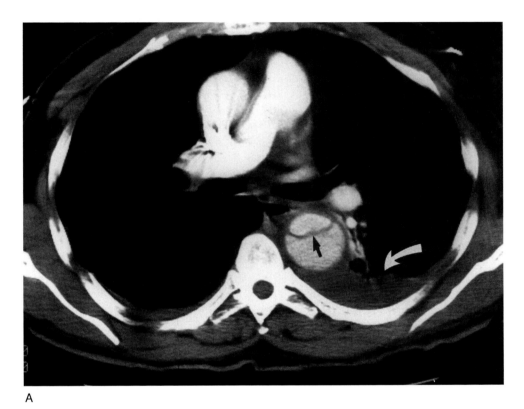

A

FIGURE 6-10A Aortic dissection. This axially displayed section was obtained as part of a helical scan acquired using five mm collimation and reconstructed with three mm spacing. A discrete intimal flap (arrow) is identified within the descending aorta. An associated left pleural effusion (curved arrow) is also identified. The intimal flap appeared to extend proximally to the level of the left subclavian artery.

intimal flap may not be seen because it is of low rather than maximum intensity. The raysum view best shows the intimal flap en face, but in our experience may also show a tortuous flap within the aortic lumen because of the relatively translucent nature of this view.

Aneurysms of the thoracic aorta are readily depicted with helical CT. The extent of clot and their relationship to the great vessels are commonly depicted on axially displayed sections. As for aortic dissection, three-dimensional rendering is only necessary in cases of confusing anatomy.

Three-dimensional rendering may be of value in patients that have confusing, anomalous, or aberrant vessels. At times it is difficult to tell the origin and nature of the vessel because of redundancy and difficulty in following the vessel from section to section. If this is the case, shaded-surface models often will allow better understanding of the vascular

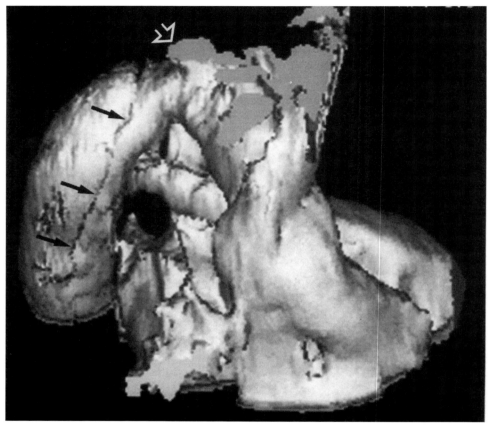

B

FIGURE 6-10B Right lateral view of shaded-surface model also shows the intimal flap (arrows) originating just beyond the origin of the left subclavian artery (open arrow). The shaded-surface display will only demonstrate the intimal flap if it extends all the way to the external surface of the vessel. If it does not, or if the model is viewed in a position which is not perpendicular to the course of the flap, the surface display may not show the abnormality.

anatomy (Figure 6-11). Because of inherent differences in contrast enhancement, MIP views may help differentiate aberrant arteries from veins.

SPLANCHNIC CIRCULATION

There are a wide variety of diseases that affect the mesenteric and portal circulations. These include atherosclerotic disease, neoplastic conditions, and inflammatory processes.

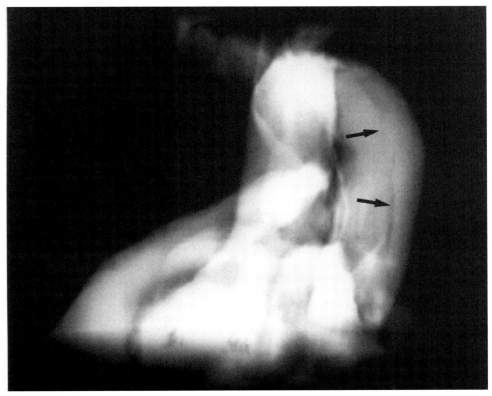

C

FIGURE 6-10C Ray-sum view in the left lateral position clearly shows the intimal flap (arrows) as a linear lucency originating just beyond the left subclavian artery. Because the ray-sum view is relatively translucent, it is often possible to see the intimal flap projecting as a lucency through the contrast-enhanced lumen of the vessel.

Because of three-dimensional rendering and scanning with high levels of contrast, helical CT is well-suited to evaluation of the splanchnic circulation.

Atherosclerotic Disease of the Superior Mesenteric Artery and Other Causes of Bowel Ischemia

To date, there is relatively little experience in the evaluation of superior mesenteric artery stenosis. In those limited cases where a specific examination of the superior mesenteric artery was requested, we perform our renal artery protocol, but position the helix at the origin of the superior mesenteric artery. More commonly, we evaluate the superior mesenteric artery in the context of a patient being evaluated for abdominal aortic aneurysm. In

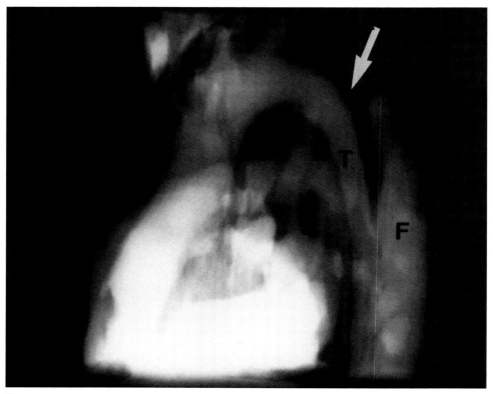

D

FIGURE 6-10D Over the ensuing several weeks, the patient's aortic dissection worsened. The fine intimal flap progressed into a true dissecting hematoma (arrow). The true (T) and false (F) channel within the dissection are apparent. By using helical CT and three-dimensional display of the CT data, patients with chronic dissection may be noninvasively followed. The vascular images have a similar appearance to conventional arteriograms, and provide a type of display with which vascular surgeons are immediately comfortable.

those cases we have made sure to begin our helical acquisition above the level of the superior mesenteric artery, and extended the helix to the iliac bifurcation as described above. Of the three patients with superior mesenteric artery stenosis that we have studied thus far, axially displayed sections visualized the stenosis in two of three cases (Figure 6-12). Three-dimensional rendering demonstrated the stenosis in all three patients (see Figure 6-1). Many of the same problems plaguing evaluation of the renal arteries also pertain to evaluation of the superior mesenteric artery. Calcified plaque may obscure stenosis on both surface model and MIP views.

There are three other common causes of bowel ischemia. These are hypotension/hypovolemia (i.e., "slow flow" syndrome), arterial emboli, and venous thrombosis. If an embolus or venous thrombus is large enough, it may be identified as a low attenuation defect within the vessel (Figure 6-13). The secondary effects of ischemia may also be seen as bowel wall thickening, thumbprinting, mesenteric collaterals, and edema in the mesenteric fat.

Neoplastic Encasement of the Splanchnic Vessels

In chapter 4 we described vascular encasement as one of the major reasons for nonresectability of pancreatic cancer. When tumor has produced frank thrombosis or high-grade stenosis of a major vessel, this is readily identified on axially displayed sections. We find that lesser degrees of stenosis or subtle flattening of one surface of a vessel is far more difficult to recognize on axial sections. This is especially true if the vessel is tortuous and is difficult to follow from section to section. Three-dimensional rendering[14] and multiplanar reformatting[15] can be helpful in detecting subtle evidence of vascular involvement by tumor.

Our technique for evaluation of the portal and superior mesenteric vessels is identical to our protocol for evaluation of the pancreas. We feel that it is important that high-quality axially displayed images be obtained for interpretation, while also obtaining the data necessary for 3-D rendering during the same examination. Utilizing five mm collimation sections reconstructed at three mm intervals is sufficient for studying the vessels in the setting of pancreatobiliary neoplasm. As we previously indicated, a 70-sec injection delay is essential for adequate portal vein opacification when using a contrast injection rate of two mL/sec.

We believe that three-dimensional rendering may result in assessment of vascular encasement which in many respects is superior to that obtainable by conventional arteriography. Both arterial and venous anatomy is clearly depicted on 3-D views (Figure 6-14). While conventional arteriography clearly demonstrates the celiac axis and superior mesenteric artery, opacification of the portal vein is indirect, via the mesenteric vein. Subtle involvement of the portal vein by tumor can easily be overlooked when this vessel is not well opacified on mesenteric arteriograms. It may especially be difficult to delineate the site and extent of portal vein involvement if multiple overlying varices are present. Not only will three-dimensional rendering visualize changes in vessel calibre, but it may also demonstrate mass effect on one surface of the vessel without frank narrowing of the vessel. We find that interpretation of the three-dimensional views in conjunction with the axial sections results in a highly accurate exam for vascular encasement. Of 22 patients studied with proven pancreatic cancer, only one error in determining vascular encasement resulted when three-dimensional rendering was used as an adjunct to interpretation of the axial section. When viewed by a panel of surgeons there were eight instances where their operative plan would have changed on the basis of viewing the three-dimensional models in this group of patients. Most often, lesions that looked potentially resectable on the axial sections demonstrated much more significant vascular encasement on the three-dimensional views.

(Text continues on page 294)

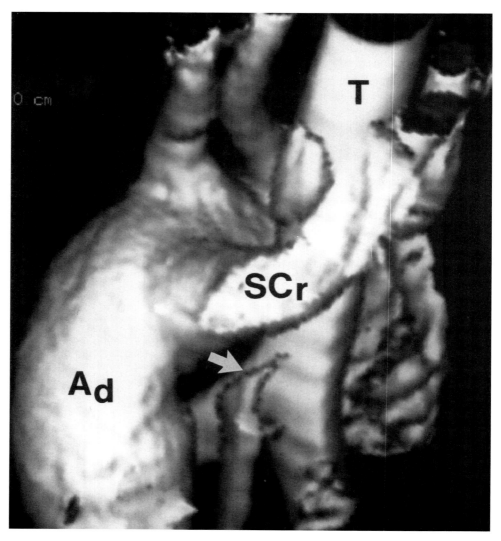

FIGURE 6-11 Aberrant right subclavian artery. Shaded-surface display was rendered from five mm collimation helical scan data reconstructed at three mm intervals. This patient had a soft-tissue mass on plane radiographs suggestive of mediastinal mass. On axially displayed sections, there appeared to be an aberrant vessel, but it was difficult to completely follow the vessel from section to section. The shaded-surface display, viewed from the posterior position, shows an aberrant right subclavian artery (SC_r) originating from the descending aorta (A_d). The other great vessels are seen in the background. As part of this study, barium was administered. Because barium is of similar attenuation to the enhanced vessels, the esophagus is identified within this model. There is abrupt impression (arrow) on the esophagus by the aberrant subclavian artery. A secondary model of the trachea (T) was also rendered, and inserted into this model as an anatomic reference point.

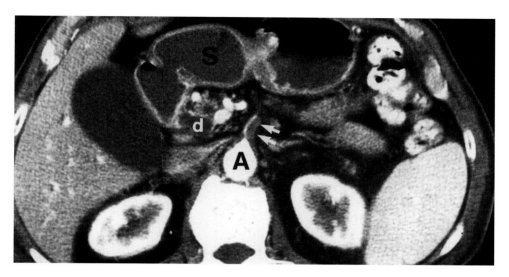

FIGURE 6-12 Atherosclerotic stenosis of the superior mesenteric artery. This axially displayed section was obtained as part of a helical scan acquired using five mm collimation. There appears to be pronounced narrowing of the superior mesenteric artery. There is either clot or thickening of the left lateral wall of the vessel (arrows). In this patient with known pancreatic cancer, it was difficult to determine whether this represented tumor invasion of the vessel or atherosclerotic disease. At surgery this proved to be the latter, without evidence of tumor spread in this region. Unfortunately the patient subsequently developed bowel ischemia. We find that high-grade stenoses are often seen on axially displayed sections, with 3-D views helpful in selected cases. (A = aorta, S = stomach, d = dilated bile duct).

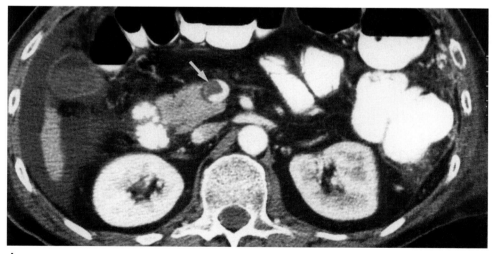

A

FIGURE 6-13A Thrombosis of the superior mesenteric vein producing bowel edema. Axially displayed section from this helical scan demonstrates low attenuation clot within the superior mesenteric vein (arrow). The patient had recently undergone bowel resection and was also believed to be hypercoagulable.

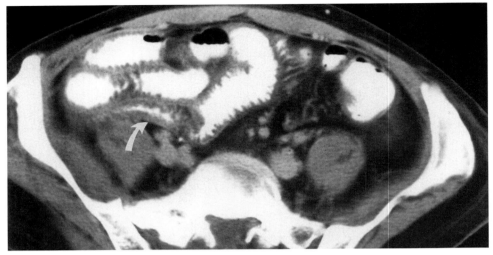

B

FIGURE 6-13B On sections obtained further caudad within the abdomen, mild small bowel dilatation is present. There also appears to be thickening of the bowel wall (curved arrow). This patient showed a marked improvement in his clinical status following anticoagulation. When thrombus is present within the portal or mesenteric vein, this is usually apparent on axially displayed sections. If it is at a branch point or in a redundant segment of the vein, three-dimensional views may be helpful in characterizing the extent of clot.

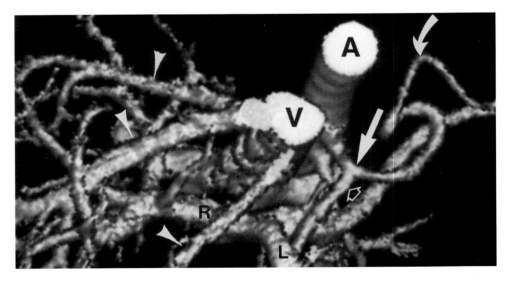

FIGURE 6-14 Normal hepatic veins, portal vein, and major arteries of the upper abdomen. Surface model based on data from helical CT viewed obliquely from above clearly shows the normal celiac axis (arrow) giving rise to the hepatic artery (open arrow) and splenic artery (curved arrow). Gastroduodenal artery is obscured in foreground by the left portal vein (L). Right portal vein (R) courses through a tangle of peripheral branches of portal and hepatic veins (arrowheads). (A = aorta, V = inferior vena cava). (*Courtesy of AJR[14] with permission.*)

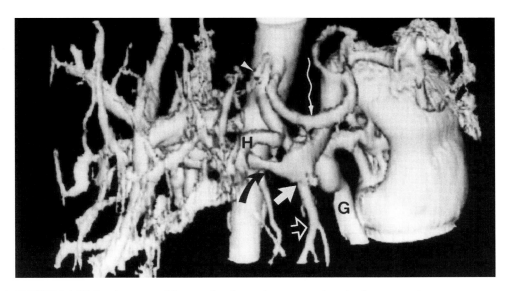

FIGURE 6-15 Involvement of the portal and superior mesenteric veins by pancreatic cancer. Surface model based on data from helical CT shows replacement of the hepatic artery (H), which shares a common trunk with the superior mesenteric artery (open arrow). The splenic artery (wavy arrow) arises from its own trunk, as does a small left hepatic artery (arrowhead). Tumor has caused amputation of the superior mesenteric vein (white arrow) just below the splenoportal confluence. The superior mesenteric artery can be seen coursing behind occluded mesenteric vein. The portal vein is also encased (black arrow) just above confluence. Although unusual, skip areas of vascular involvement may occur. The dilated gonadal vein (G) acts as a portosystemic collateral pathway. (*Courtesy of AJR*[14] *with permission.*)

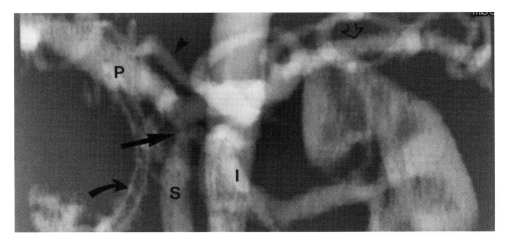

FIGURE 6-16 Encasement of the splenoportal confluence by pancreatic cancer. Anterior ray-sum projection view based on data from helical CT shows narrowing of splenoportal confluence (straight arrow) due to tumor encasement. The superior mesenteric vein (S) and inferior mesenteric vein (I) join at the confluence. (P = portal vein, open arrow = splenic vein, arrowhead = hepatic artery, curved arrow = biliary stent). (*Courtesy of AJR*[14] *with permission.*)

There is a wide range of findings that may be seen on three-dimensional rendering in patients with pancreatobiliary tumors. Anatomic variants are common and must be recognized so that aberrant arterial branches are not accidently sacrificed during surgery (See Figures 4-25 and 6-15). Ligation of a major arterial branch could jeopardize the blood supply of the common hepatic duct and result in subsequent failure of biliary-enteric anastomosis. Anomalies of the major veins also occur. The most common anomaly is the inferior mesenteric vein joining the superior mesenteric vein just below the spleno-portal confluence.

We have identified several patterns of vascular encasement by tumor. Frank caliber changes of the arteries or veins may be identified (Figure 6-15). The three-dimensional model will help display the length of the encased segment. If portal vein encasement is limited to one to two cm in length, some surgeons will consider grafting the vessel

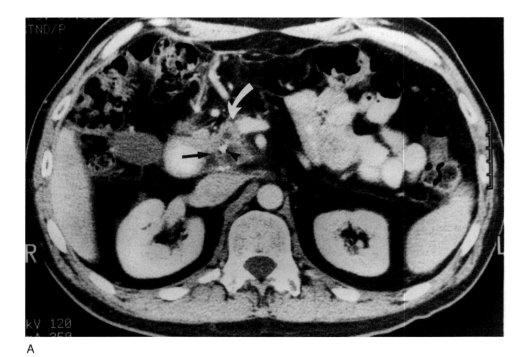

A

FIGURE 6-17A "Pad effect" on portal vein caused by tumor involvement. Axial display of helical CT scan obtained through the pancreatic head shows a pancreatic mass (straight arrow). There is subtle "flattening" of portal vein (curved arrow). Although a suggestion of a fat plane separating tumor from the vessel is present, it is difficult to say if the portal vein is encased (arrowhead = stent in bile duct).

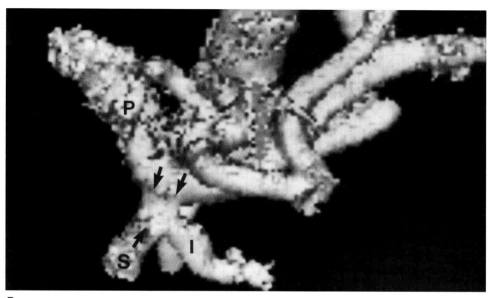

FIGURE 6-17B Anterior oblique surface model of confluence region based on data from helical CT shows a "pad effect" (arrows), with impression on the splenoportal confluence. The finding is subtle, but surgical findings confirmed it represented vascular encasement. (P = portal vein, S = superior mesenteric vein, I = inferior mesenteric vein). In pancreatic cancer, this type of pad effect has signified tumor adherence in our experience. (*Courtesy of AJR*[14] *with permission.*)

(Figure 6-16). This is technically difficult and is associated with significant morbidity and possibly even mortality. Usually if frank vessel involvement is seen, it will imply nonresectability. Mass or "pad" effect on the surface of the vessel may be subtle, but always has signified tumor adherence in our experience in dealing with pancreatic cancer (Figure 6-17). We have seen other tumors including cholangiocarcinoma and papillary-epithelial tumors of the pancreas produce similar "pad" effect and still prove resectable. We believe that the histologic nature of pancreatic carcinoma, with its lack of a well-defined capsule, makes it much more likely to adhere to adjacent vessels than well-encapsulated tumors. We are seeking to expand our experience in this area, but thus far "pad" effect implying nonresectability may only hold true for pancreatic cancer.

We find that the various methods of displaying three-dimensional models may provide complementary information in patients with pancreato-biliary tumors. The shaded-surface display excels at demonstrating subtle "pad" effect. The ray-sum view is excellent at depicting changes in vessel caliber. It is also the only view which will reliably show tumor thrombus within the vessel (Figure 6-18). Shaded-surface displays, because of their

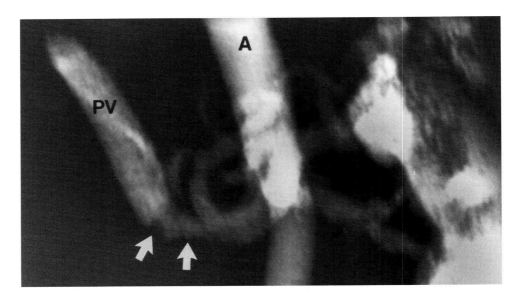

FIGURE 6-18 Tumor thrombus at splenoportal confluence. Anterior ray-sum view based on data from helical CT shows tumor invading into the lumen of the splenoportal confluence (arrows) and extending up into the portal vein (PV). The superior mesenteric vein has been obstructed by tumor. In this patient, severe bowel edema and intestinal ischemia due to venous occlusion ultimately developed. Although amputation of the superior mesenteric vein was seen on this patient's surface model, intraluminal tumor invasion was seen only on the ray-sum view. Because surface models have opaque surfaces, they may not show abnormalities within opacified vessels as well as ray-sum projections do. This method is also useful when extensive overlap of vessels occurs. Irregularity at inferior edge of left renal vein was due to overlap of vessels and was not seen after altering the model position. Celiac and mesenteric artery were seen on other views. (A = aorta). *(Courtesy of AJR[14] with permission.)*

opaque contours, do not allow depiction of the vessel interior. The MIP view is only of value in cases where it is difficult to differentiate arterial from venous structures. This is relatively uncommon.

CONCLUSION

Helical CT will play an increasing role in the evaluation of vascular abnormalities. It is less expensive and less invasive than conventional arteriography. In the setting of vascular encasement by neoplasm, it may help eliminate needless surgery on nonresectable tumors.

REFERENCES

1. Rubin GD, Walker PJ, Dake MD, et al. Three-dimensional spiral computed tomographic angiography: an alternative imaging modality for the abdominal aorta and its branches. *J Vasc Surg* 1993; **18**:656–665.
2. Rubin GD, Dake MD, Napel SA, McDonnell CH, Jeffrey RB. Three-dimensional spiral CT angiography of the abdomen: initial clinical experience. *Radiology* 1993; **186**:147–152.
3. Galanski M, Prokop M, Chavan A, Schaefer CM, Jandeleit K, Nischelsky JE. Renal arterial stenoses: spiral CT angiography. *Radiology* 1993; **189**:185–192.
4. Zeman RK, Silverman PM, Berman PM, Weltman D, Davros WJ, Gomes MN. Evaluation of abdominal aortic aneurysms: experience using variable collimation helical CT. *Radiology* 1994; **193**: 555–560.
5. Rubin GD, Dake MD, Napel S, et al. Spiral CT of renal artery stenosis: comparison of three-dimensional rendering techniques. *Radiology* 1994; **190**:181–189.
6. Polacin A, Kalender WA, Marchal G. Evaluation of section sensitivity profiles and image noise in spiral CT. *Radiology* 1992; **185**:29–35
7. Gomes MN, Davros WJ, Zeman RK. Preoperative assessment of abdominal aortic aneurysm: the value of helical and 3-D computed tomography. *J Vasc Surg*. (in press).
8. Papanicolaou N, Wittenberg J, Ferrucci JT Jr, et al. Preoperative evaluation of abdominal aortic aneurysms by computed tomography. *AJR* 1986; **146**:711–715.
9. Costello P, Ecker, Tello R, Hartnell GG. Assessment of the thoracic aorta by spiral CT. *AJR* 1992; **158**:1127–1130.
10. Costello P, Dupuy DE, Ecker CP, Tello R. Spiral CT of the thorax with reduced volume of contrast material: a comparative study. *Radiology* 1992; **183**:663–666.
11. Burns MA, Molina PL, Gutierrez IR, Sagel SS. Motion artifact simulating aortic dissection on CT. *AJR* 1991; **157**:465–467.
12. Posniak HV, Olson MC, Demos TC. Aortic motion artifact simulating dissection on CT scans: elimination with reconstructive segmented images. *AJR* 1993; **161**:557–558.
13. Sommer T, Holzknecht N, Smekal A, et al. Thin-section spiral CT in the evaluation of aortic dissection: comparison with MR imaging and transesophageal echocardiography (abstr). *Radiology* 1993; **189**(P):112.
14. Zeman RK, Davros WJ, Berman PM, et al. Three-dimensional models of the abdominal vasculature based on helical CT: usefulness in patients with pancreatic neoplasms. *AJR* 1994; **162**:1425–1429.
15. Fishman EK, Wyatt SH, Ney DR, et al. Spiral CT of the pancreas with multiplanar display. *AJR* 1992; **159**:1209–1215.

Appendix 1

Comparison of Helical/Spiral CT Scanners

William J. Davros / Robert K. Zeman

SUMMARY OF AVAILABLE HELICAL/SPIRAL SCANNERS

This appendix will summarize the comparative features of commercially available helical/spiral scanners. Every attempt was made to provide up-to-date, reliable information. Since equipment features are in constant evolution, the reader is advised to consult with their vendor's product and application specialists, as well as fellow radiologists using helical/spiral equipment, to confirm specifications and device features. By seeking input from a number of individuals, we have tried to achieve a balanced approach, which avoids comparison of apples and oranges.

Tables 1-13 summarize the relevant equipment technical features. Specific caveats may also be found in the chapter 1 text and subsequent narrative section.

Gantry Geometry

One way of characterizing helical CT scanners is by the motion of the x-ray tube relative to the detector bank. There are currently two geometric configurations of CT scanner gantries: one is called "rotate-rotate" (third generation) and the other is called "rotate-fixed" (fourth generation) (Table A-1).

In the rotate-rotate geometry, the x-ray tube central ray is lined up 180° away from the center detector of a detector bank which subtends a certain number of degrees of arc. The x-ray tube and detector bank are on a common mount. This common mount rotates about the long axis of the gantry. The x-ray tube and detector bank rotate as the mount rotates but

TABLE A-1 Geometry and detector data

Vendor	Scanner Geometry	Detector Type[c]	Number of Detectors	Detector Bank Degrees of Arc	Number of Detectors Per Degree of Arc
Elscint CT-Twin	Rotate-Rotate Dual Detector Bank[a]	SS	526[a]	43	12.0
GE HiSpeed Advantage	Rotate-Rotate Single Detector Bank	SS	852	49	17.4
Philips Tomoscan SR 7000	Rotate-Rotate Single Detector Bank	Xe	768	48	16.0
Picker PQ-2000	Rotate-Fixed[b]	SS	4800[b]	360	NA
Siemens Somatom Plus-40	Rotate-Rotate Single Detector Bank	Xe	768	42.6	18.0
Toshiba Xpress/sx	Rotate-Rotate Single Detector Bank	SS	896	49	18.3

[a]Elscint uses two banks of detectors which are juxtaposed sharing a common axis of rotation. Each of these detector banks has 526 detectors.
[b]Picker uses rotate-fixed geometry and its x-ray beam subtends 44° of arc.
[c]SS = solid state, Xe = Xenon gas ionization chamber

always with 180° of separation between them. The rotate-rotate design uses primary radiation efficiently because detector collimators are focused at the x-ray source.

In the rotate-fixed geometry the x-ray tube rotates concentrically inside a 360° ring of fixed detectors. This design limits the number of moving parts and the amount of weight that must be precisely rotated. This design also permits each detector to be calibrated on each scan because each detector is exposed to primary radiation at some point in a slice acquisition. One possible disadvantage with this design may be the technical difficulties associated with servicing a large number of detectors and associated electronics. Currently, Picker International uses the rotate-fixed geometry.

X-Ray Detectors

X-ray detectors are used in CT scanners to count the number of x-rays that are transmitted through an object. This value is used in conjunction with the number of x-rays incident on an object to compute the linear attenuation coefficient along a path traversed by the x-ray beam. Three important features to consider when comparing CT scanners on the basis of detectors are the *type* of detectors used, the *absolute number* of detectors present in the scanner, and the *concentration* of detectors per degree of irradiated arc.

The two general types of detectors used currently in helical CT scanners are solid state detectors (SS) and gas-filled ionization detectors (Table A-1). Solid state detectors, as their name implies, are made of solid materials that give off light when they are struck by x-rays. Early solid state detectors were NaI(Tl) and CsI. Later these were replaced with ceramics doped with rare earth elements. In order to collect the light signal from solid state detectors, photomultiplier tubes or photodiodes are used. These two devices convert the light signal to an electrical signal. The electrical signal acquired from solid state detectors is the amount of charge collected over a fixed time interval. Solid state detectors have the advantage of being small. They also have high x-ray-to-electrical signal conversion efficiencies. While solid state detectors are believed to harbor residual energy after exposure to photons (so-called afterglow), this does not appear to significantly degrade clinical images. If there is one weakness of solid state detectors it is the difficulty in manufacturing them. Companies that use solid state detectors include Elscint, General Electric Medical Systems, Picker International, and Toshiba America Medical Systems.

Gas-filled ionization chambers used today are filled exclusively with the inert gas Xenon. When an x-ray enters a Xenon-filled chamber it may ionize Xe atoms. If an atom is ionized, freed electrons will drift towards a positively charged collecting anode and the positively charged atom will drift towards the negatively charged outer walls of the chamber to be neutralized. The electrical signal acquired from a Xe gas detector is the amount of charge collected over a fixed time interval; this is called integral mode. They tend to be less efficient at producing an output signal for a given input signal. Their main advantage is that they are easy to manufacture, require no exotic materials, are inexpensive relative to solid state detectors, and are well understood. The two vendors that use gas-filled ionization chambers on their premium line helical CT scanners are Philips Medical Systems and Siemens Medical Systems.

The absolute number of detectors a helical CT scanner possesses is a measure of its immunity to produce artifacts from detector failure. It also is a measure of the scanners complexity. Among scanners of the rotate-rotate geometry, Toshiba Medical Systems leads in the number of detectors in a single bank with 896 solid state detectors spread over an arc of 49°. Elscint uses 1052 solid state detectors in a unique two-bank detector array, each bank having 526 detectors over an arc of 43°. Picker International, using the rotate-fixed geometry, leads the industry with a total of 4800 SS detectors in their PQ-2000 scanner. A summary of detector information is found in Table A-1.

The number of detectors per degree of arc subtended by the x-ray fan beam (detector density) is a measure of the scanner's ability to acquire independent views through an object, provided that signal can be extracted from detectors quickly. This is the angular version of equal interval sampling theory. The more views a scanner gets of an object the better, in theory, it can reconstruct the high-contrast fine structure of that object. If a vendor lacks high density of detectors per degree of arc this can be compensated for to some degree by sampling the signal with greater frequency as the x-ray exposure is made of the object of interest.

Detectors can be judged on three basic criteria. The first criterion is their *efficiency*. The second is *response time length* of a detector to a stimulus and the amount of "afterglow" or paralysis before it is ready to accept another input stimulus. The third criterion is *temporal stability*. Each of these will be discussed separately below.

The first criterion, *efficiency,* is a measure of how much signal is given out for a known number of signals in (photons incident on the detector). Ideally, this value would be 100 percent; every x-ray into the detector would cause an ionizing event that would be added to the signal integration over the readout time of the detector. The actual detector efficiency can be obtained by asking vendors for it though it is a difficult number to independently verify. Solid state detectors range from 65 to 85 percent efficient. Xenon detectors range from 40 to 65 percent efficient depending on the method of efficiency measurement and calculation. It is probably best to look at image noise, low-contrast resolution, and high-contrast spatial resolution, all taken together, to judge the performance of a CT scanner, rather than detector efficiency alone.

The second criterion is the *response time length* of a detector to a stimulus and the amount of time before it is ready to accept another input stimulus. Ideally a detector would produce an output immediately after receiving an input. It would ideally also be instantaneously ready to receive a second input. In practice neither of these is true. There is a finite amount of time needed to collect signal. There is also a finite amount of time a detector needs to "reset itself" before it can accurately record a second input. These two times added together (the recovery time) provide the theoretical limit for scanning speed. A single detector cannot be resampled more rapidly than its recovery time. Solid state detectors have longer recovery times than Xenon detectors.

The third criterion is *temporal stability*. In an ideal setting, once a detector was calibrated it would not drift from that calibration as time passed. However, all detectors do have some calibration drift. What is important when comparing detectors is to find one with minimal drift and one where the recalibration can be done quickly and easily.

Scan Time

Scan time is an important parameter when considering choices for a helical CT scanner. Many CT generators are limited in the amount of tube current that can be generated, so increasing scan time is the only way left to increase the x-ray tube current-time product (milliAmperes/sec). It is also a parameter that ideally should have some flexibility for those cases that must be done quickly; thus *scan time* should be variable from subsecond settings to at least four seconds for nonhelical scans. A one and one-half to two sec 360° rotation helical scan may be useful for generating higher milliAmperes in heavier patients. Most vendors specify scan time for two scanning scenarios: full scanning, which is the time it takes the x-ray tube to travel 360°, and partial scanning, which has a variable definition from vendor to vendor but usually is the time it takes the x-ray tube to travel the minimum number of projections to produce an acceptable image (180° + the fan beam angle).

The minimum time for a full scan is one sec. This time is found on all manufacturers' premium helical units. All vendors have additional times, usually in one-sec increments. Picker has incorporated one and one-half-sec full scanning and is the only vendor to have a noninteger scan time. There are at least two limiting factors associated with scan time. One is the mechanical strength of the x-ray tube mount. This mount is subjected to centripetal force generated by the tube mass and the velocity at which it is rotated about the gantry.

The second limiting feature is the number of x-rays the x-ray tube can produce in one revolution of the gantry. Image quality is related to the product of tube current multiplied by scan time. If scan time per image is to shorten due to rapid rotation and image quality is to remain constant, tube current must be increased. Increased tube current causes increased tube heating which can limit x-ray tube life and shorten the amount of time the x-ray tube is on for a single helical study. All vendors except Siemens use 0.6 sec for partial scanning. Siemens uses 0.7 sec for partial scanning.

Collimation

Collimation is an important feature to consider when comparing helical CT scanners (Table A-2). Helical CT scanning collimation controls effective slice thickness in combination with table speed. It does not control the location of the reconstructed image. Collimation together with pitch will dictate the amount of partial volume averaging that any object will suffer in the image. Pitch is defined as the ratio of the table velocity given in mm/sec and the collimation setting given in mm; it is expressed below as:

$$Pitch = \frac{V(mm/sec)}{C(mm)}$$

Currently, pitch is best set at between one and two for most scanners, and may be selected by the user (see Table A-6). Using a 180° linear interpolation algorithm, scans with a pitch of 1.5:1 will have a broader beam profile than 1:1 pitch scans. In some clinical situations this will be acceptable, but in others it may not.

Collimation together with pitch also will affect the amount of noise in an image which in turn will affect low-contrast object detection. The current state-of-the-art method is to scan with the smallest collimation available consistent with producing images of sufficient quality and coverage needed to make a diagnosis. A two mm collimation scan obtained at a pitch ratio of 1.5:1 will provide the same coverage as a three mm collimation scan obtained with a pitch of one. The vendor data on this differs slightly, but most agree that the spatial resolution would be better for the two mm collimation scan even though it was obtained with higher pitch. While using thinner collimation is desirable, it can only be accomplished if the x-ray tube can provide adequate x-ray output. If it cannot, the images will look photon-starved when using thinner sections.

CT scanners are being used in an increasing number of new ways since the advent of helical CT, and as such, the need for flexible collimation is paramount. Today all helical scanners offer at least four collimation settings (Elscint) and as many as eight (Picker). Most vendors offer five collimation settings. The maximum collimation for all vendors is

TABLE A-2 Collimation and gantry specifications

Vendor	Collimation Choices (mm)	Gantry Aperature Diameter (cm)	Gantry Tilt Range (degrees)	Gantry Dimensions (m) H × W × L
Elscint CT-Twin	1, 2.5, 5, 10	70	–20 to 30	1.9 × 2.2 × 1.1
GE HiSpeed Advantage	1, 3, 5, 7, 10	70	–30 to 30	
Philips Tomoscan SR 7000	1, 1.5, 3, 5, 10	70	–30 to 30	1.9 × 2.4 × 1.0
Picker PQ-2000	1, 1.5, 2, 3, 4, 5, 8, 10	70	–30 to 30	2.0 × 2.3 × 0.9
Siemens Somatom Plus-40	5 user selectable between 1 and 10 in 1 mm increments; Standard are 1, 2, 3, 5, 10	70	–25 to 25	2.1 × 2.7 × 1.0
Toshiba Xpress/sx	1, 2, 3, 5, 7, 10	72	–25 to 25	1.9 × 2.2 × 0.9

10 mm and the minimum is one mm. There is some disagreement in the range greater than or equal to two mm and less than 10 mm. All vendors agree that five mm is a useful collimator setting. Siemens is unique in permitting the user to define five collimator settings in the range one mm to 10 mm in integer increments. As a general guide to collimator choice it would be reasonable for a vendor to supply a minimum of five settings. Many studies for renal artery stenosis are performed with three mm collimation, but recently we have found that two mm collimation is superior, especially with a pitch ratio of 1.5:1. The two mm scan also gives better coverage than one mm collimation. The inclusion of two mm collimation on scanners would therefore be helpful.

Gantry Tilt Range

Gantry tilt is used in certain neuroradiological examinations where it is important to acquire true coronal imaging or in situations where certain structures such as the lenses of the eyes need to be avoided. It is also used during some biopsy procedures. The more the gantry can tilt, the more comfortable the patient will be. Gantry tilt among helical CT vendors ranges from a low of 20° to a high of 30° (Table A-2); tilt is to both sides of vertical and is usually symmetric except for Elscint, which is –20° to +30°. It is conceivable that helical scanning with Multiplanar Reformatting (MPR) will lessen the need for gantry tilt capability.

Gantry Dimensions

Gantry dimension is important in that it dictates, in part, the space that will need to be allocated for a particular scanner. The gantry is typically the tallest fixture in a system so it is wise to be mindful of what overhead fixtures will be near the gantry. These overhead fixtures may include suspension devices, power injectors, and patient monitoring equipment. Generally speaking, the more compact the gantry, the more room will be left for the patient, patient support equipment, and hospital staff. In general most gantries are approximately two m high, two and one-half m wide, and one m deep in the table travel direction. Each vendor will vary slightly from these numbers (Table A-2).

Gantry Aperture Diameter

Gantry aperture diameter is very nearly standardized to 70 cm. Having a wide aperture unit is important in that it provides plenty of space around the patient to work in, it helps the patient to feel less claustrophobic, and it permits a larger range of gantry tilt (Table A-2).

Localizing Light Source

There are two types of light localizing systems used on most helical CT scanners. The first is a system that employs incandescent light bulbs as the light source. These systems use lenses to project a light beam on the patient. Often one light source is to the left or right of the patient and a second one above the patient. Incandescent light sources are simple and relatively inexpensive. The weakness is in the amount of light output. In a room with a high ambient light level, an incandescent source may be difficult to see.

The other popular system is laser beam alignment. Laser beams are brought out of the gantry to the left and right of the patient and usually down from above the patient. Laser alignment systems are very bright and sharply focused. There is no difficulty seeing the light beam lines. They are, however, more expensive and more sensitive to misalignment.

Regardless of the light source used, a reasonable minimum requirement is that there be a set of alignment sources outside the scan plane of the gantry that are positioned relative to the scan plane in the gantry. Secondly, there should be a set of alignment lights that indicate the position of the imaging scan plane. Both are important for positioning for neuroradiologic scans, and for guidance of interventional procedures.

Patient Table

The patient table is an important feature in a CT scanner (Table A-3). The table must be able to go low enough to the floor so that a patient can get onto it easily or can be lifted on by house staff. The table must support the weight of a patient and still incrementally move accurately. It must move over a long distance so patient positioning can be accomplished easily. It must also have a long scanning distance so multiple body parts can be scanned without repositioning the patient.

The tabletop height range for any individual vendor CT line is typically fairly constant, but between vendors can vary considerably. In the current line of CT scanners, the minimum table height varied from a low of 30 cm to a high of 68 cm. The difference between the highest and the lowest table height varied from 36 cm to 70 cm.

Longitudinal travel is a measure of the absolute travel limits the table is capable of going. A unit with a long limit is less likely to incur a scan error by running up against its travel limit; it is a more forgiving device regarding patient positioning.

The scanning range is the absolute limit that the scanner can collect data over. The scanning range specified by the user must lie within the boundaries of the longitudinal travel limits for a scan to take place. Ideally, the scanning range should be larger than the

TABLE A-3 Patient table movement and load parameters

Vendor	Table Height (cm)	Height Range (cm)	Longitudinal Travel (cm)	Scannable Range (cm)	Weight Limit for Accurate Movement (kg)
Elscint CT-Twin	68–109	41	168	100	215
GE HiSpeed Advantage	51–107	56	170	135	182
Philips Tomoscan SR 7000	45–105	60	143	135	150
Picker PQ-2000	56–103	47	180	162	205
Siemens Somatom Plus-40	69–104	36	160	140	135
Toshiba Xpress/sx	30–100	70	182	100	135

coverage required for any patient needing a multiple body part exam (neck, chest, abdomen, and pelvis). If it is shorter than that the patient will need to be repositioned to complete the scan. Make sure your room is large enough to allow at least three feet of clearance around the patient table at all extremes of positioning, not just the neutral or parked position.

The weight limit specification of a patient table is the patient weight above which the table will not accurately increment to the next slice position in nonhelical mode and will not drive at a constant velocity in helical mode. Serious damage to the table's drive motors can occur causing unwanted downtime if a patient exceeds the table weight limit.

X-ray Tube

There are four features of x-ray tubes to consider: fan beam arc, heat storage, heat dissipation, and focal spot size (Table A-4). All helical CT scanners use fan beams. They are called fan beams because the sector shape of the x-ray beam resembles a fan. Fan beams are characterized by the angle at the apex of the sector. Among vendors this angle does not differ greatly; it ranges from a low of 42.6° for Siemens to a high of 49° for General Electric.

Heat storage capacity is usually reported in Heat Units (HU). It is the amount of heat an x-ray tube can hold without failure due to overheating. For three-phase and high-frequency generators, a heat unit is defined as:

$$\text{Heat Unit} = \text{tube potential} \times \text{tube current} \times \text{scan time} \times (\text{1-phase-to-3-phase correction factor})$$

$$\text{Heat Unit} = kVp \times mA \times \text{scan time(s)} \times 1.4 \text{ (for 3-phase)}$$

Example: a routine abdomen study. 120 kVp, 280 mA, 30 sec
$$HU = 120 \times 280 \times 30 \times 1.4 = 1.41 \text{ million HU}$$

Heat unit storage is generally divided up into the amount of heat the anode can hold and the amount of heat that the fluid in the outer cooling jacket can hold. One must be careful when evaluating helical CT units on the basis of heat units. The heating limit for the entire x-ray tube assembly is the heat unit capacity of the subunit with the *lowest* heat unit capacity, such as the anode focal spot track. Currently, heat unit capacities for x-ray tube anodes range from 3.4 million HU for Picker to 5.2 million HU for Philips. In the future there will be a move toward higher HU capacities as demand for long scans and higher milli-Amperes increases. Do not forget, however, to ask each vendor how long the tube can be on for, and at what milliAmperage for helical/spiral exposures of that duration. (See Table A-6.) Review images at *that* milliAmperage in patients of varying size/weight to make sure the images do not look photopenic to your eye.

Heat unit dissipation rate is an extremely important quantity when considering a unit. This value is the number of heat units that can be carried away from the anode out to the oil jacket. The higher this number, the better. As the above example demonstrated, it is

TABLE A-4 X-ray tube data

Vendor	Fan Beam Angle (degrees)	Heat Storage Capacity (MHU)*	Max. Heat Dissipation Rate (MHU/min)	Focal Spot Size (mm × mm)	Focal Spot area (sq. mm)
Elscint CT-Twin	43	5.0	0.504	1.5 × 1.4 0.75 × 1.4	2.1 1.05
GE HiSpeed Advantage	49	3.5	0.820	1.2 × 1.2 0.7 × 0.9	1.44 0.63
Philips Tomoscan SR 7000	48	5.2	0.900	1.0 × 1.2 0.5 × 0.7	1.2 0.35
Picker PQ-2000	44	3.4	0.830	0.9 × 0.9 0.6 × 1.3	1.71 0.78
Siemens Somatom Plus-40	42.6	4.3	0.613	1.3 × 1.2 0.8 × 0.9	1.56 0.72
Toshiba Xpress/sx	49	3.5	0.735	1.5 × 1.0 0.9 × 0.9	1.5 0.81

*(MHU = Million heat units)

fairly easy to generate one million heat units. It is this number that dictates how long a user will have to wait between helical studies before enough heat units have been removed from the anode to start another helical study. At present, no vendor can dissipate greater than 0.9 million heat units per minute (Philips) and the lowest dissipation rate belongs to Elscint with a dissipation rate of 0.504 million heat units. example, let us say that in the course of a day we built up 3.3 MHU on our tube and our next study would generate another 1.5 MHU. Let us also assume our limit is 3.5 MHU and our dissipation rate is 0.75 MHU/min. How long will we have to wait to do the next study?

$$3.5 - 1.5 = 2.0 \text{ MHU (This is the level we need to cool down to.)}$$

$$3.3 - 2.0 = 1.3 \text{ MHU (This is the amount of HU we need to dissipate.)}$$

$$1.3 \text{ MHU} \div 0.75 \text{ MHU per min} = 1.73 \text{ minutes or 1 minute 44 seconds.}$$

While this is not long to wait between patients, this would be an unacceptable waiting period between helices in a single patient. Furthermore, tube cooling algorithms (simulation software that tells the computer that heat has dissipated, and that another scan can be initiated) are designed to be quite conservative. Because of this algorithm, which has been designed to protect the x-ray tube, many scanners will not allow additional scanning at total heat unit levels well below the tube limits. That is why asking the vendors what milliAmperage and length of exposure is allowed by their device is so important.

The fourth important tube parameter is focal spot size. Most x-ray tubes on premium line scanners come with dual focal spots. The large focal spots range from 1.2 mm^2 to 2.1 mm^2 and the small focal spots go from 0.35 mm^2 to 1.1 mm^2. Most vendors kept a ratio of large focal spot area to small focal spot area of approximately two. Generally speaking, large focal spots cause less anode track heating because the electrons incident on the anode are spread out over a larger annular area. They suffer, however, from reduced resolution. Small focal spots permit theoretically better high-contrast spatial resolution. As with much of CT, these two competing factors need to be evaluated by the consumer as to their relative importance to a potential purchase.

X-ray Generator and Tube Output

X-ray generators are rated for the maximum safe output of their secondary transformer windings (Table A-5). If the rating is exceeded, the transformer may be damaged due to effects of overheating. Damage may include short-circuits across damaged electrical insulation and melted windings. Generator rating is expressed in units of kilowatts (kW). For

TABLE A-5 High voltage generator data

Vendor	Generator Rating (kW)	kVp Choices	mA Choices	High Frequency Generator	High or Low Voltage to Ring
Elscint CT-Twin	60	90, 120, 140	50–400 incr = 50	yes	Low
GE HiSpeed Advantage	48	80, 100, 120, 140	40–400 incr = 10	yes	Low
Philips Tomoscan SR 7000	48	100, 120, 140	50–400 incr = 25,50	yes	Low
Picker PQ-2000	30	80, 100, 120 130, 140	80–140 incr = 15–25	yes	Low
Siemens Somatom Plus-40	40	80, 120, 137	70–320 vendor selected by application	yes	Hybrid
Toshiba Xpress/sx	48	80, 100, 120, 135	50–400 incr = 10	yes	High

(incr = increments of, kW = kilowatts)

three-phase generators or high-frequency generators, kilowatt ratings are calculated according to the following equation:

$$kW = \frac{kV \times mA}{1000},$$

where kV is the potential across the x-ray tube in kiloVolts and mA is the x-ray tube current in milliAmperes. For example, unit A has a maximum kV = 140 and a maximum mA = 300 at the 140 kVp setting. This unit's generator rating is:

$$Rating\ (kW) = \frac{140 \times 300}{1000} = 42 kW.$$

Tube potential is the voltage applied across the anode-cathode space in the x-ray tube. It is the source of the acceleration force that electrons feel as they move off of the filament into the vacuum of the x-ray tube. From a CT imaging point of view, x-ray tube potential affects total counts registered by detectors, so it also affects contrast in the image. High kiloVolt peak promotes efficient use of the x-ray tube because x-ray tubes produce more x-rays per milliAmperes at high kiloVoltage compared to lower kiloVoltage. This use increases tube life. Because more x-rays are incident on the patient, more x-rays will be detected. This leads to higher counts, less image noise, and better low-contrast resolution. One also gets more counts at high-kiloVoltage because high-kiloVoltage photons have a higher probability of penetrating through the entire object without an interaction than do low kiloVolt x-rays. The problem with using high kiloVolt peak is the lower probability of k-edge absorption in iodinated contrast media of higher energy x-rays. Contrast resolution of enhanced structures may adversely be affected. This remains an unresolved issue at this time with no easy solution. The most popular kiloVoltage setting for adult CT scanning is 120 kV. Vendors of helical CT scanners are generally providing choices of tube potential in the following intervals: 70, 80, or 90 kV; 100 kV; 120 kV; and 130 to 140 kV.

Tube current is a measure of the number of electrons that are flowing through the vacuum of the x-ray tube from the cathode towards the anode. Tube current is measured in milliAmperes (mA). Maximum sustainable tube current is the most important parameter for comparing helical/spiral CT units. It is important, however, to also take into account differences in the efficiency of x-ray production. *Just because two units have the same allowable maximum milliAmpere setting does not guarantee that they will produce the same number of x-rays per second, all else being equal.* One unit may use the electrons very efficiently and have a high ratio of exposure (milliRoentgen) to tube current multiplied by time (milliRoentgen/milliAmpere sec) whereas a second unit with the same milliAmpere setting would yield a low milliRoentgen/milliAmpere sec setting (Table A-13). The vendor's use of added filtration also must be considered when looking into how milliAmperage is used. Units with large amounts of filtration may have beams with high effective energy but low counts, while other units with less filtration may have a lower effective energy beam but with higher counts.

What is important to compare when considering competing units on the basis of x-ray generators is how efficiently each produces x-rays (i.e., milliRoentgen/milliAmpere sec at a specified location, material, and kiloVolts) and what type of image is achieved at the exposure (high-contrast resolution, low-contrast detection, and image noise). The scanner should produce, at that specified technique, phantom, location, and reconstruction algorithm, either an image with superior low-contrast object detection and low noise, or for protocols demanding high spatial frequency information images with excellent high-contrast spatial resolution at the expense of increased noise. The physicist and his or her phantom studies, and the radiologist's evaluation of clinical image quality should both be considered during assessment of devices.

Helical/Spiral Scanning Capability

The ability to efficiently and routinely perform helical/spiral scans in almost all patients should be the focus of device evaluation. At the heart of helical CT are the relationships between scanned distance, scan time, kiloVolt peak, milliAmpere, milliRoentgen/milliAmpere sec, pitch, image contrast, and spatial resolution. Each vendor has a different approach to optimizing these parameters within the technical constraints of their equipment. From a user's perspective it can be a maze specifications and confusion.

There are, however, some generalizations that might help clear up some of this confusion. First, one needs to consider what types of scanning need to be done. Is it primarily abdomens where low-contrast object detection and patient coverage are important? Is it head and neck work where collimation needs to be narrow and high-contrast spatial resolution needs to be superior? Or more likely, is it a mix of cases where flexibility, overall performance, and high uptime are critical. Is it a high- or low-volume practice? Once the type of scanning is identified, one can start to evaluate each scanner on its strengths and weaknesses.

Tube Current, Scan Time, and Pitch Interrelationships

As discussed previously, the product of milliAmpere and scan time is proportional to the number of heat units produced by a scanner. The number of heat units will dictate the duration of allowable exposure, and ultimately the extent of coverage (Table A-6). For example, we may scan for 35 cm to cover the anatomy of interest. We may also want to cover this anatomy by seven mm section thickness to limit partial volume effects. Scanning at pitch = one, this scan would take 50 sec (350 mm/7 mm per sec). It may be that on the scanner we are using, the generator can supply 165 mA for the 50 sec of "on-time" needed. If 165 mA produces images that are too noisy, then compromises to the scanning protocol will need to be made. One option would be to scan at a greater pitch. This would reduce scan time. In our example, if we keep the collimation at seven mm but move the table at nine mm/sec then the pitch is 1.28. This would reduce scan time to 39 sec. Referring to a scanning technique chart we may find that at 39 sec of on-time, the generator can supply 210 mA, which would increase counts and decrease noise. Another

TABLE A-6 Helical scanning capabilities data

Vendor	Maximum time (120 kVp, ≥ 200 mA) sec	Maximum Tube Current (mA) (120 kVp, ≥ 30 sec)	Maximum Coverage (cm) at Pitch = 1[a]	Minimum Intergroup Delay (sec)	Pitches Available	Sequences Per Study
Elscint CT-Twin	32	300	60	15[e]	0.5, 0.75, 1.0, 1.5, 2.0	10
GE HiSpeed Advantage	60	330	60	3	1 to 2	6[d]
Philips Tomoscan SR 7000	50	300	50	9	1 and 2	5
Picker PQ-2000	45[b]	200[b]	70[b]	3[b]	1.0, 1.25, 1.5, 2	7
Siemens Somatom Plus-40	32	210	40	15[c,e]	0.1 to 2	2[c]
Toshiba Xpress/sx	58	250	58	5	0 to 30	5

_ to _ represents continuous or nearly continuous pitch selection inclusive with the limits shown; all other pitch data represent discreet selections. Intergroup delay is between helices or helical and nonhelical scans.
[a]With variable reduction in mA
[b]Available on future release ZAP 100
[c]Future software release
[d]Can mix scan parameters, collimation, and pitches
[e]Requires entry of second prescription

approach would be to increase collimation to 10 mm and keep pitch equal to one. This would reduce scan time to 35 sec and could increase the permitted tube current to 235 mA. While system operating software will often offer these types of alternatives to the technologist, there is no substitute for the technologist and radiologist having a working knowledge of their system limitations and range of exposure factors.

The maximum allowable milliAmperage is not as important as the milliAmperage that can be sustained for 30 sec or more. A 30-sec scan duration is necessary to efficiently use this technique in a high volume practice where most of the scans will be performed helically or spirally. For combination exams, (e.g., of the thorax and abdomen) it is also important to ask how low one would have to drop the milliAmperage if one wanted to scan beyond 30 sec. It is often effective to scan the abdomen at high milliAmperage first, and then reduce the milliAmpere for scanning the chest. The radiologist and technologist must make sure that they understand the interplay between all the scan parameters, coverage, and image quality. Noise reduction from increased milliAmperage must be balanced against reduced low-contrast object detection brought on by increased pitch. Increasing collimation and keeping the pitch ratio at 1:1 must be balanced against decreased collimation with increased pitch. More study is needed in this area to make clear what are the optimal setting for each particular exam done using helical CT.

Computer Processing

Computer processing is that part of a CT scanner that is concerned with data collection, computations needed to produce an image, reconstruction time per slice, and other functions such as being able to do two or more tasks synchronously (Table A-7). This section will briefly discuss the computers vendors use, scan field of view options, reconstruction times per slice, and the advantages of multitasking and parallel processing.

TABLE A-7 Information storage and computing speed data

Vendor	RAM (MB)	Hard Disk Drive Capacity (MB)	Number of Images (512×512)	Number of Raw Data Files	Processing Speed (MFLOPS)	Additional Memory Devices
Elscint CT-Twin	192	760	2100	400	133	FD, MT, EOD
GE HiSpeed Advantage	96	860	1800	450	170	MT, DAT, WORM
Philips Tomoscan SR 7000	132	1560	800	800	100	FD, MT, EOD
Picker PQ-2000	340	4000	2500	355	200	WORM, DAT
Siemens Somatom Plus-40	112	1200	2400	300		WORM, MT, EOD
Toshiba Xpress/sx	160	3000	1800	400		FD, EOD

(FD = floppy disk, MT = magnetic tape, DAT = digital audio tape, WORM = write once read many optical drive, EOD = erasable optical drive, MFLOP = million floating point operations/sec)

Computer CPU

One of the most important pieces of equipment in any helical CT scanner is the computer that operates the scanner. This "computer" may in fact on some systems be a group of small computers (distributed processing) working in concert to produce a viable system. Whether the system uses one computer or multiple computers, it must allow ease of use, flexibility in software and hardware upgrades, and rapid data processing. The other issue relating to the computer is how many images and raw data files can it deal with.

Reconstruction Time Per Slice

Reconstruction time (in sec) is the time it takes for the processing of data to form an image. On the surface it looks like a simple definition, but when one considers the number of choices vendors offer for reconstruction and viewing it becomes more complicated. The race to reduce reconstruction times changes almost monthly. We have not included reconstruction time data in our tables for this reason. One vendor may have two-sec reconstruction time per image but may not permit viewing until *all* image data is acquired and *all* images reconstructed. A second vendor may have five-sec reconstruction per image, but may let you view each image as it is completed; this unit may also permit asynchronous acquisition of new data while previously acquired data is being processed. From this example, even though the first unit's reconstruction time was much faster than the other, it was the "slower unit" that produced a useful image first because of the processing sequence of events (acquire continuously, reconstruct continuously, view when ready compared to acquire all, reconstruct all, view all). When comparing helical CT scanners be sure a complete description of the image processing and display sequence is clearly explained before comparisons are made.

Reasonable questions to ask the vendor include:

1. Is there simultaneous data acquisition, reconstruction, and display capability?
2. Is there a mode for rapid reconstruction to view a specific image, such as the last image in a helix?
3. Is there a mode that is a compromise between one and two?
4. Are the different modes of processing selected easily by the user?
5. Can reconstruction order and/or viewing order be specified by the user; i.e., last acquired/first seen or first acquired/first seen?

System Random Access Memory (RAM)

Random access memory (RAM) is the space the computer uses to store information it needs to perform calculations leading to a reconstructed image. This memory may be used to store programs, patient information, scanning parameters, raw data that is streaming in from a scan, and other data. Large amounts of RAM are desirable because the information it holds can be accessed very quickly by the central processing unit (CPU) or an array processor (AP). If there is a shortage of RAM then the information must be moved to another storage device such as an optical disk or a magnetic storage device (hard disk drive, floppy disk drive, or magneto-optical drive). This data movement takes time and therefore may cause unacceptable delays in processing.

Standard Hard Disk Capacity

Practically speaking, no system can have enough RAM to deal with the vast amount of data a helical CT scanner can generate. To overcome this limitation, manufactures ship systems with one or more hard disk drives to store information not immediately needed by the CPU or AP. Hard disks are specified by the number of bytes of information they can hold. Hard disks included with helical CT scanners are specified in units of million (mega) bytes (MB) or, for even larger drives, billion (giga) bytes (GB). Larger system hard disk drives offer a slight advantage because cases are on-line for review longer.

Standard Number of Images On-Line

The number of images that can be stored on the system is dictated by the size of the images in pixels being stored (1024×1024, 512×512, 340×340, or 256×256), by the partitioning of the hard disk into raw data storage space verses image storage space, and by the size of the hard disk. Table A-7 contains the size of each unit's hard drive and the number of images it can hold when the images are *not* compressed. The reader is warned to make sure to ask vendors if when compressing an image and then decompressing it, information is irreparably destroyed. Under certain circumstances the user may wish to permanently store images in uncompressed format to maintain full image integrity.

Keep in mind that stored image data and raw data are different. Raw data is necessary to apply different algorithms or reconstruct overlapping scans. Most systems keep anywhere from 300 to 800 raw data files on-line. If the radiologist is planning on reviewing a patient's images before deciding if overlapping scans should be reconstructed, the raw data files need to be preserved for at least several hours. In a busy practice that performs a high volume of body CT, availability of 400 to 450 raw data files will assure that files will be there at the end of the day for additional reconstruction if necessary.

Other Storage

Most systems have other optional storage devices that are mainly used for archival purposes. These really should not be considered optional, as they are absolutely necessary, especially if hard copy films should become lost. Available storage media include magnetic tape (MT), floppy disks (FD), write-once-read-many optical disks (WORM), erasable optical disks (EOD), digital audio tape cartridges (DAT), and additional hard disk drives (HD). Other storage devices, standard number of images, hard disk space, and

RAM are given in Table A-7. The decision whether to use WORM or EOD cartridges will vary from practice to practice. The EOD cartridges are more expensive, but if they are recycled at short (less than one year) intervals, they can be cost-effective. If electronically archived images must be kept longer (for medico-legal reasons), the WORM optical cartridges may be more cost-effective. DAT drives can be used for storing raw data because of their high capacity. They are slow, however, and should a significant number of individual cases have to be called up for transfer to the system hard disk, the process can be laborious.

Image Display Parameters

Monitor matrix size is a specification of the number of pixels a vendor uses to display an image. The monitor parameters are shown in Table A-8. These are most often specified in powers of two, such as 256, 512, or 1024. It is important for a potential customer to understand the difference between a reconstruction matrix (actual image data from x-ray projections) and a display matrix (number of pixels shown on the monitor). A reconstruction matrix is a grid of data locations in computer memory that the computer is going to calculate CT numbers for. It will calculate the CT numbers from collected projection data. A display matrix is a grid on a monitor whose brightness values are correlated to the CT

TABLE A-8 Image display device characteristics

Vendor	Display Matrix Size	Reconstruction Matrix	Black and White or Color	CT Number Range	Image Zoom Factor	Maximum # of images displayed at once
Elscint CT-Twin	1280 × 1024	340, 512, 768, 1024	Color	−1000 to 3095	10×	80
GE HiSpeed Advantage	512 × 512	256, 512	Black and White	−1024 to 3071	16×	16
Philips Tomoscan SR 7000	1024 × 1024	320, 512	Black and White	−2000 to 4000	9.9×	25
Picker PQ-2000	1024 × 1024	512	Color	−2048 to 6143	16×	25
Siemens Somatom Plus-40	1024 × 1024	512	Black and White	−1024 to 3071	16×	16
Toshiba Xpress/sx	512 × 512	512	Black and White	−1000 to 4000	4×	16

number of the data the pixel represents. It is possible to have more display pixels than reconstruction pixels. If an image is reconstructed at 512 × 512 then displayed at 1024 × 1024, *no new information is gained.* The additional display pixels are interpolated (fabricated) based on the original set of 512 × 512 reconstruction pixels. If a vendor reconstructs with a matrix larger than 512 × 512 (say 1024 × 1024), there is the potential to have much more information than an image reconstructed at 512 × 512. In general, one would want images to be reconstructed with the largest matrix possible that is consistent with acceptable processing time. Remember that a 1024 × 1024 reconstruction array has four times the number of pixels as a 512 × 512, so it will take four time as long to process. Large reconstruction matrices open the opportunity for higher spatial resolution and it is likely that as computer speed increases, reconstruction matrices will grow.

Vendors offer with their systems a monitor from which a technologist can watch images being reconstructed. This monitor is either a grayscale monitor or a color monitor. In most cases either type is fully adequate for routine work. Color monitors may add some additional cost to the system, but it is only a small amount in the context of the entire purchase price. A color monitor offers more flexibility in labeling and "colorization" of images and three-dimensional reconstructions. A black and white monitor generally renders grayscale better than a color monitor renders grayscale, but again this is a minor inconvenience at best. Which monitor gets used is in the final analysis up to the flexibility of the system and user preference.

CT number range is the range of values that can be displayed on the system. Despite quoted specifications, the practical limit for CT range is from −1000 Hounsfield units (air) to +3000 Hounsfield units (metals). Any margin on the low side is useless in that it is clinically insignificant to image materials less attenuating than air. Any margin on the top side is currently useless but may have applications in future work on metal object identification and metal artifact reduction.

Image zoom factor is a measure of how magnified the reconstructed image can be made to appear on the display device. Image magnification is done by interpolation of reconstructed data and therefore does not increase the information on the image. (New information can only be acquired if the scan field of view is reduced and the smaller acquired field is reconstructed over the entire reconstruction array.) Image zoom is often used to see structures that are normally very small on an image that is not magnified but that cannot be acquired with a smaller field of view. The image zoom factor ranges from 4 to 16 across vendor lines.

Image Quality Indicators

Helical CT images can be characterized by three measures of image quality: modulation transfer function (MTF), low contrast object detection, and noise (Tables A-9–A-12). Any one of these taken alone cannot impart to a potential buyer the entire truth about the image quality for a particular scanner. They must examined together. It must be stressed also that

(Text continues on page 322)

TABLE A-9 Modulation transfer function for highest resolution scanning mode

Vendor	50% lp/m	10% lp/cm	0% lp/cm	kVp	mA	s	S.T. (mm)	R.M.	SFOV (cm)	DFOV (cm)	Phantom	Zoom	Filter	Comment
Elscint CT-Twin	9.4	16.7	20	120	200	1	2.5	512	25		Acrylic/air	2	detail	
GE HiSpeed Advantage	8.5	13	15	120	340	1	10	512	25		MFT of PRF from Tungsten pin		edge	
Philips Tomoscan SR 7000	10.1	12.7	14.5	120	175	1	1.5	512	16		AAPM CATPHAN MARK5	13	2H	
Picker PQ-2000	10.5	18	21			1		512			MTF of PRF from Tungsten pin			Maximum Spatial Resolution
Siemens Somatom Plus 40	10	13	15											High Resolution Inner Ear
Toshiba Xpress/sx	9.5	12.2	18.0	120	250	1	2	512	24		Toshiba Standard		FC80	

(lp/cm = line pairs per cm, MTF = Modulation transfer function, PRF = Point response function)

TABLE A-10 Modulation transfer function for standard body scanning mode

Vendor	50% lp/m	10% lp/cm	0% lp/cm	kVp	mA	s	S.T. (mm)	R.M.	SFOV (cm)	DFOV (cm)	Phantom	Zoom	Filter	Comment
Elscint CT-Twin	5.4	8.5	11	120	300	1	10	512	43	24	acylic/air bars		detail	Standard mode
GE HiSpeed Advantage	4.0	6.0	8.0	120	340	1	10	512	25	25	FFT of PRF from .05 mm dia. Tungsten wire			Standard algorithm
Philips Tomoscan SR 7000	4.5	7.8	10	120	250	1	10	512	25	25			F1	Normal resolution mode
Picker PQ-2000	4.0	7.5	>9	130	200	1	10	512	48					Abdomen standard algorithm
Siemens Somatom Plus 40	4.3	7.2	10											
Toshiba Xpress/sx	3.4	7.0	12										FC20	

(FFT = Fast Fourier Transform)

TABLE A-11 Noise data at abdominal scanning techniques

Vendor	% Noise	50% MTF Standard Mode	kVp	mA	s	S.T. (mm)	R.M.	SFOV (cm)	DFOV (cm)	Filter	Dose (mGy)	Phantom
Elscint CT-Twin	0.32	8.5	120 120	300 200	1 1	10 2.5	512	25		Standard	30	Elscint Phantom 21.6 cm dia. water equivalent
GE HiSpeed Advantage	0.33	6.0	120	340	1	10	512	25				21.6 cm dia. AAPM water
Philips Tomoscan SR 7000	0.30	7.8	120 120	250 175	1 1	10 1.5	512				40	16 cm dia.l AAPM water
Picker PQ-2000	0.36	7.5	140 130	200	1	10	512	48				21.6 cm dia AAPM water
Siemens Somatom Plus 40	0.36	7.2	120	290	1	10	512	50		AB7555		16 cm dia. water
Toshiba Xpress/sx	0.50	7.0	120	300	1.5	10	512	24		FC70		24 cm dia. water

(MTF = Modulation Transfer Function, s = sec, S.T. = slice thickness, R.M. = reconstruction matrix, SFOV = scan field of view, DFOV = display field of view, mGy = milliGray

TABLE A-12 Low contrast object detection data at abdominal scanning techniques

Vendor	Low Contrast Measure	50% MTF Standard Mode	kVp	mA	s	S.T. (mm)	R.M.	SFOV (cm)	DFOV (cm)	Filter	Dose (mGy)	Phantom
Elscint CT-Twin	0.25% @ 3 mm	8.5	120	300	1	2 × 10	512	25		Standard	30	16 cm AAPM with ATS insert
GE HiSpeed Advantage	0.25% @ 2.5 mm	6.0	120	400	1	2.5	512	25				16 cm AAPM with ATS insert
	0.35% @ 5 mm		120	340	1	10	512	25				CATPHAN
Philips Tomoscan SR 7000	0.5% @ 2 mm		120	250	1	10	512			F0	40	16 cm AAPM with ATS insert
	0.25% @ 4 mm		120	250	1	10	512			F0	40	
		7.8	120	175	1	1.5	512					
Picker PQ-2000	0.35% @ 2 mm		130	200	1	10	512	48		Standard		6 in CATPHAN
	0.35% @ 4 mm		130	200	1	10	512	48		Standard		8 in CATPHAN
	0.4% @ 3.5 mm		130	200	1	10	512	48		Standard		16 cm AAPM with ATS insert
		7.5	130	200	1	1	512	48				
Siemens Somatom Plus 40	0.3% @ 2.5 mm	7.2	120	290	1	10	512	50				16 cm AAPM with ATS insert
Toshiba Xpress/sx	0.25% @ 2.5 mm		120	200	2	10	512	24		FC20		Toshiba Standard
	0.3% @ 2.0 mm		120	200	2	10	512	24		FC20		Toshiba Standard
		7.0	120	300	1.5	10	512	24		FC70		

(see Abbreviations Table A-11)

they are affected by the kiloVolt peak, milliAmperage, section thickness, scan field of view, reconstruction matrix, reconstruction algorithm, interpolator, pitch, and scan time. When comparing two units, one must be careful that scanning techniques were similar. As an example of this, if a scanner has a relatively noisy image the noise could stem from low counts or it could stem from the fact that the data was processed with a reconstruction algorithm that has a high MTF value at high spatial frequencies. In the latter case the noise value may be acceptable if that type of imaging technique were used for procedures demanding high-contrast, small-object resolution.

Image quality cannot be divorced from the task the scanner is asked to do. If subtle low-contrast liver tumors need to be detected then a scanner with an algorithm resulting in a low noise value and superior low-contrast object detection is what is needed; high-value, high spatial frequency MTF is only needed here secondarily to demarcate tumor edges, and extremely high value, high frequency MTF is not wanted or needed. If on the other hand very fine bone fractures need to be seen then a scanner having an algorithm that embodies MTF high value at high spatial frequencies is absolutely needed. Here noise and low-contrast object detection mean little.

Modulation Transfer Function (MTF)

MTF is a curve that describes the ability of an imaging system to faithfully record information. An MTF of one is perfect: all of the information transmitted has been recorded. An MTF of zero means that none of the information transmitted has been recorded. MTF curves for CT scanners are scaled in the spatial frequency direction in line pairs per centimeter (lp/cm) (Figure A-1). They have two typical shapes. In one, the MTF value is a maximum at zero lp/cm and decreases slowly to MTF = zero at about 10 lp/cm. This type of curve would be typical for a standard body algorithm where a compromise between superior low-contrast object detection and high-contrast object detection has been reached. A second characteristic MTF is one that has a peak value of MTF in the three to nine lp/cm region then decreases gradually to zero at greater than 13 lp/cm. This type of curve is used to augment structures of clinical significance in the region of the MTF curve where the boost of MTF greater than one occurs.

Low Contrast (Resolution) Object Detection

Low-contrast resolution is a measure of a system's ability to detect objects that vary only slightly from their surroundings (Table A-12). A typical low contrast object in CT is on the order of two to five mm in diameter and has a contrast 0.2 percent to 0.5 percent different from its background. Low-contrast object detection is a function of how much noise there is in the image, how large the object is, and how different it is from its background. If image noise is low, then small objects that differ only slightly in contrast from their background are likely to be seen. On the other hand, if the image noise is high, then low contrast objects could be obscured unless they are fairly large. Low contrast can be quoted by a vendor as 0.xx percent contrast at y mm. This means that one can see an object y mm in diameter if its contrast difference is 0.xx percent greater than or less than the background.

Noise

Noise is a measure of statistical fluctuation in CT values in a region of interest on an image of a uniform object such as a water phantom (Table A-11). If all scanning techniques are equal and one scanner has a lower noise value than another, it may be that the lower noise unit is using available transmission x-rays more efficiently. This comparison in practice is difficult to make because one would have to be sure that the MTF in both cases was the same; that would be unlikely. It remains, though, that if a phantom is scanned under recommended techniques for a particular study such as adult abdomen and the images are reconstructed using a recommended algorithm, then the unit with the lowest noise will have a clinical advantage for low contrast objects.

When comparing units for purchase it is important to have a qualified medical imaging physicist scan phantoms at clinical techniques to analyze low-contrast object detection, high contrast object resolution, and noise. It is only through self-testing that one can make an informed purchase of helical CT equipment. Certainly for acceptance testing, once a unit has been purchased, these same parameters should be analyzed to make sure they comply with the vendor's published specifications. For more information on testing, of CT units refer to a recent report by the National Council on Radiation Protection and Measurement (NCRP) Report Number 99 entitled *Quality Assurance for Diagnostic Imaging*.

Radiation Dosimetry

For a helical scanner to provide low noise images it must be able to sustain high radiation output for the required number of seconds to scan the anatomy of interest. One measure of

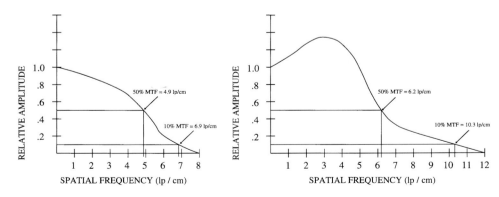

FIGURE A-1

a device's output is the amount of absorbed dose at two locations in a standard phantom. These values must be reported by law and are provided by each vendor. They are called *Computed Tomography Dose Index* (CTDI) values. They are always given at specific techniques and are accompanied by tables that give factors to correct for other techniques. Measurements are done in a 32 cm diameter polymethyl-methacrylate phantom described in the *Code of Federal Regulation 21 §1020.33 (6) "CT dosimetry phantom."* Table A-13 contains a listing of CTDI for each vendor. The technique used varies, as there is yet no standard methodology for testing or reporting. The column labeled "center" refers to the dose at the geometric center of the phantom. The column labeled "edge" refers to the dose one cm in from the outer surface of the phantom. The values are specified for body scanning at techniques given in the table. An effective scanner will have the ability to output the radiation levels needed to produce images that are diagnostically useful to the user at the combination of kiloVolt peak, milliAmpere, and time selected. From the above table it is clear why one cannot simply compare milliAmperes per second between units as a measure of output. For the same milliAmpere setting, different vendor units could have widely differing outputs. Therefore it is not safe to assume that just because a unit scans at a low milliAmpere it produces noisy images; this may be true, but not necessarily.

TABLE A-13 Body scanning dose data

Vendor	kVp	mA	s	Slice Thickness (mm)	Center (mRad/mAs)	Average edge (mRad/mAs)	Comments
Elscint CT-Twin	140	340	1	2 × 10	5.9	11.5	403° overscan
GE HiSpeed Advantage	120	170	2	10	3.2	5.9	Standard Algorithm, 35 cm SFOV
Philips Tomoscan SR 7000	120	250	1	10	5.2	10.2	
Picker PQ-2000	130	200	1	10	5.5	10.5	Filter 1
	130	200	1	10	7.0	15.5	Filter 2
Siemens Somatom Plus-40	120	290	1	10	4.1	9.6	0.2 mm Cu filtration
Toshiba Xpress/sx	120	200	2	10	6.7	11.8	Large SFOV

(s = sec, SFOV = scan field of view, Cu = copper)

Index

Index

Abdomen
  abscesses of, 158
  biopsy of, 158
  CT examination of trauma, 158, 159, 208, 209
Acetabulum, 249, 250
Adenocarcinoma
  of kidney, 212–216
  of lung, 116, 117
  of pancreas, *See* pancreas, carcinoma of
Adenoma
  of kidney. *See* oncocytoma
Adenopathy
  of mediastinum, 120
  of retroperitoneum, 195
Algorithms, reconstruction, 2–6
Aneurysm
  Abdominal aortic
    CT Scanning for, 274–280
    Multiplanar reformation of, 278
    Scanning technique for, 274–276
    3-D rendering of, 277–280
    Intracranial, 52–58

  Thoracic aortic, 124–129, 281–286
Angiography
  CT, 22, 29–82, 107–110, 121–131, 199, 200, 265–297
Ankle
  trauma to, 247, 248
Aorta
  aneurysms of 19, 124–129, 274–280
  arch of, 121–130
  anomalies of, 121–123
  dissections of, 284–286
    CT of, 130, 131
Arch of aorta, 121–130, 281–286
Arteriovenous malformation of lung, 118–120
Artery
  aortic, 124–130, 274–286
  carotid, 29–48
  hepatic
    anatomy, 199–200
  iliac
    calcification of, 279, 280
    extension of aneurysm, 276–280
  pulmonary, 131–139, 282

Artery *(Cont.)*:
   renal
      stenosis of, 22, 266–274
      three-dimensional rendering of, 266–274
   subclavian aberrant right, 290
   superior mesenteric, 195–200, 287, 288, 291
Arthrography
   CT, 243–245, 252–255
Artifacts
   aliasing, 155
   metal, 257–259
   misregistration 1, 105, 154, 222
   pseudothrombosis of
      inferior vena cava, 167–169
      superior mesenteric vein, 167–169
      superior vena cava, 106
   pulsation, 123, 283–284
   stair step, 4–6, 8, 84

Bile duct
   common, 172
   obstruction of, 193–194
   Tumors of
      CT of, 198, 203–205
Biopsy
   CT-directed, 158, 242, 243, 251, 252
Bladder
   contrast opacification of, 158
Bone
   exostosis of 230, 281
   giant cell tumor of, 228, 229
   prosthesis of, 260, 261
   trauma of, 222
Bowel, small
   ischemia of, 287–289, 291, 292
   thickened folds of, 292
Brain
   arteriovenous malformation of CT scan of, 69, 80, 82–85
   helical scanning of, 82–88
   hematomas of, 83, 84

Breast
   metastatic carcinoma of, 178, 184, 185
Bronchi
   abnormalities of, 141, 142
   anatomy of, 139
   hamartoma of, 141–144
Bronchogenic carcinoma
   CT scan for, 111–115, 120
   CT scan of, 120
   hilar involvement in, 120
   lymph node staging of, 120
   metastatic to hila, CT of, 120
   pleural invasion, 120–122
Bronchus, *See* Bronchi

Calcium
   CT detection of, 115
   MIP 3D views of, 19, 31, 40, 271, 273
Carcinoma. *See also* Tumor(s), and under specific organs
   bronchogenic. *See* Bronchogenic carcinoma
   islet cell, 201, 202
      metastases to liver, 182, 183
   of bile duct, 198, 202–204
   of breast metastatic to liver, 178, 184, 185
   of colon metastatic to liver, 178–181
   of kidney. *See* Renal cell carcinoma
   of lung. *See* bronchogenic carcinoma
   of pancreas, 193–202
Carotid artery
   calcification of 40, 41
   CT examination of 29–48
   stenosis, 31–41
   three-dimensional rendering of 29–48
Cholangiocarcinoma
   focal hepatic mass in, 203
   obstructive jaundice due to, 202–204
   of bile duct, 198
   of common hepatic duct, 202–204
   staging of, 202–205

Circle of Willis
    CT angiography of, 48–62
Collimation, 9–11, 303, 304
Colon
    metastases from, 178–181
Computed axial tomography. *See*
        Tomography, computed
Contrast media
    administration of
        intravenous bolus, 172–179
    for CT angiography, 266
    intravenous infusion
        limitations of
            for hepatic CT, 173–175
    ionic vs nonionic, 160
    volume of, 179
Cyst(s)
    of kidney, 210, 211
    of liver, 182
    partial volume effect of, 182, 210
Cystic neoplasm of pancreas, 201

Data
    raw image, 1, 313–315
Detectors, 300–302
Diaphragm, 139
Dosimetry, radiation, 222, 223, 324
Dual phase examination
    of liver, 178–183
    of pancreas, 189–191
Duct
    bile, 172, 193, 194
    pancreatic, 171–173

Embolism, pulmonary
    CT of, 107, 131–139
Esophagus
    vascular anatomic relationships of, 290

Facial bones
    three-dimensional rendering of, 88–92
Femur
    trauma to, 236–239

Fistula
    bronchopleural, 145
Fracture(s)
    of cervical spine, 96–99

Gastrointestinal tract. *See* specific parts
Gleoid labrum, 243
Graft
    coronary artery, 130

Hamartoma, pulmonary, 114
Hemangioma
    of liver, 187
Hemorrhage
    subarachnoid, 52–62
Hepatic artery
    anatomy of, 199, 200
    encasement of, 199, 200
Hepatic attenuation, 176, 177
Hepatoma
    contrast enhancement of, 182
Hip
    CT of, 249–251
Humerus, 230, 231, 252, 253

Image quality, 17–18, 317–324
Image noise, 3, 324
Inferior vena cava
    pseudothrombosis of, 167–169
    renal cell carcinoma invasion of,
        213–216
    thrombosis of, 214, 215
Interpolation, 2–6
Iohexol
    administration strategies for
        scan of abdomen, 159, 160,
            172–179
        scan of chest, 108, 109
    carotid evaluation, 30
    circle of Willis evaluation, 50
Ischemia
    of small bowel, 287–289, 291, 292

Joint
    ulnar-trachlear 254, 255,

Kidney
    adenocarcinoma of, 212–216
    carcinoma of, 212–216
    corticomedullary enhancement of, 207–210
    cysts of, 210–211
    hematoma of, 208–209
    masses in CT criteria of, 210, 211
    oncocytoma of, 210–212
    renal artery stenosis of, 266–274
    renal vein thrombosis of, 213
    scanning technique for, 207–210
    3-D rendering of, 215

Larynx
    three-dimensional rendering of, 92–96

Liver
    adenoma of, 187
    contrast enhancement of, 172–179
    dual-phase scan of, 178–183
    fatty infiltration of, 187
    hemangioma of, 187
    hypervascular metastasis of, 182, 183
    scanning technique for, 161
    three-dimensional rendering of 185, 186
    tumors of
        metastatic, 179–183
        primary, 812, 183–187
        vasculature of, 187

Lungs
    adenocarcinoma of, 116, 117
    anatomy of, 110
    arteriovenous malformation of, 116
    bronchogenic carcinoma of, 120
    embolism of
        acute, 107, 131–139
        chronic, 107, 137, 139
        metastases to, 115–118
        nodules in, 111–115
    scanning techniques for, 108, 109
    transplant of, 145

Lymph nodes
    celiac, 194, 195
    mesenteric, 194, 195
    of mediastinum, 120
    paraortic, 213

Lymphadenopathy
    celiac, 194, 195
    mesenteric, 194, 195
    of mediastinum, 120
    paraaortic, 213

Maximum intensity projection, 18–21, 52, 110, 268, 269
Mediastinum, 120, 121
Medulla of kidney, 170
Mesenteric artery,
    superior, 195, 196
Mesentery
    lymph nodes of, 194
    lymphadenopathy of, 194
Metastatic disease
    of liver, 179–183
    of lung, 115–118
Modulation tranfer function, 317–322
Musculoskeletal system
    biopsy of, 242, 243, 251, 252
    CT of, 221–263
    neoplasms of, 228–232
    trauma of, 222, 232–242
    three-dimensional rendering of, 226–228
Multiplanar reformatting, 18–24, 216, 223, 230, 233, 242–255, 278
Myoma
    of uterus
        enhancement of, 216–217

Nodule
    pulmonary, 111–115

Oncocytoma
  of kidney
    CT of, 210–212
Osler-Weber-Rendu
  syndrome, 116, 118–120
Osteochondoma, 141
Osteoid osteoma, 232, 233
Osteomyelitis, 232–235
Ovary, 217

Pancreas
  adenocarcinoma of, 193–202
  carcinoma of
    bile duct dilatation due to, 193, 194
    contrast enhancement of, 188–193
    dual phase scanning of, 189–191
    duodenal invasion, 189
    extension of, 189–197
    pancreatic duct dilatation due to 193, 194
    vascular encasement due to, 191, 192, 194–200
  duct of, 171–173, 193, 194
  islet cell tumor of, 201, 202
    metastases from, 182, 183
  scanning technique for, 188–193
  three dimensional rendering of, 199, 200, 289, 293–296
Pancreatitis
  acute
    contrast enhancement of, 202
Pelvis
  CT of, 216–217
Pitch ratio, 9–11, 267, 303, 304, 311, 312
Pleura, 120, 122
Pott's disease, 232–235
Prosthesis
  three-dimensional rendering of, 260, 261
Pseudothrombosis
  of inferior vena cava, 167–169
  of portal vein, 167–169, 190
Pulmonary artery
  embolus of, 131–139

Pulmonary embolus. See embolism, pulmonary

Ray-Sum projection, 19, 268, 269, 274
Reconstruction
  algorithms for, 2–5
  overlapping, 1, 11–13, 107, 170, 171, 192, 193
  spacing, 11–13
Reformatting, multiplanar, 18–24, 223
Region of interest
  of renal masses, 211
Renal artery stenosis, 266–274
Renal cell carcinoma
  attenuation value of, 211
  CT scan of, 212–216
  metastatic to liver, 179–182
  metastatic to bronchus, 146
  scanning technique for, 207–210
  staging of, 213
Renal pelvis
  delayed views for visualization, 208
Rendering, three-dimensional, 18–24
Retroperitoneum
  adenopathy of, 195, 213

Scanner(s), CT
  design features, 299–324
  Elscint Twin, 17, 300–324
  General Electric HiSpeed, 15 17, 300–322
  Philips Tomoscan SR 7000, 17, 300–322
  Picker PQ 2000, 16, 17, 300–324
  Siemens Somatom, 15, 17, 300–324
  Slip-ring gantry for, 14, 15, 299, 300
  Toshiba X-press, 15, 17, 300–324
  Technical specifications for, 13–18, 299–324
Scanning protocol
  for abdominal aorta, 276
  for carotid, 28
  for cervical spine, 98

Scanning protocol *(Cont.)*:
  for Circle of Willis, 29
  for kidney, 163
  for liver, 161
  for pancreas, 162, 188–192
  for routine abdomen, 159
  for thorax, 108, 109
  for whole head, 72
  metastatic survey, 160
  musculoskeletal, 227
Shaded surface display, 18, 19, 52, 110, 268, 269
Section sensitivity profile, 4–6
Spine
  cervical
    CT of, indications for, 96
      trauma of, 99, 237, 239, 246
    CT scan of, 96–99
      fracture of, 99
Splanchnic vessels, 286–296

Thorax
  abnormalities of, 111–152
  CT of, 105–152
  scanning strategies for
Three-dimensional rendering. *See* specific sites
Threshold, 30, 267
Thromboembolic disease
  pulmonary, 131–139
Thrombosis
  basilar tip, 74–76
  of renal vein, 212
  of superior mesenteric vein, 199, 293–296
Thymoma, 123
Tomography, computed
  helical
    detectors for, 16–17
    exposure direction, 6, 9, 154
    for routine head studies, 82–88
    selecting equipment, 13–18

technical principles, 1–26
Trachea, 139–147
Trauma
  facial, 240–243
  musculoskeletal, 232–242
  to abdomen, 158
  to kidney, 208–209
  to spine, 99, 237, 239, 246
Tumor(s). *See also* carcinoma(s)
  and specific body parts
  cholangiocarcinoma, 198, 202–205
  giant cell, 228, 229
  islet cell, 182, 183, 201, 202
  metastatic
    to liver, 179–183
    of bone, 228–232
    of kidney
      adenocarcinoma, 212–216
    of liver, 179–187

Uterus
  enhancement of, 216, 217
  leiomyoma of, 216, 217
  myoma of, 216, 217

Vagina
  enhancement of, 216, 217
Vasospasm, 61
Vein

Vein *(Cont.)*:
  hepatic, 185–187
  renal, 213
  portal, 184–185
  superior mesenteric, 190–192, 194–199, 293–296
Vena Cava
  inferior
    pseudothrombosis of, 168, 169
    thrombosis of, 213–216
  superior
    enhancement of, 107